Tactile Aids for
the Hearing Impaired

Practical Aspects of Audiology

Series Editor: Michael Martin, OBE, Royal National Institute for the Deaf, London

Audiology is a relatively new discipline, formed over the last 50 years. As with all new disciplines, the pace of research is high and standardisation or acceptance of agreed procedures and norms has been low. Examples of this may be seen in the work of the International Standards Organisation (ISO) which only in recent years has produced standards for basic audiometric test methods and given levels for masking signals in pure-tone audiometry.

While much is written on audiology, a great deal of the material concentrates on research aspects of the work. The aim of this series of books is to emphasise the practical aspects of audiology and to set out clearly current practice and ways in which research might be applied.

Furthermore, an international perspective will be given to the series, in order to spread the information that is available on a world-wide scale. This will bring to the attention of practitioners and students ideas and procedures that may appear novel in their own countries but which are widely used in other parts of the world. Today, audiology is an international subject, and recognition must be given to this fact in our thinking. With the move to international standardisation, particularly in instrumentation, it is essential that we are aware of the different approaches being used.

Speech Audiometry, edited by Michael Martin, Royal National Institute for the Deaf, London.

Paediatric Audiology, *0–5 years*, edited by Barry McCormick, Nottingham General Hospital, UK.

Manual of Practical Audiometry, Volume 1, edited by Stig Arlinger, Swedish Audiometry Methods Group.

Manual of Practical Audiometry, Volume 2, edited by Stig Arlinger, Swedish Audiometry Methods Group.

Cochlear Implants: A Practical Guide, edited by Huw Cooper, Royal Ear Hospital, London.

Tactile Aids for the Hearing Impaired, edited by Ian Summers, University of Exeter.

Tactile Aids for the Hearing Impaired

Edited by

Ian R. Summers

Medical Physics Group,
Department of Physics, University of Exeter

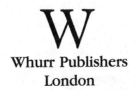

Whurr Publishers
London

© Whurr Publishers Ltd, 1992
19B Compton Terrace, London N1 2UN, England

Reprinted 1996

British Library Cataloguing in Publication Data

Tactile aids for the hearing impaired.
  I. Summers, Ian
  617.8

  ISBN 1-870332-17-2

Composition by Scribe Design, Gillingham, Kent

Foreword

Tactile sensation is generally taken for granted, and most people are really aware of it only when hurt or receiving pleasure. It is therefore not surprising that little attention has been paid to tactile stimulation as a means of giving an awareness of sound.

Deaf people are a group who, as a result of their personal experience, understand the value of the sense of touch for receiving acoustic information, but this has been largely ignored by workers in the field of deafness.

In recent years a few groups of workers scattered around the world have appreciated this potential for the tactile sense. Their work has not had the high profile of the research into cochlear stimulation, but offers considerable benefit to totally and profoundly deaf people, many of whom may never have the opportunity of receiving the very costly cochlear implants. In some cases, tactile devices may complement the use of implants or hearing aids.

Tactile stimulation requires no surgery. It *does* require appropriate user training to achieve benefit, and the development of proper methods of providing this is necessary. Careful research is needed to optimise devices in terms of what can be recognised through a limited information channel.

This book brings together, for the first time I believe, a wide range of information relating to this area. The current position forms a basis for progress which, as well as adding to our general level of knowledge, could mean considerable improvements to the well-being of large numbers of deaf people.

M.C. Martin, OBE
Series Editor
Royal National Institute for the Deaf

Preface

Perhaps one in a thousand* of the population are potential tactile aid users. This book presents current thinking on tactile aids and brings together a wide range of relevant material, previously available only in a very dispersed form throughout the scientific literature, concerning the design of tactile devices and their use to benefit the hearing impaired.

Although the earliest recorded work is as far back as the sixteenth century, research into tactile communication has attracted a relatively small number of scientists over the years. However, the past decade has seen increased activity, with a greater understanding of the sense of touch and a more accurate assessment of the strengths and weaknesses of tactile aids, together with the commercial availability of several devices. There are now an impressive number of high-quality research groups worldwide, the great majority of these being represented in this volume.

I have asked the author(s) of each chapter to cover a specific topic, although there is sometimes, of course, a little overlap of material.

The first three chapters cover the basics of tactile stimulation: Ron Verrillo and George Gescheider review the large body of research which has now been accumulated on perception via the sense of touch; Brian Brown and John Stevens discuss electrical stimulation and the practical problems which must be overcome to provide safe and effective stimuli; Roger Cholewiak and Michael Wollowitz consider how best to satisfy the conflicting design requirements for vibrotactile transducers, and present an interesting case study.

Chapters 4, 5 and 6 consider the design of tactile aids: Jan Weisenberger discusses the acoustic features which may usefully be communicated by a tactile device, and the effectiveness of existing devices in transmitting

---

*Figure based on Thornton's 1986 survey (*Br. J. Audiol.* **20**, 221–229) in which he estimates that the hearing impaired represent 0.0712 of the British population, and of these 1.56% have a better-ear, average threshold $\geqslant 100$ dB HTL

these; in my contribution I consider the various strategies available for coding such information within the limited capacity of a single-channel output; Jim Mason and Barrie Frost present an equivalent analysis for multichannel systems which attempt to take advantage of the full range of spatiotemporal perception available through the skin.

It now seems clear that a significant amount of user training is necessary before the full potential of a tactile device can be realised. In Chapter 7, Geoff Plant suggests criteria for selection of subjects and discusses the types of training which are most appropriate for adults and children.

Although the situation has improved in recent years, there is still a dearth of aid evaluations whose results are presented in such a way that an easy comparison is possible across different studies. Lynne Bernstein considers the evaluation of tactile aids – the reliability of various tests and their relation to 'real life' performance – in Chapter 8.

The development of cochlear implants has provided new impetus to research into tactile aids, not least because it has made deaf persons more aware of the possibilities that present-day electronic technology can offer. Peter Blamey and Bob Cowan have extensive experience with cochlear implants, and have also been involved in the development of an electrotactile aid. They are thus particularly qualified – perhaps uniquely so – to assess the relative merits of implants and tactile devices (Chapter 9). It is, of course, particularly important to make a comparison in terms of potential benefit and cost-effectiveness in order to give appropriate advice to potential users of either type of device.

There is another important strand to our discussion: The 'natural' method of Tadoma, used by some deaf-blind individuals, provides an impressive demonstration of the extent to which effective tactile communication is possible. As editor, I found some difficulty in finding the best position in the sequence of chapters for the contribution by Charlotte Reed, Nat Durlach and Lorraine Delhorne which covers Tadoma and related techniques. It appears as Chapter 10, but contains material relevant to many of the other chapters.

In the final chapter (Chapter 11), Roger Thornton and Andy Philips present the results of their major comparative trial of four commercially available aids: Tactaid II, TAM, Minifonator and Minivib. It is disappointing to find that the Tactaid II, Minifonator and Minivib – all designed to improve speech reception – were ranked lower overall in this trial than the TAM, whose design limits it to being little more than an environmental aid.

Having worked with tactile aids to a greater or lesser extent for most of my scientific career, I have always found the multidisciplinary nature of the topic to be particularly exciting. I hope that readers of this volume will experience something of this excitement, and that the information presented will lead to the more effective use of tactile aids in the next few years, not just in the research laboratory but – the aim of all authors in this volume – to benefit the hearing impaired in the wider community on a day-to-day basis.

Ian Summers, Exeter
May 1991

Contents

Contributors

Lynne E. Bernstein, Center for Auditory and Speech Sciences, Gallaudet University, Washington DC, USA

Peter J. Blamey, Human Communication Research Centre, Department of Otolaryngology, University of Melbourne, East Melbourne, Victoria, Australia

Brian H. Brown, Department of Medical Physics and Clinical Engineering, University of Sheffield, Sheffield, UK

Roger W. Cholewiak, Department of Psychology, Princeton University, Princeton, New Jersey, USA

Robert S. C. Cowan, Human Communication Research Centre, Department of Otolaryngology, University of Melbourne, East Melbourne, Victoria, Australia

Lorraine A. Delhorne, Research Laboratory of Electronics, Massachusetts Institute of Technology, Cambridge, Massachusetts, USA

Nathaniel I. Durlach, Research Laboratory of Electronics, Massachusetts Institute of Technology, Cambridge, Massachusetts, USA

Barrie J. Frost, Department of Psychology, Queen's University, Kingston, Ontario, Canada

George A. Gescheider, Psychology Department, Hamilton College, Clinton, New York, USA

James L. Mason, Department of Electrical Engineering, Queen's University, Kingston, Ontario, Canada

Andrew J. Phillips, MRC Institute of Hearing Research, Royal South Hants Hospital, Southampton, UK

Geoff Plant, National Acoustic Laboratories Central Laboratory, Chatswood, NSW, Australia

Charlotte M. Reed, Research Laboratory of Electronics, Massachusetts Institute of Technology, Cambridge, Massachusetts, USA

John C. Stevens, Department of Medical Physics and Clinical Engineering, University of Sheffield, Sheffield, UK

Ian R. Summers, Medical Physics Group, Department of Physics, University of Exeter, Exeter, UK

A. Roger D. Thornton, MRC Institute of Hearing Research, Royal South Hants Hospital, Southampton, UK

Ronald T. Verrillo, Institute for Sensory Research, Syracuse University, Syracuse, New York, USA

Janet M. Weisenberger, Central Institute for the Deaf, St Louis, Missouri, USA (Present address: Department of Speech and Hearing Science, Ohio State University, Columbus, Ohio, USA)

Michael Wollowitz, Engineering Design and Analysis, Somerville, Massachusetts, USA

Chapter 1
Perception via the Sense of Touch

RONALD T. VERRILLO and GEORGE A. GESCHEIDER

Human speech is the most complex, sophisticated and subtle form of communication that we know. The wealth of information conveyed by speech is unparalleled in the animal kingdom, and the inability to use it effectively imposes a severe handicap. In natural acquisition of speech, there must be a feedback system between the ear and the apparatus used for the production of sounds. People who are profoundly deaf at a prelingual age are doubly handicapped; they are unable to hear and, because the feedback loop is incomplete, they are at a severe disadvantage in learning to produce the sounds that are necessary to communicate with the world of the hearing. Signing by hand alleviates the problem between deaf people, and speech and language therapy is employed to ease the problem of communication between the deaf and the hearing. In spite of these efforts, effective auditory communication for the prelingually deaf child is at best marginal. One of the goals of research on tactile systems has been to further the development of devices to help alleviate this problem.

It was once believed that the tactile sense was inadequate for the task of transmitting and processing complex information. This view has changed dramatically over the past four decades as sophisticated electronic measuring devices have found their way into tactile research, inherited primarily from the auditory laboratory. It is the intention in this chapter to outline the results of investigations that provide basic information about the response characteristics of vibrotactile receptor systems. An understanding of the functional characteristics that define the capabilities and the limitations of tactile sensation is essential for the development of efficient, effective, sensory aids for the hearing impaired.

The chapter is divided according to the major factors that affect responses to tactile stimuli, namely temporal domain, spatial domain, intensity effects, complex stimuli, subject variables and underlying receptor mechanisms.

1

Temporal Domain

Frequency

One of the most fundamental sensory characteristics of a mechanoreceptive system is its response to different frequencies of sinusoidal stimulation. Such data become particularly important if we hope to develop a
channel of communication to substitute for hearing. Early studies have
established that the skin is, indeed, differentially sensitive to different
frequencies of vibration (Gilmer, 1935; Hugony, 1935; Setzepfand, 1935;
von Békésy, 1939; Sherrick, 1953). In order to determine the sensitivity
of the skin to different frequencies, measurements were made in our
laboratory on the thenar eminence of the right hand using a wide variety
of contactor sizes (Verrillo, 1963, 1966a). The results shown in Figure 1.1
reveal that when a large contactor is used to vibrate the skin the
(displacement) threshold response is independent of frequency at low
frequencies (25 and 40 Hz), but as the frequency is increased the threshold improves at a rate of about 12 dB/octave until maximal sensitivity is
reached in the range 200–300 Hz. At higher frequencies, up to about

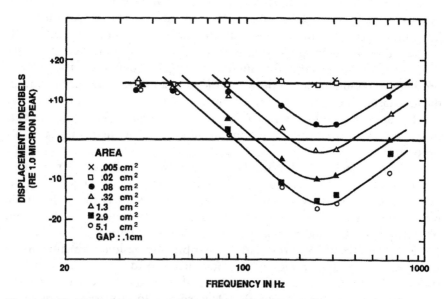

Figure 1.1 Thresholds for the detection of vibrotactile stimuli measured as a function of
sinusoidal frequency at the thenar eminence of the right hand. Contactor size is the parameter. A
gap of 0.1 cm is imposed between the circular contactor and the rigid surround that prevents
surface waves from spreading across the skin. Note that for contactors larger than 0.02 cm², the
threshold characteristic is flat at low frequencies and U-shaped at higher frequencies, with a
maximal sensitivity at about 250 Hz. The threshold for very small contactors is independent of
frequency. (From Verrillo, 1963.)

1000 Hz, sensitivity decreases rapidly. It is unlikely that valid thresholds can be determined above this frequency.

Thus it is evident that the threshold curve for large contactors is composed of two limbs: a flat portion at low frequencies where differences in frequency have no effect on the detectability of the signal, and a U-shaped limb at higher frequencies. In contrast, where very small contactors are used, a flat curve extending across all frequencies is seen, indicating that when small contactors are used the threshold response is independent of frequency. A double-limbed curve obtained in measurements of biological systems often indicates the presence of two underlying mechanisms, and in this case each limb is determined by a separate cutaneous receptor system (Verrillo, 1963). We shall discuss this in greater detail below.

Frequency discrimination

Being able to detect stimuli at different frequencies is important, but is only a small part of the problem of utilizing the skin as a communication channel. Of equal importance is the ability to discriminate differences between frequencies when stimuli are presented at intensities above the detection threshold. The auditory system is exquisitely designed to make these discriminations, but the skin is quite limited and very few studies addressing this question has been published. Mowbray and Gebhard (1957) found that discrimination was fairly good at low frequencies but deteriorated rapidly as frequency increased (Figure 1.2). Their subjects detected vibrations through a pulsating rod held between the fingers. Goff (1967) reported a difference limen of about 30% between frequencies; a rather poor showing when compared with the ear which can discriminate frequency differences of the order of 0.3%.

As a preliminary step towards the development of a tactile vocoder, experiments were performed on the volar forearm and the finger using sinusoids, Gaussian and non-Gaussian pulses, and 'warble' (time-varying frequency) tones, with careful matching of the subjective magnitude of the frequencies being compared (Rothenberg et al., 1977). The results (shown in Figure 1.2) show that pulses produce better discrimination than do sine waves and that the difference limen for constant-frequency stimuli is better at low than at high frequencies, which is consistent with the findings of Goff (1967). Discrimination at higher frequencies was improved by using warble tones (Figure 1.2, solid lines), when subjects were asked to detect small frequency fluctuations about a center frequency.

In a follow-up study, Rothenberg and Molitor (1979), using the same equipment, studied the ability of eight hearing and five deaf subjects to identify the stress pattern in a short sentence from variations in voice fundamental frequency. The results supported the hypothesis that there is

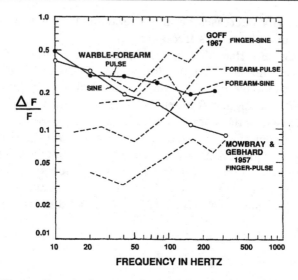

Figure 1.2 Difference limen for frequency discrimination of pulses and sinusoids measured on the volar forearm and finger (- - - -). The results are plotted as the Weber fraction ($\Delta F/F$). In general, the ability to discriminate between frequencies diminishes as frequency increases, however the opposite is true for detection of whether stimuli are frequency modulated (warble tones on the forearm: ——). (From Rothenberg et al., 1977.)

an association between perceived vibrotactile frequency and auditory pitch, and that intonation patterns with moderate to strong stress patterns could be discriminated on the skin by hearing and deaf subjects alike. The five prelingually, profoundly deaf subjects evidenced a deficit in the perception of vibrotactile pitch, but this deficit could be overcome by training (using amplified sound when some residual hearing exists).

These studies indicate that the skin is rather poor at discriminating frequency differences and that its limited ability to do so decreases as frequency increases. There is an anecdotal observation made by several investigators, however, that may be of some value. The *quality* of sensation is quite different at lower (below 100 Hz) frequencies than at higher frequencies. Subjects report a sensation of periodicity or 'buzzing' at low frequencies and a more diffuse, 'smooth' sensation at higher frequencies. This difference in sensory quality may be useful to the designers of tactile aids.

Stimulus duration

An important parameter to consider when attempting to understand any sensory system is the effect of stimulus duration upon sensation. There is usually a trade-off between the duration of the stimulus and the intensity necessary to perceive it. Such information also provides clues to the functional characteristics of the nervous system as a whole and to the levels within it where information processing takes place. Since stimulus duration is an important component of word recognition by the auditory system, in all likelihood it will be an important consideration for the development of auditory substitution devices.

Figure 1.3 depicts threshold shift referred to the threshold at 1000 ms as a function of stimulus duration in milliseconds, with contactor size as the parameter (Verrillo, 1965). It is clear that when the area of the contactor is large (2.9 cm^2), a short signal is more difficult to detect than a long one, and that the improvement in detectability is a very orderly function of signal duration. It is noteworthy that the rate of decline in thresholds of 3 dB per doubling of duration for durations up to approximately 200 ms indicates that the tactile system is capable of temporally integrating stimulus energy over a limited period of time. That function is described in Figure 1.3 by the solid curve, which is the prediction of threshold shift made by Zwislocki's theory of temporal summation (Zwislocki, 1960). Zwislocki's theory also predicted accurately the threshold response as a

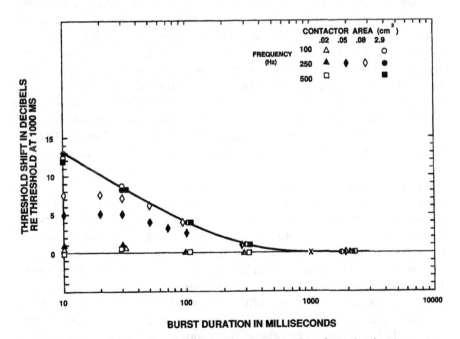

BURST DURATION IN MILLISECONDS

Figure 1.3 Vibrotactile detection thresholds plotted as a function of stimulus duration measured at the thenar eminence. The reference duration is 1000 ms. Contactor size is the parameter. The curve represents predicted values based on Zwislocki's (1960) theory of temporal summation. Note that the data conform to the prediction when a large contactor (2.9 cm^2) is used, but departures from the prediction occur as the size of the contactor is reduced. The very small contactor resulted in data that are independent of burst duration, indicating no temporal summation. (From Verrillo, 1965.)

function of pulse repetition rate and the number of pulses in a stimulus burst. The fact that temporal summation does not occur when a very small contactor (0.02 cm²) is used is suggestive of the duplex nature of tactile sensation that will be discussed later. Gescheider (1976) found that temporal summation is absent for low frequencies of vibration, a finding that also has implications for theories of neural mechanisms responsible for temporal summation.

Gap detection

The temporal resolution capabilities of people with hearing disorders is commonly assessed by measuring their ability to detect the silent temporal interval (gap) between two auditory stimuli. Although gap detection has received considerable attention in auditory laboratories (Plomp, 1964; Buunen and Van Valkenburg, 1979; Fitzgibbons, 1983, 1984) the literature concerning this measurement is very scanty for the sense of touch. Gescheider (1966, 1967) measured the minimum detectable separation between a pair of tactile clicks as a function of click intensity and found that gap detection improves as a function of the time interval separating the clicks and the intensity of the clicks. Gap detection thresholds were found to be about 10 ms, but may be as low as 5 ms for highly damped mechanical pulses (Gescheider, 1974; Sherrick, 1982). Van Doren, Gescheider and Verrillo (1990) studied the effect of age on the ability to detect temporal gaps between bursts of sinusoids and bursts of band-limited noise in subjects ranging from 8 to 75 years. The gap became easier to detect as its duration increased, and gaps between sinusoidal bursts were significantly easier to detect than those between bursts of noise. The data from noise stimuli in this experiment agree well with the data obtained using clicks (Gescheider, 1967). Subjects reported that the sinusoids felt 'smooth' and perceived the gap as a small click in the stimulus; the noise, however, felt 'rough' and the gap was perceived as a modulation of stimulus amplitude. These subjective observations are similar to those reported in Weisenberger's (1986) study of vibrotactile amplitude modulation and they suggest that different strategies may be employed in the detection of gaps in sinusoidal and noise stimuli. Tactile gap detection thresholds are substantially higher than auditory thresholds measured under comparable conditions and therefore much of the temporally modulated information in speech may fail to be transmitted in tactile communication systems. Further research is needed to define these limitations.

Amplitude modulation

Although amplitude modulation refers to variations in the amplitude of the envelope of the stimulus, it is used as an index of temporal sensitivity because it measures the detection thresholds of the modulation amplitude as a function of the rate of modulation. It has proven to be a useful method for assessing the temporal sensitivity of both the auditory (Zwicker, 1952; Viemeister, 1979) and visual systems (Kelly, 1972). The response of the vibrotactile system to amplitude-modulated stimuli has been investigated in relation to the rhythmic aspects of speech (Geers, 1986; Goldstein and Proctor, 1985), but only Lamoré, Muijser and Keemink (1986) and Weisenberger (1986) have made systematic measurements. Lamoré et al. modulated high-frequency sinusoids (1000–2000 Hz) that are beyond the normal range of sensitivity on the skin. They found that by using amplitude modulations of 10–500 Hz they were able to replicate the U-shaped portion of the curve shown in Figure 1.6. The implications of this finding are discussed by the authors in terms of the filter characteristics of the tissues involved. Weisenberger (1986), on the other hand, modulated sinusoidal carrier frequencies within the range of human sensitivity as well as wide band and narrow band noise carriers. The results show that the perception of amplitude modulation using sinusoids is superior to that with wide or narrow band noise. Maximal sensitivity occurred at modulation frequencies of 20–40 Hz. Weisenberger concluded that, although not as sensitive to amplitude modulation as the auditory system, the vibrotactile system can reasonably be expected to resolve temporally varying waveforms that can be utilized for processing speech information by the skin.

Temporal order

Another aspect of temporal perception is the ability to count successive multiple stimuli on the skin. In this regard, tactile performance has been found to be inferior to auditory but superior to visual performance when the rate of presentation was 2–8 pulses per second (Lechelt, 1974a,b, 1975; Lechelt and Tanne, 1976). Sherrick (1982) concluded that Lechelt's data indicate that the numerosity judgements require short-term memory. Hirsh and Sherrick (1961) found the threshold for temporal-order judgments to be about 20 ms between the onsets of two brief stimuli. This threshold, however, was found to increase progressively as the number of stimuli increases beyond two (Sherrick, 1982). When the number of stimulus elements is increased to five or six, the stimulus onset intervals needed for correct identification of the temporal sequence may be nearly 500 ms. It is clear that tactile communication systems that require absolute identification of the temporal order of several sequentially presented stimuli presented to different body sites would require very slow rates of presentation of information if it is to be effectively used; too slow for the perception of speech in real time. On the other hand, if the task is simply to discriminate between two temporal sequences with no requirement to identify temporal order, increasing the number of stimulus elements has little effect on performance and discrimination thresholds are generally below 100 ms (Sherrick, 1982).

When the problem of cutaneous temporal relations is investigated for complex displays in which many areas of the skin are stimulated in various temporal sequences, cognitive factors such as short-term memory, attention ar/d pattern recognition become increasingly important. Advances in our understanding of these complex cognitive processes as they relate to tactile perception should correlate with significant improvements in tactile communication systems.

Spatial Domain

Contactor size

Although auditory stimuli can be translated into a given area of stimulation upon the basilar membrane, we do not normally think in terms of an area of stimulation for the sense of hearing. In vision and taction, which are more spatially oriented sensory systems, the amount of stimulation, in spatial terms, becomes very important. In taction such information can be documented in terms of contactor area, and in vision in terms of visual angle.

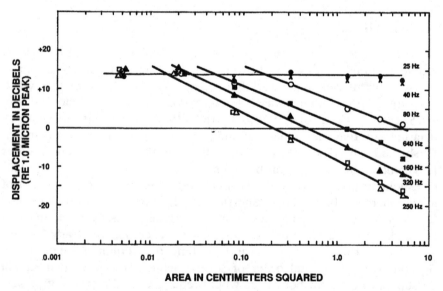

Figure 1.4 Vibrotactile detection thresholds at different frequencies as a function of contactor size. At the higer frequencies (above 40 Hz), complete spatial summation of energy is indicated by the 3-dB improvement of threshold for each doubling of area. No spatial summation occurred at the low frequencies (25 and 40 Hz). (From Verrillo, 1963.)

It is apparent from Figure 1.1 that as the size of the contactor is decreased the sensitivity to vibration in the U-shaped segment of the curve is also diminished in an orderly fashion, so that the results form a nest of curves. Also, when very small contactors are used the threshold response is independent of frequency. These data are replotted in Figure 1.4 as a function of contactor size in order to show the effect of the area of stimulation (Verrillo, 1963, 1966a). At the higher frequencies (80–320 Hz) sensitivity increases directly with the size of the vibrating surface, at the rate of approximately 3 dB per doubling of contactor area. More specifically, the 3 dB decrease in threshold produced by every doubling of contactor size corresponds exactly to a constant amount of energy integrated over space needed for detecting the stimulus. This indicates that there is spatial summation on the skin and that the system is capable of spatially integrating all of the energy that is delivered to the skin surface. However, at low frequencies (40 Hz and below) the size of the contactor has no effect on the detection threshold: there is no spatial summation. These results, obtained from glabrous skin of the hand, were replicated on the hairy skin of the volar forearm (Verrillo, 1966b).

It also has been demonstrated that spatial summation occurs at suprathreshold levels of stimulation. The magnitude of sensation has been shown to increase as contactor size increases (Verrillo, 1974) and also as the number of vibrating elements increases in a multi-contactor matrix (Cholewiak, 1979).

Body site

The study of tactile sensation on different parts of the body is important because of differences in threshold sensitivity, suprathreshold function, the potential interference or confusion of signals delivered to different sites and the cosmetic considerations of wearing a tactile communication device. Many investigators, dating from the classic studies of Weber (1835), to the more recent ones of Katz (1925) and Weinstein (1968), have dealt with the sensitivity of the skin at different body sites. Most studies, however, suffered from problems of instrumentation, which were inadequate to produce a precise quantification of results.

The experiments performed in the authors' laboratories involved threshold and suprathreshold responses at several sites on the body and the interactive effects of stimulation at different sites. The data shown in Figure 1.5 represent measurements of threshold detectability at three body sites: the volar forearm (Verrillo, 1966b), the middle fingertip (Verrillo, 1971) and the thenar eminence (Verrillo, 1963). All measurements were made under identical experimental conditions. It is evident that the forearm is by far the least, and the fingertip the most, sensitive of the three sites tested. Any communication device designed for use on the forearm would

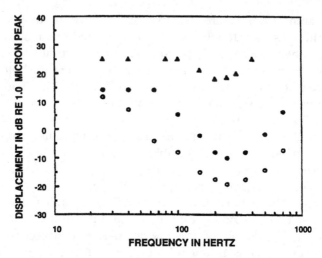

Figure 1.5 Comparison of detection thresholds as a function of sinusoidal frequency measured at the volar forearm (▲), the thenar eminence (●) and the distal pad of the middle finger (○). Contactor size 0.28 cm². All show the characteristic U-shaped curve at higher frequencies. The greatest sensitivity exists at the fingertip and the least on the forearm.

have higher energy requirements than one designed for the fingers or the palm of the hand.

Other experiments involved the measurement of the growth of subjective magnitude at the same three sites (Verrillo and Chamberlain, 1972; Verrillo, 1974). It is important to consider not only the absolute sensitivity of the skin at the particular site where a tactile communication device might be applied, but also the rate at which the subjective intensity of the signal grows with amplitude of vibration. The method used to measure subjective magnitude was a combination of absolute magnitude estimation (Zwislocki and Goodman, 1980) and magnitude production, a method called *numerical magnitude balance* by Hellman and Zwislocki (1961, 1963). The curves in Figure 1.6 show that the subjective magnitude ('loudness') of the stimulation increases as the physical intensity of the vibration is increased (Verrillo and Chamberlain, 1972; Verrillo, 1974). Steeper curves indicate a more rapid increase in psychological magnitude. The subjective intensity of vibration appears to grow most rapidly on the volar forearm and least rapidly at the finger pad, with the thenar eminence in the middle position. The steepness of these curves is inversely related to the number of sensory receptors located in the skin at the various sites (Verrillo, 1974). Similarly, Cholewiak (1979) has reported a rapid growth magnitude of sensation for stimulation of the thigh, a site that has relatively few sensory receptors.

Gilson (1968, 1969a,b, 1974) performed a series of experiments in which he determined the effect of stimulus on one body site upon the

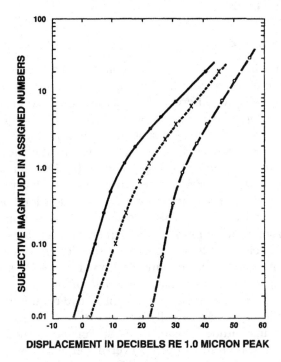

Figure 1.6 The growth of subjective magnitude as a function of vibration amplitude measured by the method of numerical magnitude balance. The steepness of the curves increases as sensitivity decreases from finger to forearm, indicating that subjective intensity increases more rapidly on areas of the body that have low sensitivity. ●—●, Finger; x—x, thenar; O—O, forearm. (From Verrillo and Chamberlain, 1972, by permission of the Psychonomic Society, Inc.)

sensation experienced from a stimulus applied to a different site. He used up to 11 different sites on ipsilateral and contralateral sides of the body, some closely spaced and some widely spaced. In general, he found a substantial elevation in thresholds, a suppression of sensation, when several body sites were stimulated simultaneously. He concluded that the effects of the interactions were due to central (rather than to peripheral) neural activity and that differential time delays observed in these effects are due to differing neural distances between the sites of stimulation and a central processing center. The designer of a tactile communication device that uses multiple sites of stimulation must be alert to the possibility that a stimulus delivered by one stimulator may degrade the response to a stimulus applied to another site on the body.

In addition to changes in threshold sensitivity and in the growth of sensation, there are other ways in which the sensation at one body site may be altered by the application of a stimulus to another site. This phenomenon will be discussed more fully in the section below.

Intensity Effects

Subjective magnitude

Because stimuli will be applied to the skin at suprathreshold levels, the developer of tactile aids will have to consider not only the absolute (threshold) sensitivity to different frequencies of vibration, but also the differences in subjective intensity produced by equal-amplitude suprathreshold vibrations at different frequencies. Such an effect of frequency was first observed in hearing and led to the measurement in the auditory system of equal-loudness curves by Fletcher and Munson (1933) and others. These curves show the physical intensity that a tone must have at any given frequency in order to sound as loud as a specified tone at a different frequency. This information is important when it is necessary to balance or emphasize the perceived intensities of stimuli at difference frequencies and it is essential for the design of telephones and other devices used for vocal communication. It is no less important a consideration for communication via the sense of touch.

Because loudness is a term used for the subjective magnitude of auditory signals, the tactile curves are usually referred to as curves or contours of equal sensation magnitude (Stevens, 1968; Verrillo, Fraioli and Smith, 1969). The curves shown in Figure 1.7 (Verrillo et al., 1969) were derived from data obtained by the method of numerical magnitude balance (Hellman and Zwislocki, 1961, 1963). Measurements were made at ten

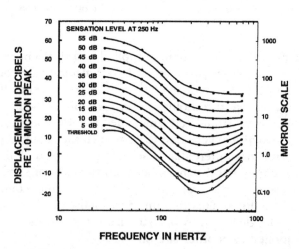

Figure 1.7 Curves of equal sensation magnitude plotted as a function of frequency. Each curve describes the combinations of frequency and intensity that result in judgements of equal subjective intensity. Measurements were made by the method of numerical magnitude balance on the thenar eminence. (From Verrillo, Fraioli and Smith, 1969, by permission of the Psychonomic Society, Inc.)

stimulus intensities and ten frequencies. Each curve defines the combinations of frequency and intensity that result in judgments of equal sensation magnitude. From these curves it can be determined how intense a vibration must be to equal the subjective intensity of a vibration at any other frequency. It is obvious that, at suprathreshold levels, the higher frequencies require a lower level of displacement to equal the subjective magnitude of a low-frequency signal. An important difference between these curves and those for hearing is that the hearing curves flatten as intensity increases (which tends to make high-intensity sounds appear equally loud regardless of frequency), whereas the vibration contours at various intensities are almost parallel.

Intensity discrimination

The ability to make intensity discriminations in the auditory system has been the subject of intense investigation by hearing scientists for many years (see Viemeister, 1988 for a review). The auditory system is remarkable for the enormous range of intensities that it is capable of processing, up to 130 dB above the detection threshold. It is also able to discriminate relatively small intensity differences at 115 dB above threshold. By comparison the vibrotactile system is rather limited, with an intensity range of about 55 dB above the detection threshold, beyond which the vibrations become very unpleasant or painful. Also, our knowledge of vibrotactile intensity relationships is much less extensive than that of the auditory system.

The smallest detectable intensity difference in tactile stimulation (0.4 dB) was reported by Knudson in 1928 and the highest value (2.3 dB) was reported by Sherrick in 1950 (Sherrick, C.E., unpublished data). Other studies have reported values between these extremes (Schiller, 1953, unpublished data; Craig, 1972, 1974; Fucci, Small and Petrosino, 1982). Because the methodologies and experimental conditions vary between laboratories, it is difficult to make direct comparisons of the results reported in these studies.

In a more recent study (Gescheider et al., 1990), the difference threshold for the detection of changes in the amplitude of vibration was measured on the thenar eminence as a function of the stimulus intensity and frequency. One of the purposes was to compare results obtained by three different methods of stimulus presentation. The best intensity discriminations were made when an intensity increment was imposed upon a continuous background 'pedestal' of vibration rather than on pedestals of brief duration. Subjects were able to detect amplitude increments of as small as 0.7 dB and there appeared to be no significant differences between the results using wide-band noise, narrow-band noise or sinusoids of various frequencies, which suggests that the ability to detect amplitude differences on the skin is independent of the power spectrum and frequency of the stimulus. The value of the relative-difference threshold, expressed in decibels, was found to decrease slightly as intensity level increased, indicating a near-miss to Weber's law. This effect is very similar to that observed when listening to pure tones, but is different from that observed for auditory noise, which does obey Weber's law.

Effects of multiple stimulation

It is well known that the presence of one stimulus in close temporal proximity to another (target) can affect the perceived intensity of the target stimulus. The types of perceptual phenomena that have been measured have been defined as follows:

- *Masking* is the reduced ability to detect the target signal in the presence of a background, or masking stimulus. The effect can be observed when the signal and masker occur simultaneously (simultaneous masking), when the signal precedes (backward masking) or follows (forward masking) the masker by a brief time interval (Gescheider, Bolanowski and Verrillo, 1989).
- *Enhancement* occurs when the presence of a brief stimulus causes a second stimulus to appear to be of greater intensity than when it is presented alone (Verrillo and Gescheider, 1975).
- *Summation* refers to the total or combined sensation magnitude of two stimuli occurring close together in time (Verrillo and Gescheider, 1975).
- *Suppression* occurs when the presence of one stimulus decreases the ability of the subject to detect a second stimulus when the two stimuli are delivered to different places on the surface of the skin (Verrillo and Gescheider, 1975). In a sense, suppression may be considered to be masking from a remote site.

We will consider first the capacity of one tactile stimulus to reduce (*mask*) the detectability of another vibration. Many of the early studies were performed in an effort to provide information basic to the development of tactile communication devices, including the effects of masker location and temporal relationship of the masker to the signal (Sherrick, 1964; Gilson, 1969a), the number of maskers (Gilson, 1969b) and the psychophysical method employed (Gescheider, Herman and Phillips, 1970; Snyder, 1977; Gilson, 1974). In time, masking studies focused on underlying neural mechanisms of vibrotactile functioning (Verrillo and Capraro, 1975; Craig, 1976b; Ferrington, Nail and Rowe, 1977; Hamer, Zwislocki and Capraro, 1978; Labs et al., 1978; Hamer, Verrillo and Zwislocki, 1983). It is clear from these and many other studies that the detectability of one vibrotactile stimulus can be decreased by the presence of another.

The functional characteristics of vibrotactile masking were detailed in a series of studies designed to elucidate the effects of frequency, intensity, and timing (Verrillo and Capraro, 1975; Gescheider and Verrillo, 1979; Gescheider, Verrillo and Van Doren, 1982; Hamer, Verrillo and Zwislocki, 1983; Verrillo et al., 1983; Gescheider, O'Malley and Verrillo, 1983). Basic masking functions measured on the skin of the hand are shown in Figure 1.8 (Gescheider, Verrillo and Van Doren, 1982). When a narrow-band noise centered at 275 Hz was used to mask the detection of a 300-Hz sinusoid (solid circles) the effect was robust; masking increased as a linear function of the intensity of the masker. When the masker is placed in the high-frequency region (275 Hz) and the signal at low frequencies (15, 50, 80 Hz), there is a plateau in the function indicating a cessation in the masking increment. This phenomenon occurs when masker and signal excite different mechanoreceptor systems located in the skin (see section on Receptor Mechanisms below). Within certain intensity limits the presence of high frequencies does not affect the detection of low frequencies and vice versa.

The interaction of several stimuli presented to the skin can result in other changes in sensation. When the presence of one stimulus causes another to appear more intense, *enhancement* occurs. This phenomenon has been well documented in hearing (Zwislocki et al., 1974; Zwislocki

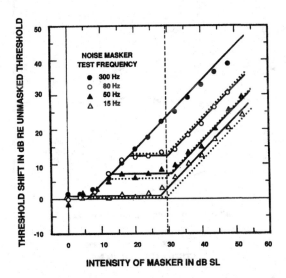

Figure 1.8 Vibrotactile masked thresholds as a function of the intensity of the masker. The masker was narrow-band noise centered at 275 Hz and the test stimuli were sinusoids at 15, 50, 80 and 300 Hz. The dotted lines are predicted from threshold data and the solid lines are linear regression fits to the data. Masking occurs only when both signal and masker are confined to a single mechanoreceptor system (the rising slope portions of the curves), but none results when the signal and masker excite different receptor systems (plateau portions of the curves). (From Gescheider, Verrillo and Van Doren, 1982.)

and Sokolich, 1974), and in vibrotaction (Verrillo and Gescheider, 1975, 1979; Gescheider et al., 1977) studies, where subjects were asked to judge the subjective intensity of the second of a pair of short bursts on the skin at various intervals between the first and second bursts. The judgment was made by adjusting the intensity of a third burst so that it matched the subjective magnitude of the second. The adjusted intensity of the third burst was used as a measure of enhancement. The results shown in Figure 1.9(a) demonstrate that enhancement occurs when the two stimuli are within 500 ms of each other and that the effect is a decreasing function of the inter-stimulus time interval (Verrillo and Gescheider, 1975). Enhancement is evoked at both high and low frequencies (300 and 25 Hz), but disappears when high and low frequencies are mixed in the same stimulus presentation (25–300–300 Hz).

Figure 1.9(b) shows the results when the subject is asked to judge the combined subjective intensity of both stimuli in the pair. The result is *summation*, which is more robust when the frequencies are more widely spaced, and is the opposite of the enhancement effect. The underlying

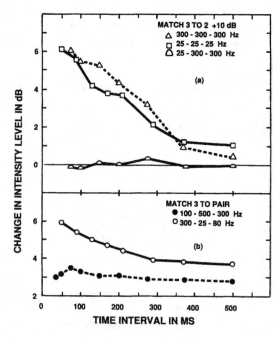

Figure 1.9 The effects of enhancement (a) and summation (b) in the pacinian and non-pacinian vibrotactile systems. Enhancement occurs when the stimulus frequencies in the first and second of a pair of bursts activate a single system (△, □). When both systems are activated by a combination of high and low frequencies (◒), no enhancement occurs. Summation results when the paired stimuli activate both systems (○), but is absent when the frequencies of the pair are confined to a single system (●). (From Verrillo and Gescheider, 1975, by permission of the Psychonomic Society, Inc.)

mechanism of these psychophysical phenomena has not been identified, but the effects on the skin parallel those found in hearing. It has been suggested that they are loosely analogous to presenting stimuli with sufficient frequency differences to be in different critical bands in the auditory system. The amount of summation measured when the frequencies of the two stimuli greatly differ is consistent with the hypothesis that perfect summation of sensation magnitude occurs under this condition (Verrillo and Gescheider, 1975). The results of Marks (1979) who, using magnitude estimation, found summation of sensation magnitude when two components are not similar in frequency, support this. Marks found energy summation when the components are similar in frequency.

The close temporal proximity of two short stimuli does not always result in an increase of perceived magnitude. When the two stimuli of the pair are separated on the body, even contralaterally, there is a marked loss of sensation for the second stimulus at short inter-stimulus time intervals. Figure 1.10 (Verrillo and Gescheider, 1976) shows the loss of sensation at short time intervals followed by an enhancement effect that is maximal at 150 ms. These measurements were made on the thenar eminence and middle fingertip of the right hand. Similar results were obtained between the thenar eminences of both hands and between the thigh and thenar

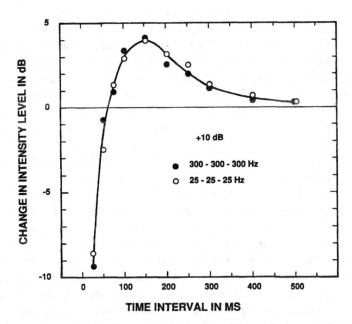

Figure 1.10 Suppression effects observed when the first and second of a pair of stimuli are delivered to different parts of the body (ipsilateral finger and thenar) separated by short time intervals (less than 75 ms). The effect is followed by enhancement at longer time intervals and can be observed in both pacinian (●) and non-pacinian (○) receptor systems. (From Verrillo and Gescheider, 1976, by permission of the Psychonomic Society, Inc.)

eminence on the same side of the body. The designer of a tactile communicator that employs multiple stimulation at different body sites should be aware of the possible consequences of such stimulus patterning.

Adaptation

The growth of sensation magnitude during approximately the first one second of vibrotactile stimulation is attributed to temporal summation (Gescheider and Joelson, 1983); the subsequent decrement in sensory magnitude and in the detection threshold following more prolonged stimulation is attributed to sensory adaptation. The absolute threshold for detecting a test stimulus increases following intense stimulation of the test site, with recovery over time (Cohen and Lindley, 1938; Wedell and Cummings, 1938). Changes in the subjective magnitude of suprathreshold stimuli have also been recorded (von Békésy, 1959; Berglund and Berglund, 1970; Gescheider and Wright, 1968, 1969; Hahn, 1966, 1968a). Sensation magnitude declines during the exposure to the adapting stimulus and then gradually recovers to the preadaptation level during the postadaptation period; recovery time ranges from a few seconds to several minutes depending on duration and intensity of exposure.

There are several possible explanations of adaptation: Tapper (1965), and Nafe and Wagoner (1941) cited stimulus failure in the case of steady-state pressure stimuli; von Békésy (1959) cited changes in the state of the receptor system; Hahn (1966) cited mechanical alteration of the tissue lying between the stimulator and the receptor; Gescheider and Wright (1969) proposed a two-factor hypothesis in which the total reduction in sensation magnitude is accounted for by a combination of mechanical and neural changes; and O'Mara, Rowe and Tarvin (1988) provided evidence that adaptation is largely a central process. Whatever the basic mechanisms of adaptation, it is important because of the magnitude of its effects at both threshold and suprathreshold levels. It must be seriously considered when designing tactile communication systems.

Wedell and Cummings (1938) were the first to discover that the extent of adaptation depends on the frequency relationship between the test and adapting stimuli. Hahn (1968b) later showed substantial adaptation effects when the test and adapting stimuli were at the same frequency (either 10 or 200 Hz), but not when the adapting and test stimuli were at 10 and 200 Hz respectively. This is consistent with the notion of separate neural channels, pacinian and non-pacinian, for detecting high- and low-frequency vibrations respectively (Verrillo, 1963, 1968). Since Hahn's study, the results of several other studies on cross-frequency adaptation have supported the hypothesis that adaptation within one tactile channel does not affect the sensitivity of others (Verrillo and Gescheider, 1977; Gescheider, Frisina and Verrillo, 1979; Hollins et al., 1990).

The fact that it is possible to selectively adapt a single tactile channel has provided an experimental technique for separating channels so that their characteristics can be examined independently (e.g. Gescheider, Frisina and Verrillo, 1979; Hollins et al., 1990; Verrillo and Gescheider, 1977; Verrillo and Schmiedt, 1974). An adapting stimulus is used that will substantially elevate the thresholds of all channels except the one under study: because the psychophysical detection threshold is always determined by the channel with the lowest threshold, the characteristics of the unadapted channel are revealed simply by measuring psychophysical thresholds while maintaining other channels in an adapted state by selecting an appropriate adapting stimulus.

In most natural situations, including those where tactile aids are used, stimuli of moderate to high intensity (often with several frequency components) do not result in selective adaptation but adapt all channels to varying degrees. Thus, conditions in which the skin is exposed to vibration containing a broad band of frequencies could result in a substantial amount of adaptation, since each of the vibrotactile channels may become adapted through exposure to stimulation within its own frequency range.

Complex Stimuli

Patterns

It is likely, although not certain, that vibrotactile stimuli that will function as a substitute for hearing will impose upon the skin a complex spatial pattern of stimulation rather than the simple single-contactor stimulation favored in most basic research laboratories. Although there are a number of multicontactor devices being marketed that vary in complexity of display, a current favorite is the Optacon (Bliss, 1974; Craig, 1976b), which was developed as a reading aid for the blind.

An impressive body of research on the identification and discrimination of vibrotactile spatial patterns generated by the Optacon has been reported by Craig (1976a,b, 1977, 1978, 1982a,b, 1983a,b, 1985, 1988, 1989; Horner and Craig, 1989). Because any system of tactual speech comprehension must involve sequential and simultaneous stimulation of the skin, an important factor to consider is masking. The masking effects of unpatterned stimuli have already been considered, but it is probable that speech information will be conveyed to the skin in the form of a pattern or array. Craig (1976a,b, 1978, 1980) has determined that the perception of patterned stimuli (letters) is interfered with by other patterns imposed upon the skin of the finger before or after the target stimulus. Performance in letter recognition was degraded more when the target stimulus preceded the masking stimulus (backward masking) than when it followed the masker (forward masking), and the identification of the pattern stimulus improved as the time between masker and target was increased. Unfortunately, any identification of speech by way of tactile patterns will be time-bound by the speech pattern of the speaker; there will be little or no control over the speed of stimulus presentation, in contrast to the situation when reading printed matter. To complicate matters further, Craig (1982a, 1983a) found that maskers configured in a pattern had a worse effect than did unpatterned maskers: it is assumed that patterns derived from speech will be patterned. The effects of forward and backward temporal masking could cause serious problems in tactual speech perception and should be factored into design considerations.

Craig (1983b) also compared static (long display times) and scanning (transient display times) modes of presentation and found significantly better recognition of letters and three-letter words under static conditions. The fact that pattern recognition is diminished with decreasing display time is yet another complicating factor for recognizing speech patterns on the skin.

Spatiotemporal relationships

Do changes in the spatial parameters of stimulation affect temporal tuning of the tactile system? Do changes in the temporal parameters of stimulation affect spatial tuning? Van Doren, Pelli and Verrillo (1987) concluded that, in both pacinian and non-pacinian I channels, temporal and spatial tuning are independent. This conclusion was based on measurements of detection thresholds for spatial sinusoidal patterns of vibration of variable temporal frequency that drifted across the skin. The authors found that changing the temporal frequency of the stimulus may change the overall sensitivity but does not change the spatial tuning curve, and vice versa.

Van Doren (1990) pointed out that this 'spatial-temporal independence hypothesis' should be valid for both sinusoidal and non-sinusoidal spatial stimuli, and referred to Verrillo's (1963) demonstration of spatiotemporal independence for the pacinian channel using circular contactors. As seen in Figure 1.1 the temporal tuning, as determined by threshold measurements at various frequencies, does not change in the U-shaped portion of the function as contactor size changes (although sensitivity level changes dramatically because of spatial summation). Verrillo (1966b) reported similar findings for stimulation of the volar surface of the forearm.

Van Doren (1990) has further demonstrated that the spatial and temporal tuning characteristics of the non-pacinian I channel are independent for non-sinusoidal changes in the spatial configuration of the stimulus. Psychophysical thresholds as a function of frequency were measured without a rigid surround, and with a rigid surround with a 1 mm gap between it and the perimeter of a 0.72 cm² contactor. When the surround is used, the stimulus is confined to the immediate region of the contactor, but when it is not the vibratory stimulus is free to spread over an extensive region. Removal of the surround elevated thresholds uniformly by about 10 dB at all low frequencies demonstrating that, although changing the spatial configuration of the stimulus substantially changes the sensitivity of the non-pacinian I system, it has no effect on its temporal tuning.

Van Doren (1989) proposed a model similar to that of Phillips and Johnson (1981), from which it was possible to accurately predict the spatial tuning of both the pacinian and non-pacinian I channels. According to the model, which is based on calculated strains in the tissue, the spatial tuning of the channels is a function of the tissue surrounding the receptors whereas the temporal tuning is an intrinsic property of the receptors.

The tactile analogy of auditory sound localization provides us with another aspect of spatiotemporal relations on the skin. Sound localization is possible because the ears, being spatially separated, provide the brain with information in terms of binaural differences in time of stimulation and intensity of stimulation, that is, correlated with the location of a sound source. Von Békésy (1955, 1957) reported that, with training, subjects can accurately localize sound sources when stimulation is exclusively tactile. In his experiments, acoustic stimuli activated two spatially separated microphones and the signals from each were amplified separately to drive two tactile stimulators, one attached to each forearm. This arrangement presented to the two forearms the temporal and intensive differences in stimulation known to play important roles in auditory localization. Using a similar system, in which the fingertips were stimulated, Gescheider (1965) found that accuracy of sound localization was nearly the same for the skin as for the ears – average errors of localization for click stimuli were 8.0° for ears, 9.0° for ring and index fingertips of the same hands, and 10.3° for the index fingertips of the left and right hands.

In the first few training sessions, Gescheider's subjects reported that when the sound source location was changed, the relative intensity of vibration on the two fingertips also seemed to change and that this served as a cue for localization. In later sessions, however, many observers reported that tactile sensations were projected out into space between the two fingertips to a position corresponding to the sound source. Such a phenomenon is not unlike what we experience in auditory localization of sound and visual localization of objects. Stimulation occurs at the receptors, yet the experience may be projected out into the environment to correspond more closely with the source of stimulation.

Independent manipulation of intensity and temporal difference cues revealed that, although auditory localization is influenced by both types of cue, tactile sound localization depends mainly on intensity differences (see also Alles, 1970). For example, Gescheider (1974) reported that when the stimulation time delay is systematically manipulated, subjects judge that the maximum displacement of the sensation from the midline occurs at delays of 1.0 ms for the ears and 4.0-6.0 ms for the skin.

When the time interval between brief stimuli is made so long that the localized sensation is shifted completely to the ear or skin area first stimulated, further increases eventually lead to the image breaking up into two images perceived successively – one in each ear or at each skin site. In binaural stimulation, when two equally intense clicks are separated, fusion is lost for intervals of more than about 1.5-2.0 ms; in contrast, tactile sensations remain fused until the time interval between stimuli exceeds 5-10 ms, at which point successive sensations are perceived (Gescheider, 1966, 1967, 1974).

The phenomenon of apparent motion on the skin may emerge at inter-stimulus intervals greater than the fusion threshold of 5-10 ms and the temporal order threshold of 20 ms. When the time interval between tactile stimuli applied to spatially separated sites is 75-150 ms, the sensation is perceived as moving rapidly from the first to the second test site in a way reminiscent of the phi phenomenon in vision (Sherrick and Rogers, 1966; Kirman, 1974). Sherrick and Rogers found that, at various stimulus durations, the optimal inter-stimulus intervals for apparent motion were virtually identical for visual, tactile and electrocutaneous stimuli. A fundamental feature of apparent motion is that the sensation seems to move in a continuous uninterrupted path from the first to the second stimulated site.

A different phenomenon of spatiotemporal interaction, but involving similar ranges of interstimulus intervals, was discovered by Geldard and Sherrick in 1972, which they referred to as the cutaneous 'rabbit'. This is a perceptual illusion, first noted when mechanical pulses delivered to the forearm produced sensations that were not always localized under the contactors. If the intensity and temporal sequence of pulses delivered to multiple sites on the forearm are in the correct configuration, the sensation is a smooth progression of taps at and between the stimulators, not unlike a rabbit hopping along a straight line. The cutaneous rabbit (now referred to as 'saltation') was originally discovered by accident when Geldard and Sherrick became interested in repeating some of the work of Helson and King (1931) who had demonstrated the 'tau effect', in which perceived distance between two tactile sensations is positively related to the temporal interval between stimulation of the two sites. Since then sensory saltation has been extensively studied (Cholewiak, 1976; Geldard, 1975, 1976, 1977, 1982, 1985), and has been demonstrated to be a general principle that also occurs in hearing (Sherrick, 1982; Geldard, 1984) and vision (Geldard, 1975, 1976).

Geldard and Sherrick also examined the spatial limits of saltation on different body sites in a study of the neural basis of cutaneous saltation (Geldard and Sherrick, 1983). The areas within which saltation can occur averaged 145.7 cm², 31.0 cm² and 2.28 cm² for the volar forearm, palm and index fingertip respectively. The sizes and shapes of saltatory areas at different body sites are correlated with the sizes and shapes of the receptive fields of single neurons in the somatosensory cortex. They concluded that each saltatory area must involve many cortical neurons with overlapping receptive fields; however, the specific neural mechanism of saltation remains unknown.

Subject Variables

The eventual user of tactile aids will have certain biological characteristics over which we have no control. Omitting variables caused by injury or disease that can result in peripheral (or central) neuropathies, the two features of our species over which we have little or no control are *gender* and *age*. If these have any effect on the functional characteristics of vibrotaction that have been discussed, we must know what they are.

Gender

Are men different from women in their sensitivity to vibration on the skin? Goff et al. (1965) reported a gradual loss of sensitivity with increasing age for women, starting in the late teens; other studies (Plumb and Meigs, 1961; Steinberg and Graber, 1963; Verrillo and Ecker, 1977) report no gender differences. Figure 1.11 shows a comparison of vibrotactile detection thresholds on the hands of men and women of comparable age (Verrillo, 1979a): It is clear that vibrotactile sensitivity on the hand is the same in both sexes. Women's sensitivity varies over the duration of the menstrual cycle (Gescheider et al., 1984): sensitivity at high frequencies (250 Hz) was lowest 12–13 days after the onset of menstruation and then gradually improved, reaching maximal sensitivity just before menstruation. For a few days before menstruation women are more sensitive to high-frequency vibration than are men.

Another important consideration in making sensory comparisons between groups is the rate at which sensation grows with increasing physical intensity of the stimulus. Men and women of comparable age were tested by the method of numerical magnitude balance (Hellman and Zwislocki, 1963). The results (shown in Figure 1.12) indicate that, because sensation magnitude grows more rapidly in women than in men, the perceived sensation of suprathreshold stimuli is greater for women (Verrillo, 1979a). The experiment was repeated using a visual stimulus (line length) in order to rule out possible biases by women in their use of numbers. With visual stimuli men and women did not differ, indicating that vibratory stimuli at suprathreshold levels are felt more intensely by women.

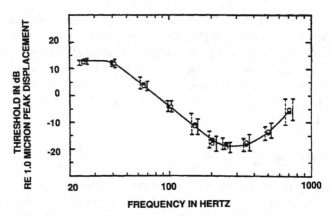

Figure 1.11 Vibrotactile thresholds of detectability measured in men (●) and women (○). The vertical bars represent one standard deviation. There is no apparent gender difference in the vibrotactile sensitivity for averaged data. (From Verrillo, 1979a, by permission of the Psychonomic Society, Inc.)

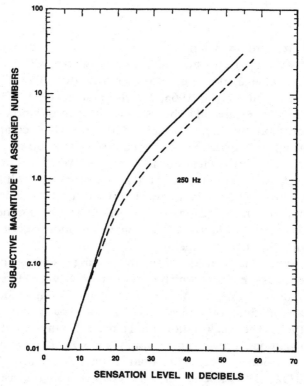

Figure 1.12 Curves of numerical magnitude balance of women (——) and men (- - - -). Although the threshold (−18.2 dB) and slope of the power functions are the same in both groups, the higher position of the curve for women indicates that they feel the same amplitude of vibration as subjectively greater than do men. (From Verrillo, 1979a, by permission of the Psychonomic Society, Inc.)

Age

The other variable worthy of careful consideration is the age of the subject. It has been well documented that to some extent all sensory systems decline in function with age, including vibrotactile sensitivity (Cosh, 1953; Plumb and Meigs, 1961). Studies have shown a progressive loss of sensitivity at high frequencies, with little or no change at the lower frequencies (Frisina and Gescheider, 1977; Verrillo, 1977, 1979b, 1982). The results of Verrillo (1979b) (shown in Figure 1.13) indicate that if higher frequencies are used in a tactile communication system, the age of the user must be taken into account. The loss of sensitivity in the high-frequency region of the curves reflects age-related changes that occur in the structure and number (decreased) of pacinian corpuscles.

There are also changes with advancing age at suprathreshold levels. The growth of the subjective-magnitude function at a frequency of 250 Hz was significantly steeper at 66 years of age than that from a group of 25-year-olds. This finding parallels results from tests of patients with symptoms of cochlear pathology in the auditory system.

Sensory persistence is a phenomenon measured in aging subjects. It occurs when a sensation is prolonged psychologically beyond the stimulus, and could result in inability to distinguish two stimuli closely spaced

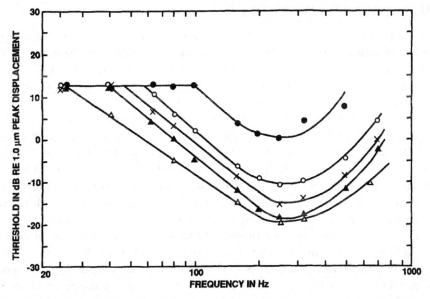

Figure 1.13 Detection thresholds of vibrotaction measured in five age groups ($\triangle$, 10; $\blacktriangle$, 20; $\times$, 35; $\bigcirc$, 50; $\bullet$, 65 years). Vibrotactile sensitivity decreases with age in the U-shaped portion of the curve, where the pacinian corpuscle system determines the response. The non-pacinian systems (flat portion of the curves) do not appear to be affected by age. (From Verrillo, 1979b, © Gerontological Society of America.)

in time. Older subjects (mean age 66 years) could not differentiate two tactile pulses when they were separated by less than 100 ms, a task easily performed by a group of 22-year-olds (Verrillo, 1982). Similarly, the ability to detect temporal gaps in vibration is adversely affected by age (Van Doren, Gescheider and Verrillo, 1990).

It may be concluded that tactile sensation at threshold and suprathreshold levels of stimulation in both the frequency and temporal domains are negatively affected by advancing age. The effect of age must not be overlooked by the designers of tactile communication systems.

Handedness

Another subject variable over which no control can be exercised is hand preference, or handedness. No sensitivity difference was found between the hands of right handed, left handed or ambidextrous subjects (Verrillo, 1983); however, when the task involved the enhancement or suppression effect of *contralateral* stimuli, only the ambidextrous subjects showed no cross-body influences. Sensations on one hand of ambidextrous persons appear to be independent of sensory input to the other hand, whereas pronounced enhancement and suppression effects were observed in subjects having a strong preference for either hand.

Receptor Mechanisms

Human skin contains at least four different, morphologically distinct, receptor end organs that are involved in tactile sensations arising from the mechanical disturbance of its surface. It is important to know what they are and what their functional characteristics are if the surface of the skin is to be efficiently used as a channel of communication.

The four primary receptors located in glabrous cutaneous tissues are the pacinian corpuscle, the Meissner corpuscle, the Merkel cell neurite ending, and the Ruffini ending. It has been the goal of many laboratories over many years to identify specific sensations with specific receptors located. At different times, scientists have vacillated between the extremes of a single-receptor system that mediated *all* cutaneous sensations and 34 different receptors that signaled the many fine nuances of tactile sensation.

In the early 1960s Verrillo proposed that tactile sensation was mediated by at least two cutaneous mechanoreceptor systems (Verrillo, 1963, 1965). One of these was identified as having the pacinian corpuscle as its end organ (Verrillo, 1966c,d, 1968) and the other was an unspecified, non-pacinian, system. The identification of the two systems was based on the findings that the detection-threshold characteristic had two limbs; a flat portion at low frequencies and a U-shaped portion at high frequencies (Figure 1.1): the correspondence of the U-shaped psychophysical curve with published data of recordings from pacinian corpuscles (Sato, 1961) led to the identification of one of the two cutaneous mechanoreceptor systems. A group of investigators led by Montcastle (Talbot et al., 1968) came to a similar conclusion a few years later, based on a psychophysical experiment in humans and electrophysiological experiments in monkeys. It was also shown that the pacinian system is capable of integrating energy over time and space, whereas the non-pacinian system could not (Verrillo, 1963, 1968). An extensive series of experiments established that the two systems constituted independent channels of communication to the central nervous system.

The knowledge accumulated from psychophysical experiments over a period of 28 years has been integrated with anatomical and physiological data to confirm that tactile sensations are mediated by four receptor systems: the pacinian and three non-pacinian (Bolanowski et al., 1988). Furthermore, the physiological responses of each of the four receptor types, identified most conclusively by Johansson and colleagues (Johansson, 1976, 1978; Johansson, Landström and Lundström, 1982), have been linked by Bolanowski and colleagues to functional psychophysically measured characteristics. It was obvious at an early stage that the flat portions (non-pacinian) of the curves shown in Figure 1.1 were the product of more than one receptor system. It became necessary to measure vibrotactile thresholds at very low frequencies (0.4 Hz) before responses from all four systems could be elicited. Figure 1.14 compares the physiological data of Johansson et al. (1982), represented by data points and solid lines, with psychophysically measured threshold-frequency characteristics, represented by dashed lines. The top panel shows the frequency response characteristic of the Meissner corpuscle, which is found only in glabrous skin. The psychophysical response was obtained by using a very small contactor (0.01 cm^2) and holding the skin temperature at 30°C. This channel has been designated the non-pacinian I (NPI) system in the psychophysical literature.

The responses of the pacinian channel are shown in Figure 1.14B. The psychophysical data were obtained with a large contactor (2.9 cm^2), and 30°C skin temperature. Figure 1.14C shows the results of recording from fibers that innervate Merkel cell neurite receptors, found in both hairy and glabrous skin, and psychophysical measurements using maskers of 0.7, 10, 20 and 100 Hz and a large contactor. The physiological response of the Ruffini endings is shown in Figure 1.14D along with the psychophysical response curve (Capraro, Verrillo and Zwislocki, 1979; Gescheider et al., 1985; Verrillo and Bolanowski, 1986).

The complete four-channel model is represented in Figure 1.15, showing the overlapping sensitivities of the channels which combine to mediate tactile perception. The absolute sensitivity at a particular frequency is determined by the channel having the lowest threshold at that frequency. The

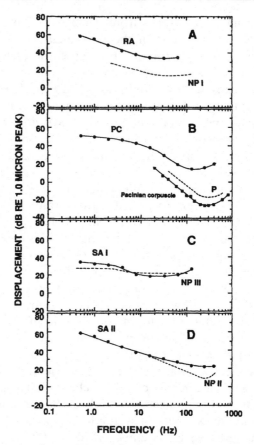

Figure 1.14 The frequency characteristics of the four receptor systems found in glabrous skin. The data points and solid lines (●—●) represent data obtained by neurophysiological measurements from nerve fibers. Physiological recordings were made from rapidly adapting (RA), pacinian (PC), and slowly adapting type I (SA I) and type II (SA II) nerve fibers. The dashed lines (- - - -) represent results from psychophysical experiments. A, the curves produced by activity in Meissner corpuscles; B, curves obtained from pacinian corpuscles (■—■), responses of six corpuscles measured in the author's laboratory); C, results of activating the Merkel cell neurite receptors; D, curves resulting from activation of the Ruffini endings. (From Bolanowski et al., 1988.)

exact position of the curves may be influenced by stimulus conditions such as contactor size, skin surface temperature (Bolanowski and Verrillo, 1982) and stimulus duration. Thus, the four-channel model of vibrotaction includes the response of Merkel endings at very low frequencies, with the Meissner corpuscles dominating the response in the mid frequencies, and the domain of the pacinian corpuscle in the U-shaped portion of the curve. The frequency response of the Ruffini system is U-shaped as is that of the pacinian corpuscle, but at such a reduced sensitivity that it would require a stimulus of considerable intensity to activate it.

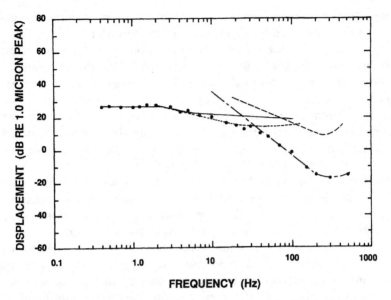

Figure 1.15 The four-channel model of vibrotaction. Shown are the threshold-frequency characteristics of the pacinian (— · —, Bolanowski and Verrillo, 1982); NPI (- - - -, Verrillo and Bolanowski, 1986); NP II (- - - -, Gesheider et al., 1985); and NP III (——) channels, as determined by psychophysical measurements. The data points (●) represent psychophysically measured detection thresholds. (From Bolanowski et al., 1988.)

A considerable amount of research will be necessary in order to convert this knowledge into practical applications in the design of a tactile communication system. Spatial discriminability of the elements of the display is of central importance. In this regard, it is significant that Sherrick, Cholewiak and Collins (1990) reported that 25-Hz stimuli on the hand, predominantly exciting non-pacinian receptors, are only slightly more accurately localized than 250-Hz stimuli, exclusively exciting the pacinian channel. They suggested that spatial acuity is as dependent on receptor density and its gradient as it is on receptor types and their corresponding receptive field sizes.

Summary

It is clear that a multitude of hurdles must be overcome before an effective device for utilizing the skin as a surrogate for hearing speech communication can be produced. Technology does not seem to be the problem. Although substantial advances have been made in recent years, not enough is known about the psychophysical characteristics of skin. Compared with the volume of research on the visual and auditory systems, the research on cutaneous mechanoreception has been relatively small.

One very important aspect of communication systems in general concerns their information carrying capacity. In order to design an effective, efficient device for tactile communication, quantitative estimates of the information transfer or information transfer rate which is available via the skin must be determined. The basic information, including the frequency response of tactile receptor systems and the just noticeable intensity differences is known, but the determination of information transfer capacity is rather complex because we are dealing with a non-linear system with multiple channels. Investigators at the Institute for Sensory Research are currently working on the problem.

Another major problem that exists within the context of what is known about tactile sensory characteristics is the masking of one sensation by another when the two stimuli are presented in close temporal or spatial proximity. Masking occurs maximally when the two stimuli are simultaneous, but also occurs when the target stimulus precedes or follows the masker. It can be reduced by increasing the temporal or spatial separation of the stimuli, but this opens the door to other problems. Speech is a time-bound stimulus and even if the time sequences were lengthened artificially, the rate at which information could be transmitted would be reduced considerably. Spatial separation of stimuli on the body is not a suitable solution because it might easily result in confusion of the locus of stimulation and would necessitate the integration of information fed centrally from spatially distant sites, presenting a formidable problem to the user. In spite of these problems, a number of devices have been developed, and governmental funding agencies now recognize that an effective device would ease the burden and expense of those who suffer from hearing deficits. Although the source of support for research tends to be cyclic, it is the principal hope for maintaining an effective research effort, basic and applied, towards the goal.

Acknowledgments

This work was supported in part by funds from Grants PO 1 DC 00380 and RO 1 DC 00098 from the National Institutes of Health, US Department of Health and Human Services.

References

ALLES, D.S. (1970). Information transmission by phantom sensations. *IEEE Trans. Man–Machine Systems* **11**, 85–91.

BÉKÉSY, G. VON (1939). Über die Vibrationsempfindung. *Akust. Zeits.* **4**, 316–334.

BÉKÉSY, G. VON (1955). Human skin perception of traveling waves similar to those on the cochlea. *J. Acoust. Soc. Am.* **27**, 830–841.

BÉKÉSY, G. VON (1957). Sensations on the skin similar to directional hearing, beats, and harmonics of the ear. *J. Acoust. Soc. Am.* **29**, 489–501.

BÉKÉSY, G. VON (1959). Synchronism of neural discharges and their demultiplication in pitch perception on the skin and in hearing. *J. Acoust. Soc. Am.* **31**, 338-349.

BERGLUND, U. and BERGLUND, B. (1970). Adaptation and recovery in vibrotactile perception. *Percept. Mot. Skills* **30**, 843-853.

BLISS, J.C. (1974). Summary of three Optacon-related cutaneous experiments. In: Geldard, F.A. (ed.), *Cutaneous Communication Systems and Devices*. Austin, TX: The Psychonomic Society, pp. 84-94.

BOLANOWSKI, S.J. JR and VERRILLO, R.T. (1982). Temperature and criterion effects in the somatosensory system: A neurophysiological psychophysical study. *J. Neurophysiol.* **48**, 837-856.

BOLANOWSKI, S.J. JR., GESCHEIDER, G.A., VERRILLO, R.T. and CHECKOWSKY, C.M. (1988). Four channels mediate the mechanical aspect of touch. *J. Acoust. Soc. Am.* **84**, 1680-1694.

BUUNEN, T.J.F. and VAN VALKENBURG, D.A. (1979). Auditory detection of a single gap in noise. *J. Acoust. Soc. Am.* **65**, 534-537.

CAPRARO, A.J., VERRILLO, R.T. and ZWISLOCKI, J.J. (1979). Psychophysical evidence for a triplex system of cutaneous mechanoreception. *Sens. Proc.* **3**, 334-352.

CHOLEWIAK, R.W. (1976). Satiation in cutaneous saltation. *Sens. Proc.* **1**, 163-175.

CHOLEWIAK, R.W. (1979). Spatial factors in the perceived intensity of vibrotactile patterns. *Sens. Proc.* **3**, 141-156.

COHEN, L.H. and LINDLEY, S.B. (1938). Studies in vibratory sensibility. *Am. J. Psychol.* **51**, 44-63.

COSH, J.A. (1953). Studies on the nature of vibration sense. *Clin. Sci.* **12**, 131-150.

CRAIG, J.C. (1972). Difference threshold for intensity of tactile stimuli. *Percept. Psychophys.* **11**, 150-152.

CRAIG, J.C. (1974). Vibrotactile difference thresholds for intensity and the effect of masking noise. *Percept. Psychophys.* **15**, 123-127.

CRAIG, J.C. (1976a). Attenuation of vibrotactile spatial summation. *Sens. Proc.* **1**, 40-56.

CRAIG, J.C. (1976b). Vibrotactile letter recognition: The effect of a masking stimulus. *Percept. Psychophys.* **20**, 317-326.

CRAIG, J.C. (1977). Vibrotactile pattern perception: Extraordinary observers. *Science* **196**, 450-452.

CRAIG, J.C. (1978). Vibrotactile pattern recognition and masking. In: Gordon, G. (ed.), *Active Touch*. Oxford: Pergamon, pp. 229-242.

CRAIG, J.C. (1980). Modes of vibrotactile pattern perception. *J. Exp. Psychol.* **6**, 151-166.

CRAIG, J.C. (1982a). Vibrotactile masking: A comparison of energy and pattern maskers. *Percept. Psychophys.* **31**, 523-529.

CRAIG, J.C. (1982b). Temporal integration of vibrotactile patterns. *Percept. Psychophys.* **32**, 219-229.

CRAIG, J.C. (1983a). Some factors affecting tactile pattern recognition. *Int. J. Neurosci.* **19**, 47-58.

CRAIG, J.C. (1983b). The role of onset in the perception of sequentially presented vibrotactile patterns. *Percept. Psychophys.* **34**, 421-432.

CRAIG, J.C. (1985). Tactile pattern recognition and its perturbations. *J. Acoust. Soc. Am.* **77**, 238-246.

CRAIG, J.C. (1988). The role of experience in tactual pattern recognition: A preliminary report. *Int. J. Rehab. Res.* **11**, 167-183.

CRAIG, J.C. (1989). Interference in localizing tactile stimuli. *Percept. Psychophys.* **45**, 21-30.

FERRINGTON, D.G., NAIL, B.S. and ROWE, M. (1977). Human tactile detection threshold: Modification by input from specific tactile receptor classes. *J. Physiol.* **272**, 415-433.

FITZGIBBONS, P.J. (1983). Temporal gap-detection in noise as a function of frequency, band width, and level. *J. Acoust. Soc. Am.* **74**, 67-72.

FITZGIBBONS, P.J. (1984). Temporal gap resolution in masked normal ears as a function of masker level. *J. Acoust. Soc. Am.* **76**, 67-70.

FLETCHER, H. and MUNSON, W.A. (1933). Loudness, its definition, measurement and calculation. *J. Acoust. Soc. Am.* **5**, 82-108.

FRISINA, R.D. and GESCHEIDER, G.A. (1977). Comparison of child and adult vibrotactile thresholds as a function of frequency and duration. *Percept. Psychophys.* **22**, 100-103.

FUCCI, D., SMALL, L.H. and PETROSINO, L. (1982). Intensity difference limens for lingual vibrotactile stimuli. *Bull. Psychonom. Soc.* **1**, 54-56.

GEERS, A.E. (1986). Vibrotactile stimulation: Case study with a profoundly deaf child. *J. Rehab. Res. Dev.* **23**, 111-117.

GELDARD, F.A. (1975). *Sensory Saltation: Metastability in the Perceptual World*. Hillsdale, NJ: Erlbaum.

GELDARD, F.A. (1976). The saltatory effect in vision. *Sens. Proc.* **1**, 77-86.

GELDARD, F.A. (1977). Cutaneous stimuli, vibratory and saltatory. *J. Invest. Dermatol.* **69**, 83-87.

GELDARD, F.A. (1982). Saltation in somesthesis. *Psychol. Bull.* **92**, 136-175.

GELDARD, F.A. (1984). Is there a lesson for audition in tactile localization? In: Münster, M.H. (ed.), *Advances in Audiology, vol. 1*. Basel: S. Karger, pp. 117-127.

GELDARD, F.A. (1985). The mutability of time and space on the skin. *J. Acoust. Soc. Am.* **77**, 233-237.

GELDARD, F.A. and SHERRICK, C.E. (1972). The cutaneous 'rabbit': A perceptual illusion. *Science* **178**, 178-179.

GELDARD, F.A. and SHERRICK, C.E. (1983). The cutaneous saltatory area and its presumed neural basis. *Percept. Psychophys.* **33**, 299-304.

GESCHEIDER, G.A. (1965). Cutaneous sound localization. *J. Exp. Psychol.* **70**, 617-625.

GESCHEIDER, G.A. (1966). The resolving of successive clicks by the ears and skin. *J. Exp. Psychol.* **71**, 378-381.

GESCHEIDER, G.A. (1967). Auditory and cutaneous temporal resolution of successive brief stimuli. *J. Exp. Psychol.* **75**, 570-572.

GESCHEIDER, G.A. (1974). Temporal relations in cutaneous stimulation. In: Geldard, F.A. (ed.), *Cutaneous Communication Systems and Devices*. Austin, TX: The Psychonomic Society, pp. 33-37.

GESCHEIDER, G.A. (1976). Evidence in support of the duplex theory of mechanoreception. *Sens. Proc.* **1**, 68-76.

GESCHEIDER, G.A. and JOELSON, J.M. (1983). Vibrotactile temporal summation for threshold and suprathreshold levels of stimulation. *Percept. Psychophys.* **33**, 156-162.

GESCHEIDER, G.A. and VERRILLO, R.T. (1979). Vibrotactile frequency characteristics as determined by adaptation and masking procedures. In: Kenshalo, D.R. (ed.), *Sensory Functions of the Skin of Humans*. New York: Plenum, pp. 183-205.

GESCHEIDER, G.A. and WRIGHT, J.H. (1968). Effects of sensory adaptation on the form of the psychophysical magnitude function for cutaneous vibration. *J. Exp. Psychol.* **77**, 308-313.

GESCHEIDER, G.A. and WRIGHT, J.H. (1969). Effects of vibrotactile adaptation on perception of stimuli of varied intensity. *J. Exp. Psychol.* **81**, 449-453.

GESCHEIDER, G.A., BOLANOWSKI, S.J. JR. and VERRILLO, R.T. (1989). Vibrotactile masking: Effects of stimulus-onset asynchrony and stimulus frequency. *J. Acoust. Soc. Am.* **85**, 2059-2069.

GESCHEIDER, G.A., FRISINA, R.D. and VERRILLO, R.T. (1979). Selective adaptation of vibrotactile thresholds. *Sens. Proc.* **3**, 37-48.

GESCHEIDER, G.A., HERMAN, D.D. and PHILLIPS, J.N. (1970). Criterion shifts in the measurement of tactile masking. *Percept. Psychophys.* **8**, 433-436.

GESCHEIDER, G.A., O'MALLEY, M.J. and VERRILLO, R.T. (1983). Vibrotactile forward masking: evidence for channel independence. *J. Acoust. Soc. Am.* 74, 474-485.

GESCHEIDER, G.A., VERRILLO, R.T. and VAN DOREN, C.L. (1982). Prediction of vibrotactile masking functions. *J. Acoust. Soc. Am.* 72, 1421-1426.

GESCHEIDER, G.A., VERRILLO, R.T., CAPRARO, A.J. and HAMER, R.D. (1977). Enhancement of vibrotactile sensation magnitude and predictions from the duplex model of mechanoreception. *Sens. Proc.* 1, 187-203.

GESCHEIDER, G.A., VERRILLO, R.T., McCANN, J.T. and ALDRICH, E.M. (1984). Effects of the menstrual cycle on vibrotactile sensitivity. *Percept. Psychophys.* 36, 586-592.

GESCHEIDER, G.A., SKLAR, B.F., VAN DOREN, C.L. and VERRILLO, R.T. (1985). Vibrotactile forward masking: Psychophysical evidence for a triplex theory of cutaneous mechanoreception. *J. Acoust. Soc. Am.* 78, 534-543.

GESCHEIDER, G.A., BOLANOWSKI, S.J. JR., VERRILLO, R.T., ARPAJIAN, D.J. and RYAN, T.F. (1990). Vibrotactile intensity discrimination measured by three methods. *J. Acoust. Soc. Am.* 87, 330-338.

GILMER, B. VON H. (1935). The measurement of the sensitivity of the skin to mechanical vibration. *J. Gen. Psychol.* 13, 42-61.

GILSON, R.D. (1968). Some factors affecting the spatial discrimination of vibrotactile patterns. *Percept. Psychophys.* 3, 131-136.

GILSON, R.D. (1969a). Vibrotactile masking: Some spatial and temporal aspects. *Percept. Psychophys.* 5, 176-180.

GILSON, R.D. (1969b). Vibrotactile masking: Effects of multiple maskers. *Percept. Psychophys.* 8, 433-436.

GILSON, R.D. (1974). Vibrotactile masking. In: Geldard, F.A. (ed.), *Cutaneous Communication Systems and Devices*. Austin, TX: The Psychonomic Society, pp. 53-56.

GOFF, G.D. (1967). Differential discrimination of frequency of cutaneous mechanical vibration. *J. Exp. Psychol.* 74, 294-299.

GOFF, G.D., ROSNER, B.S., DETRE, T. and KENNARD, D. (1965). Vibration perception in normal man and medical patients. *J. Neurol. Neurosurg. Psychiat.* 18, 503-509.

GOLDSTEIN, M.H. JR. and PROCTOR, A. (1985). Tactile aids for profoundly deaf children. *J. Acoust. Soc. Am.* 77, 158-265.

HAHN, J.F. (1966). Vibrotactile adaptation and recovery measured by two methods. *J. Exp. Psychol.* 71, 655-658.

HAHN, J.F. (1968a). Tactile adaptation. In: Kenshalo, D.R. (ed.), *The Skin Senses*. Springfield, IL: C.C. Thomas, pp. 322-330.

HAHN, J.F. (1968b). Low-frequency vibrotactile adaptation. *J. Exp. Psychol.* 78, 655-659.

HAMER, R.D., VERRILLO, R.T. and ZWISLOCKI, J.J. (1983). Vibrotactile masking of Pacinian and non-Pacinian channels. *J. Acoust. Soc. Am.* 73, 1293-1303.

HAMER, R.D., ZWISLOCKI, J.J. and CAPRARO, A.J. (1978). Vibrotactile masking: Evidence for a peripheral threshold. *J. Acoust. Soc. Am.* 63 (Suppl. 1), 575.

HELLMAN, R.P. and ZWISLOCKI, J. (1961). Some factors affecting the estimation of loudness. *J. Acoust. Soc. Am.* 33, 687-694.

HELLMAN, R.P. and ZWISLOCKI, J. (1963). Monaural loudness function at 1000 cps and interaural summation. *J. Acoust. Soc. Am.* 35, 856-865.

HELSON, H. and KING, S.M. (1931). The Tau effect: An example of psychological relativity. *J. Exp. Psychol.* 14, 202-217.

HIRSH, I.J. and SHERRICK, C.E. (1961). Perceived order in different sense modalities. *J. Exp. Psychol.* 62, 423-432.

HOLLINS, M., GOBLE, A.K., WHITSEL, B.L. and TOMMERDAHL, M. (1990). Time course and action spectrum of vibrotactile adaptation. *Somatosens. Motor Res.* 7, 205-221.

HORNER, D.T. and CRAIG, J.C. (1989). A comparison of discrimination and identification of vibrotactile patterns. *Percept. Psychophys.* 45, 21-30.

HUGONY, A. (1935). Über die Empfindung von Schwingungen metells des tastsinnes. *Z. Biol.* 96, 548-553.

JOHANSSON, R.S. (1976). Receptive sensitivity profile of mechanosensitive units innervating the glabrous skin of the human hand. *Brain Res.* 104, 330-334.

JOHANSSON, R.S. (1978). Tactile sensibility of the human hand: Receptive field characteristics of mechanoreceptive units in the glabrous skin. *J. Physiol.* 281, 101-123.

JOHANSSON, R.S., LANDSTRÖM, U. and LUNDSTRÖM, R. (1982). Responses of mechanoreceptive afferent units in the glabrous skin of the human hand to sinusoidal skin displacements. *Brain Res.* 244, 17-25.

KATZ, D. (1925). Der Aufbau der Tastwelt. *Z. Psychol., Ergänzungsband* 11, 1-270.

KELLY, D.H. (1972). Flicker. In: Jameson, D. and Hurvich, L.M. (eds), *Handbook of Sensory Physiology, Vol. 7, Part 4: Visual Psychophysics.* Berlin: Springer, pp. 273-302.

KIRMAN, J.H. (1974), Tactile apparent movement: The effects of interstimulus onset interval and stimulus duration. *Percept. Psychophys.* 15, 1-6.

KNUDSON, V.O. (1928). Hearing with the sense of touch. *J. Gen. Psychol.* 1, 320-352.

LABS, S.M., GESCHEIDER, G.A., FAY, R.R. and LYONS, C.H. (1978). Psychophysical tuning curves in vibrotaction. *Sens. Proc.* 2, 231-247.

LAMORÉ, P.J.J., MUIJSER, H. and KEEMINK, C.J. (1986). Envelope detection of amplitude-modulated high-frequency sinusoidal signals by skin mechanoreceptors. *J. Acoust. Soc. Am.* 79, 1082-1985.

LECHELT, E.C. (1974a). Pulse number discrimination in tactile spatio-temporal patterns. *Percept. Mot. Skills* 39, 815-822.

LECHELT, E.C. (1974b). Stimulus intensity and spatiality in tactile numerosity discrimination. *Perception* 3, 297-302.

LECHELT, E.C. (1975). Temporal numerosity discrimination: Intermodal comparisons revisited. *Br. J. Psychol.* 66, 101-108.

LECHELT, E.C. and TANNE, G. (1976). Laterality in the perception of successive tactile pulses. *Bull. Psychonom. Soc.* 7, 452-454.

MARKS, L.E. (1979). Summation of vibrotactile intensity: An analog to auditory critical bands. *Sens. Proc.* 2, 188-203.

MOWBRAY, G.H. and GEBHARD, J.W. (1957). Sensitivity of the skin to changes in the rate of intermittent mechanical stimuli. *Science* 125, 1297-1298.

NAFE, J.P. and WAGONER, K.S. (1941). The nature of pressure adaptation. *J. Gen. Psychol.* 25, 323-351

O'MARA, S., ROWE, M.J. and TARVIN, R.P.C. (1988). Neural mechanisms in vibrotactile adaptation. *J. Neurophys.* 59, 607-622.

PHILLIPS, J.R. and JOHNSON, K.O. (1981). Tactile spatial resolution. III. A continuum-mechanics model of skin predicting mechanoreceptor responses to bars, edges and gratings. *J. Neurophysiol.* 46, 1204-1225.

PLOMP, R. (1964). Rate of decay of auditory sensation. *J. Acoust. Soc. Am.* 36, 277-282.

PLUMB, C.S. and MEIGS, J.W. (1961). Human vibration perception: Part I. Vibration perception at different ages. *Arch. Gen. Psych.* 4, 611-614.

ROTHENBERG, M. and MOLITOR, R.D. (1979). Encoding voice fundamental frequency into vibrotactile frequency. *J. Acoust. Soc. Am.* 66, 1029-1038.

ROTHENBERG, M., VERRILLO, R.T., ZAHORIAN, S.A., BRACHMAN, M.L. and BOLANOWSKI, S.J. JR. (1977). Vibrotactile frequency for encoding a speech parameter. *J. Acoust. Soc. Am.* 62, 1003-1012.

SATO, M. (1961). Response of Pacinian corpuscles to sinusoidal vibration. *J. Physiol.* 159, 391-409.

SETZEPFAND, W. (1935). Frequenzabhangigkeit der Vibrationsempfindung des Menchen. *Z. Biol.* 96, 236-240.

SHERRICK, C.E. JR. (1953). Variables affecting sensitivity of the human skin to mechanical vibration. *J. Exp. Psychol.* **45**, 273-282.

SHERRICK, C.E. (1964). Effects of double simultaneous stimulation of the skin. *Am. J. Psychol.* **77**, 42-53.

SHERRICK, C.E. (1982). Cutaneous Communication. In: Neff, W.D. (ed.), *Contributions to Sensory Physiology, vol. 6.* New York: Academic, pp. 1-43.

SHERRICK, C.E. and ROGERS, R. (1986). Apparent haptic movement. *Percept. Psychophys.* **1**, 175-180.

SHERRICK, C.E., CHOLEWIAK, R.W. and COLLINS, A.A. (1990). The localization of low- and high-frequency vibrotactile stimuli. *J. Acoust. Soc. Am.* **88**, 169-179.

SNYDER, R.E. (1977). Vibrotactile masking: A comparison of psychophysical procedures. *Percept. Psychophys.* **22**, 471-475.

STEINBERG, F.V. and GRABER, A.L. (1963). The effect of age and peripheral circulation on the perception of vibration. *Arch. Phys. Med. Rehab.* **44**, 645-650.

STEVENS, S.S. (1968). Tactile vibration: Change of exponent with frequency. *Percept. Psychophys.* **3**, 223-228.

TALBOT, W.H., DARIAN-SMITH, I., KORNHUBER, H.H. and MOUNTCASTLE, V.B. (1968). The sense of flutter-vibration: Comparison of the human capacity with response patterns of mechanoreceptive afferents from the monkey hand. *J. Neurophysiol.* **31**, 301-334.

TAPPER, D.N. (1965). Stimulus-response relationships in the cutaneous slowly adapting mechanoreceptor in hairy skin of the cat. *Exp. Neurol.* **13**, 364-385.

VAN DOREN, C.L. (1989). A model of spatiotemporal tactile sensitivity linking psychophysics to tissue mechanics. *J. Acoust. Soc. Am.* **85**, 2065-2080.

VAN DOREN, C.L. (1990). The effects of a surround on vibrotactile thresholds: Evidence for spatial and temporal independence in the non-Pacinian I (NP-I) channel. *J. Acoust. Soc. Am.* **87**, 2655-2661.

VAN DOREN, C.L., GESCHEIDER, G.A. and VERRILLO, R.T. (1990). Vibrotactile temporal gap detection as a function of age. *J. Acoust. Soc. Am.* **87**, 2201-2205.

VAN DOREN, C.L., PELLI, D.G. and VERRILLO, R.T. (1987). A device for measuring tactile spatiotemporal sensitivity. *J. Acoust. Soc. Am.* **81**, 1906-1916.

VERRILLO, R.T. (1963). Effect of contactor area on the vibrotactile threshold. *J. Acoust. Soc. Am.* **35**, 1962-1966.

VERRILLO, R.T. (1965). Temporal summation in vibrotactile sensitivity. *J. Acoust. Soc. Am.* **37**, 843-846.

VERRILLO, R.T. (1966a). Effect of spatial parameters on the vibrotactile threshold. *J. Exp. Psychol.* **71**, 570-575.

VERRILLO, R.T. (1966b). Vibrotactile thresholds for hairy skin. *J. Exp. Psychol.* **72**, 47-50.

VERRILLO, R.T. (1966c). Vibrotactile sensitivity and the frequency response of the Pacinian corpuscle. *Psychonom. Sci.* **4**, 135-136.

VERRILLO, R.T. (1966d). Specificity of a cutaneous receptor. *Percept. Psychophys.* **1**, 149-153.

VERRILLO, R.T. (1968). A duplex mechanism of mechanoreception. In: Kenshalo, D.R. (ed.), *The Skin Senses.* Springfield, IL: C.C. Thomas, pp. 139-159.

VERRILLO, R.T. (1971). Vibrotactile thresholds measured at the finger. *Percept. Psychophys.* **9**, 329-330.

VERRILLO, R.T. (1974). Vibrotactile intensity scaling at several body sites. In: Geldard, F.A. (ed.), *Cutaneous Communications Systems and Devices.* Austin, TX: The Psychonomic Society, pp. 9-14.

VERRILLO, R.T. (1977). Comparison of child and adult vibrotactile thresholds. *Bull. Psychonom. Soc.* **9**, 197-200.

VERRILLO, R.T. (1979a). Comparison of vibrotactile threshold and suprathreshold responses in men and women. *Percept. Psychophys.* **26**, 20-24.

VERRILLO, R.T. (1979b). Change in vibrotactile thresholds as a function of age. *Sens. Proc.* **3**, 49-59.

VERRILLO, R.T. (1982). Age related changes in the sensitivity to vibration. *J. Gerontol.* **35**, 185-193.

VERRILLO, R.T. (1983). Vibrotactile subjective magnitude as a function of hand preference. *Neuropsychologia* **21**, 383-395.

VERRILLO, R.T. and BOLANOWSKI, S.J. JR. (1986). The effects of skin temperature on the psychophysical responses to vibration on glabrous skin and hairy skin. *J. Acoust. Soc. Am.* **80**, 528-532.

VERRILLO, R.T. and CAPRARO, A.J. (1975). Effect of extrinsic noise on vibrotactile information processing channels. *Percept. Psychophys.* **18**, 88-94.

VERRILLO, R.T. and CHAMBERLAIN, S.C. (1972). The effect of neural density and contactor surround on vibrotactile sensation magnitude. *Percept. Psychophys.* **11**, 117-120.

VERRILLO, R.T. and ECKER, A.D. (1977). Effects of root or nerve destruction on vibrotactile sensitivity in trigeminal neuralgia. *Pain* **3**, 239-255.

VERRILLO, R.T. and GESCHEIDER, G.A. (1975). Enhancement and summation in the perception of two successive vibrotactile stimuli. *Percept. Psychophys.* **18**, 128-136.

VERRILLO, R.T. and GESCHEIDER, G.A. (1976). Effect of double ipsilateral stimulation on vibrotactile sensation magnitude. *Sens. Proc.* **1**, 127-137.

VERRILLO, R.T. and GESCHEIDER, G.A. (1977). Effect of prior stimulation on vibrotactile thresholds. *Sens. Proc.* **1**, 292-300.

VERRILLO, R.T. and GESCHEIDER, G.A. (1979). Psychophysical measurements of enhancement, suppression and surface-gradient effects in vibrotaction. In: Kenshalo, D.R. (ed.), *Sensory Functions of the Skin of Humans*. New York: Plenum, pp. 153-181.

VERRILLO, R.T. and SCHMIEDT, R.A. (1974). Vibrotactile poststimulatory threshold shift. *Bull. Psychonom. Soc.* **4**, 484-486.

VERRILLO, R.T., FRAIOLI, A.J. and SMITH, R.L. (1969). Sensation magnitude of vibrotactile stimuli. *Percept. Psychophys.* **6**, 366-372.

VERRILLO, R.T., GESCHEIDER, G.A., CALMAN, B.G. and VAN DOREN, C.L. (1983). Vibrotactile masking: Effects of one- and two-site stimulation. *Percept. Psychophys.* **33**, 379-387.

VIEMEISTER, N.F. (1979). Temporal modulation transfer functions based upon modulation thresholds. *J. Acoust. Soc. Am.* **66**, 1364-1380.

VIEMEISTER, N.F. (1988) Psychophysical aspects of auditory intensity coding. In: Edelman, G.M., Gall, W.E. and Cowan, W.M. (eds), *Auditory Function*. New York: Wiley, pp. 213-241.

WEBER, E.H. (1835). Über den Tastsinn. *Archiv. für Anat. Physiol. Wissenschaft. Med.*, 152-160.

WEDELL, C.H. and CUMMINGS S.B. (1938). Fatigue of the vibratory sense. *J. Exp. Psychol.* **22**, 429-438.

WEINSTEIN, S. (1968). Intensive and extensive aspects of tactile sensitivity as a function of body part, sex, and laterality. In: Kenshalo, D.R. (ed.), *The Skin Senses*. Springfield, IL: C.C. Thomas, pp. 195-222.

WEISENBERGER, J.M. (1986). Sensitivity to amplitude-modulated vibrotactile signals. *J. Acoust. Soc. Am.* **80**, 1707-1715.

ZWICKER, E. (1952). Die Grenzen der Hörbarkeit der Amplitudenmodulation und der Frequenzmodulation eines Tones. *Acustica* **2**, 125-133.

ZWISLOCKI, J. (1960). Theory of temporal summation. *J. Acoust. Soc. Am.* **32**, 1046-1060.

ZWISLOCKI, J.J. and GOODMAN, D.A. (1980). Absolute scaling of sensory magnitude. *Percept. Psychophys.* **28**, 28-38.

ZWISLOCKI, J.J. and SOKOLICH, W.G. (1974). On loudness enhancement of a tone burst preceding a tone burst. *Percept. Psychophys.* **16**, 87-90.

ZWISLOCKI, J.J., KETKAR, I., CANNON, M.W. and NODAR, R.H. (1974). Loudness enhancement and summation in pairs of short sound bursts. *Percept. Psychophys.* **16**, 91-95.

Chapter 2
Electrical Stimulation of the Skin

BRIAN H. BROWN and JOHN C. STEVENS

The idea of using direct electrical stimulation of tissue as a means of communication for the profoundly deaf is very old. Lindner (1937) was a teacher of deaf mutes who studied the use of electrical stimulation for training purposes. His 'teletactor' used audio filters to present high frequency (>1500 Hz) and low frequency (<1500 Hz) electrical stimulation to two fingers. He also applied simultaneous mechanical vibration to two fingers and found that the deaf mutes could learn to discriminate between vowels.

The last three decades have seen a reawakening in this area of research, with many suggested designs and many trials of electrotactile devices. Gilmer (1961), Hawkes (1961) and Foulke (1964) found that several intensities of stimulation could be discriminated. More recent contributions to the field will be discussed later in this chapter.

Sensory input through the skin is usually by direct stimulation of receptors for heat, pain or pressure. These receptors are located in the dermis. However, when electrical stimulation is directly applied to skin, interaction might be directly with the sensory receptors but can also be with the terminal nerve fibres or by stimulation of fibres in large nerve trunks. Which effect predominates depends upon the size of the electrode through which the electrical stimulus has been applied and its position relative to the receptors and nerve fibres. A small active electrode will give rise to high current densities directly underneath the electrode, which can stimulate individual receptors (Bishop, 1943). However, larger electrodes will not give rise to such high localised current densities and so will stimulate nerve fibres at a greater distance from the electrode. Neural stimulation has been the objective of recent electrotactile devices, as stimulation of individual receptors can be painful.

In this chapter the way in which nerve fibres can be electrically stimulated will be looked at in some detail, before considering what sites on the body might be available for the input of electrotactile information. The rate at which information might be transmitted via an electrical stimulus must then be estimated, and the practical problems of attaching electrodes to the body and of generating stimuli considered. Some of the published single and multichannel systems will be discussed with a view to assessing what the limiting value of electrotactile devices might be.

There is a wide literature on electrical stimulation. An excellent, although now rather old, review is that of Pfeiffer (1968). Some more recent material is given by Kaczmarek (1991).

Mechanism of Neural Stimulation

If a nerve is to be electrically stimulated electrical current must flow through tissue. This current will be carried by ionic charge carriers such as Na^+, K^+ and Cl^-. However, current applied to the body is most likely to be an electronic current, hence an electrode is required both to make electrical connection to the body and to allow for the exchange of electrons and ions. This is commonly achieved by a Ag/AgCl electrode coupled to the skin by a NaCl gel. The electrochemistry involved in understanding the exchange of electrons and ions at an electrode/tissue interface is beyond the scope of this book. Geddes (1972), Pethig (1979), Donaldson (1986) and McAdams (1987) are useful starting references on the subject of electrodes.

Applying currents

Current applied to the body through an electrode will spread out in three dimensions (Figure 2.1). Assuming the body is infinite and homogeneous the current from a point electrode will spread out radially and it is easy to show that the current density at a distance r from the electrode will be given by

$$\text{current density} = I/2\pi r^2 \tag{2.1}$$

where I is the current applied.

By integration the potential difference between points at radial distances r_1 and r_2 is calculated by

$$\text{potential difference} = I(r_1 - r_2)/2\pi r_1 r_2 \sigma \tag{2.2}$$

where σ is the electrical conductivity of the tissue. A typical value will be 0.33 Sm^{-1} but tissues vary widely (Barber and Brown, 1984).

It has been found that current is proportional to voltage over a wide range of values, i.e. Ohm's law applies. The current densities and potential gradients for finite-sized electrodes or for more than one electrode can therefore be determined by superimposing field patterns as shown in Figure 2.1. However, if the finite size of the body and the inhomogeneity

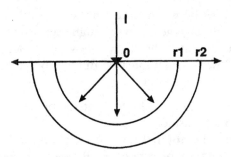

Figure 2.1 Current I applied to the body through a point electrode.

of tissue are to be taken into account then the field calculations are very much more difficult.

Neural stimulation

In order to initiate a nerve impulse the transmembrane potential of a nerve fibre must be changed. The nerve fibre shown in Figure 2.2 is myelinated, and current can only enter or leave the axon via the nodes of Ranvier.

The transmembrane potential is normally negative with respect to the outside of the nerve; therefore if this potential is to be reduced in order to initiate a propagating action potential the outside of the nerve must be made more negative with respect to the inside.

In Figure 2.2 the nodes of Ranvier are shown as areas where there is no myelin. There is still, however, a membrane surrounding the nerve axon and this will give rise to an electrical capacitance across the node. A typical value for this capacitance is 1 pF. Any stimulus current applied must persist long enough to change the voltage across this capacitance before an action potential is generated. Because the membrane is not a perfect insulator there will also be a leakage resistance associated with the node.

Nodes of Ranvier occur at regular intervals along a nerve fibre with a typical spacing of 1 mm for a 10 μm diameter fibre. As electrical current can only enter and leave the axon via the nodes, the potential gradient

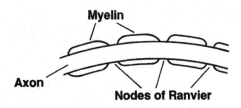

Figure 2.2 A myelinated nerve fibre.

along the nerve fibre between nodes must be sufficient to give rise to nodal transmembrane changes large enough (several tens of millivolts) to generate an action potential. From the above considerations three conditions can be laid down, which must be fulfilled before an electrical stimulus will initiate an action potential:

1. The applied current must make the outside of the nerve more negative with respect to the inside.
2. The current must be applied for sufficient time to reduce the voltage across the capacitance of a node of Ranvier by several tens of millivolts.
3. The applied current must be sufficient to cause a potential drop between adjacent nodes of several tens of millivolts. In order to produce such a potential the applied current must have a component along the nerve.

These three conditions are illustrated in Figure 2.3.

Some simple calculations will allow estimation of the amplitudes and durations of current flow required to cause nerve stimulation. A current is required to flow along the nerve: the simplest way to achieve this is to use two electrodes as illustrated in Figure 2.3. If a potential drop of 50 mV is required between nodes spaced 1 mm apart, from an electrode 10 mm from the nerve then, from equation (2.2), the required current is 10.5 mA. (A conductivity of 0.33 S m^{-1} has been assumed for the tissue.) The current flow from both electrodes must also be taken into account when calculating the potential drop along the nerve; equation (2.2) is only for one electrode. However, the difference is quite small.

The current of 10 mA will have to flow for sufficient time to reduce the voltage across the nodal capacitance by the few tens of mV noted previously. The current flow between the nodes has to pass through the

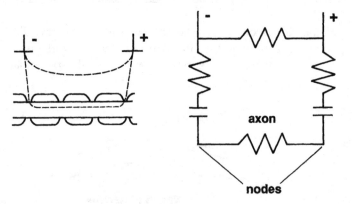

Figure 2.3 Two electrodes used to stimulate a nerve action potential by depolarising a node of Ranvier. An approximate equivalent circuit is shown on the right.

resistance of the axon (typically $5 \times 10^7 \ \Omega$) which provides a time constant of 50 μs with the nodal capacitance of 1 pF. Therefore, a current of 10 mA should be applied for 50 μs if a myelinated nerve fibre is to be stimulated at a depth of 10 mm. We have shown that threshold depends on the depth of the nerve fibre (equation 2.2). It will also depend on the size of the fibre, as large fibres conduct more rapidly and have a lower threshold than small fibres. A wide variation is therefore to be expected in subjective thresholds of electrical stimulation. An excellent account of the derivation of threshold is given by McNeal (1976).

Strength–duration curves

If the amplitude of a single stimulus at the threshold of stimulation is measured for a range of stimulus durations then a curve such as that shown in Figure 2.4 is obtained. It is often referred to as a strength–duration curve. The shape of the curve is what would be expected from our understanding of the process of nerve stimulation. Because charge must be removed from the capacitance at the node of Ranvier, if the pulse duration is reduced the current amplitude must be increased if the same charge is to flow. This is illustrated in Figure 2.4 where the charge required for stimulation is also plotted. This charge is constant at short pulse durations; at longer durations more charge is needed. This increase in charge arises because of leakage across the membrane at the node and also because low currents do not provide suffi- cient potential gradient between nodes to initiate an action potential.

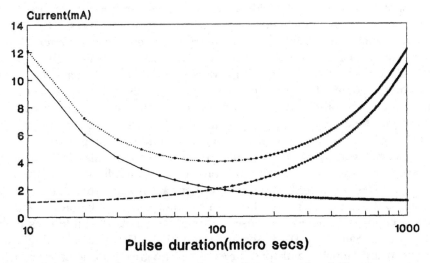

Figure 2.4 Typical strength–duration curve for a myelinated nerve (——). The energy per pulse is also shown (......) and the charge (- - -).

A third curve is shown in Figure 2.4: this shows the energy required at stimulation threshold and it can be seen that there is a pulse duration for which the energy is a minimum. For a large myelinated nerve fibre the duration where minimum energy is required for stimulation is about 100 µs. A theoretical derivation of these curves is given by Geddes and Bourland (1985). See also Butikofer and Lawrence (1978).

Convenient Sites for Electrical Stimulation

Electrotactile aids aim to stimulate nerve fibres rather than sensory receptors. Does this give any guidance as to which sites will be more suitable than others for the input of electrotactile information? Perhaps the most obvious site is the cochlea because a stimulus seems most likely to be perceived as a sound if it arises from within the ear. Whilst this may well be true there are also disadvantages to cochlear stimulation. The cochlea is inaccessible and so surgery is required to place the electrodes. Additionally the space available for processing electronics is very limited unless long connecting wires are accepted. In any case, cochlear stimulators will not be considered further, as they are distinct from electrotactile aids.

If nerve trunks are to be stimulated then the upper limbs offer several possible sites. The ulnar and median nerves run relatively superficially at the wrist and have been used by some workers (Dodgson et al., 1983) to input electrotactile stimuli. Applying a stimulus at the wrist has the advantage that people are used to wearing devices on the wrist. One disadvantage of stimulating a major nerve trunk is that both afferent and efferent fibres can be stimulated, with the result that muscle stimulation may accompany the sensory input.

There are two ways of avoiding efferent nerve stimulation. The first is to find nerve trunks which do not contain any efferent fibres. The digital nerves which run at the base of the fingers are almost free of efferent fibres and they also run superficially; another advantage of using digital nerve stimulation is that the fingers offer several sites so that multichannel devices can be considered. However, the fingers have the disadvantage that they are used for many other purposes and the electrodes used for electrotactile input may be a nuisance to the patient; also the processing electronics will probably have to be placed elsewhere, at the end of trailing wires.

A second way to avoid efferent stimulation is to stimulate the terminal nerve fibres supplying sensory end organs. An example of this is the use of electrodes on the abdomen, where there are no superficial large nerve trunks and so sensory nerve fibres can be stimulated well before the stimulus strength is sufficient to cause motor contractions. Multiple sites have been used (Saunders, 1973; Sparks et al., 1979). There are also disadvantages to abdominal stimulators, for example the greater difficulty of attaching electrodes and the problem of microphone location.

Information Transfer Rates

Many stimulation waveforms can be used to electrically stimulate a nerve. It is certainly possible simply to amplify an audio waveform to such a magnitude that direct neural stimulation will occur, which has the virtue of simplicity and has been used by some workers. However, it is certainly more efficient in terms of electrical power to stimulate using pulses of current. If pulses are used then the amplitude and frequency of the pulse train can be modulated by the audio signal in order to transmit information to the subject. The question then arises as to the rate at which information can be transmitted by this means.

The information rate of the communication channel can be considered as depending on:

1. the number of discriminable levels of pulse amplitude;
2. the number of discriminable pulse frequencies;
3. the maximum rate of change in amplitude or frequency which can be discerned.

It is arguable that pulse width could also be changed and give rise to information transfer. However, as neural stimulation depends upon the electrical charge transfer it seems likely that either pulse width or amplitude could be modulated but that it will not be possible to separate one from the other in terms of sensation.

A problem in computing the information transfer rate lies in the extent to which amplitude modulation of pulses can be distinguished from frequency modulation. Dodgson et al. (1983) asked subjects to compensate for amplitude changes by changing frequency and plotted the results as 'isofeels' (Figure 2.5). They concluded that subjects were able to compensate in this way but that large changes in frequency could be discerned independently of the pulse amplitude. There are limits to the frequency of stimulation: below about 20 pulses per second individual pulses can be felt and above about 400 pulses per second the interval between pulses is insufficient for the nerve to recover to respond to the next stimulus. The nerve is said to have a *refractory period*, during which it does not respond as normal. Between 20 and 400 pulses per second, typically three broad frequency bands could be defined, between which there was a qualitative change in sensation. This suggests that whilst amplitude and frequency changes are not completely independent, there is something to be gained by using both frequency modulation (FM) and amplitude modulation (AM).

Dodgson and co-workers found that the number of discriminable pulse amplitude levels between threshold and the point at which the stimulus becomes uncomfortable is typically six over an amplitude range of 1.6:1, i.e. 4 dB. If three frequency bands can also be discriminated then there are 18 (3 × 6) possible discriminable combinations. This corresponds to about 4

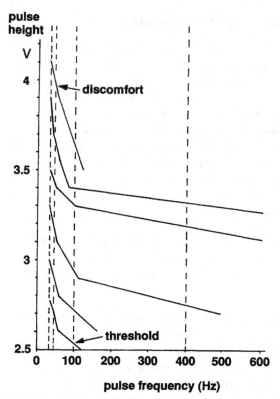

Figure 2.5 Typical 'isofeel' results showing how pulse frequency and amplitude can be changed to give a similar level of sensation. The dotted bands show frequency regions which still gave a different quality of sensation (after Dodgson, 1982).

bits of binary information. Dodgson (1982) argues, and quotes Gescheider (1974) to show, that the maximum discernible rate of change of amplitude and frequency is two times each second so that we arrive at an information rate of 8 bits s⁻¹. This is probably an optimistic estimate as in a practical situation noise will cause confusion between amplitude and frequency levels.

Pfeiffer (1968) gives an excellent review of electrical stimulation through skin electrodes and quotes several workers to support a figure of 2–6% as the minimum amplitude change which produces a just-noticeable change in sensation. (Six levels over a range of 1.6:1, used above, corresponds to 8% change per step.) Pfeiffer also says that more levels can be discriminated at higher stimulus levels close to the tolerance level and that adaptation occurs so that the apparent sensation changes with time.

Figure 2.6 shows similar results obtained in the authors' laboratory, with measurements obtained using vibrotactile stimulation for comparison. Figure 2.7 shows a comparison of electrotactile and vibrotactile frequency discrimination.

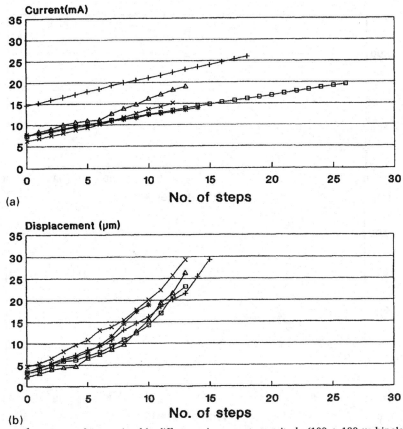

(a)

(b)

Figure 2.6 (a) Steps of just-noticeable difference in current magnitude (100 + 100 µs bipolar pulses via wrist electrodes) for five subjects. For each subject the lowest value of current corresponds to detection threshold and the highest to just below discomfort threshold; (b) steps of just-noticeable difference in vibration magnitude (1 ms Gaussian pulses on the wrist) for the same five subjects. For each subject the lowest vibration level corresponds to detection threshold and the highest to just below the maximum output available from the vibrator.

It is clear from the calculation of information transfer rate that there is a benefit from using both amplitude and frequency modulation of pulses although, from the data quoted, amplitude appears to carry more information as there are more discriminable levels. From a single channel system up to 8 bits per second of information may be transmitted. Multichannel input should certainly offer an increased capacity but there does not appear to be any published data to allow quantitation of this increase. It is also possible that modulation of pulse width, waveform, site of stimulation and field pattern might increase the potential information transfer rate, but again there appear to be no published data on this.

Having reached the conclusion that a single channel system can transmit up to 8 bits per second, it is interesting to compare this with the information

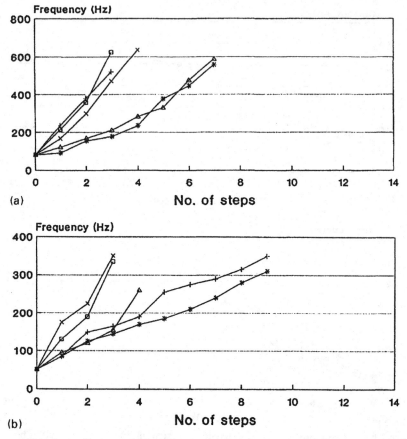

Figure 2.7 (a) Steps of just-noticeable difference in frequency (100 + 100 μs bipolar electrotactile pulses via wrist electrodes) for five subjects. The starting point for each sequence of steps was 80 Hz; (b) steps of just-noticeable difference in frequency (1 ms Gaussian vibrotactile pulses on the wrist) for the same five subjects. The starting point for each sequence of steps was 50 Hz.

rate required to transmit speech. Dodgson (1982) estimates that if speech could be transmitted as phonemes then a capacity of 50 bits s^{-1} would be required. However he notes that, due to the difficulty of extracting phonemes from speech, even efficient real-time speech transmission systems require a capacity of about 2400 bits s^{-1} (Rabiner and Shafer, 1978).

Practical Problems

The development of an electrotactile aid exposes a number of problems specific to electrical input, in addition to those which also arise with vibrotactile devices. The size and cosmetic appearance of the device are important whatever the method of sensory input; electrode problems are specific to electrotactile input.

Electrodes and their equivalent circuits

Electrodes are the means by which an electronic stimulator is interfaced to the body to produce an ionic current flow. The electrode can be thought of as a transducer which converts electrons to ions.

A comprehensive description of electrodes is outside the scope of this chapter. Brown and Smallwood (1981) give an introduction to the subject, Geddes (1972) a more comprehensive coverage and McAdams (1987) an in-depth study.

Many different materials have been used for the electrodes in electro-tactile devices. Although the materials which can be used in implanted devices need to be chosen with care, the restrictions on those which can be used in surface electrodes are less severe. Skin compatibility is impor-tant (as indeed it is in the choice of material for watch straps, where the constraints are very similar). Examples of suitable materials are stainless steel and conductive rubbers.

All electrodes, when attached to the skin, present a load to the electronic stimulator which can be described in terms of an equivalent circuit. The simplest form of this equivalent circuit and its impedance as a function of frequency are given in Figure 2.8. The resistance R_s is largely a function of the resistivity of the underlying tissues whereas R_p and C_p are determined by the electrode-tissue interface; C_p will increase and R_p decrease with increasing electrode area; R_s will be much smaller than R_p. An approximate value for R_s can be obtained from the following equation, obtained by integrating over the current flow from a surface electrode to infinity:

$$R_s = 1/\sigma\sqrt{(2\pi a)} \tag{2.3}$$

where a is the area of the electrode and σ the conductivity of the tissue. Conductivity σ will depend upon the tissue underneath the electrode but will normally lie between 0.5 S m^{-1} (for muscle) and 0.06 S m^{-1} (for fat). The calculated resistance is for one electrode with respect to a distant, much larger, electrode. This resistance is sometimes referred to as a spreading resistance. Note from equation (2.3) that an increase in the electrode size reduces the spreading resistance.

The values used to plot the graph in Figure 2.8 are typical for a pair of stainless steel electrodes each of area 100 mm^2 placed on the forearm (unabraded skin, no coupling material).

Obviously the stimulator must be able to drive the stimulation currents into the impedance presented by the electrodes. If 10 mA (as estimated earlier in this chapter) is required, then the necessary voltage would be at least 20 V for the equivalent circuit of Figure 2.8.

It is useful to have in mind the frequency components contained in a train of stimulation pulses so that the effect the impedance presented by the electrodes will have can be seen. Figure 2.9 shows two types of pulse

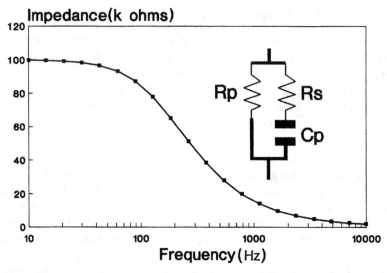

Figure 2.8 The equivalent circuit for a pair of electrodes placed on the forearm. Typical values for the components are R_s 1 kΩ, R_p 100 kΩ and C_p 10 nF. Impedance as a function of frequency for the equivalent circuit is plotted.

train and their associated frequency spectra. The Fourier series coefficients (complex exponential form) for a train of monopolar (monophasic) pulses of duration τ and repetition period T are given by:

$$\frac{V \sin(n\pi\tau/T)}{n\pi} \tag{2.4}$$

where V is the pulse amplitude.

For a train of bipolar (biphasic) pulses of overall duration 2τ, the magnitudes of the Fourier series coefficients are given by:

$$\frac{V[1-\cos(2n\pi\tau/T)]}{n\pi} \tag{2.5}$$

It can be seen that the two spectra are very different with less low-frequency energy in the bipolar pulse. However, in practice (see below) monopolar pulses would be used with a.c. coupling which would reduce the low frequency components*. In both cases most of the energy is above 5 kHz.

Editor's note. Strictly speaking, rectangular pulses become bipolar after a.c. coupling. However, such pulses may be quite accurately described as monopolar if the time constant of the a.c. coupling is long and the mark/space ratio is low. If the time constant is short the resulting pulses, with an exponentially decaying second phase of significant amplitude, are best described as bipolar.

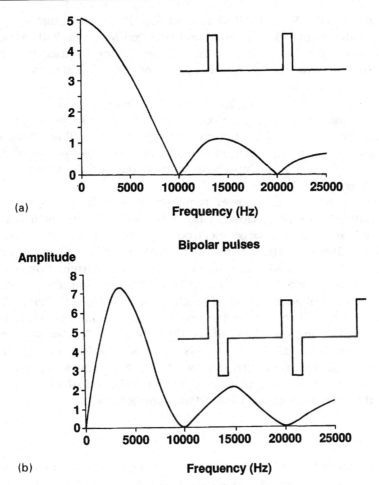

(a)

Frequency (Hz)

Bipolar pulses

Amplitude

(b)   **Frequency (Hz)**

Figure 2.9 (a) A train of monopolar pulses and their equivalent Fourier spectrum. The pulse duration is 100 μs and the repetition period 20 ms; (b) a train of bipolar pulses where each phase has the same duration as in (a). The repetition period is again 20 ms.

Power requirements

One of the potential benefits of electrical as opposed to vibratory input is the smaller range of power levels required from threshold to maximal acceptable stimulation. An approximate calculation of the power required can be made.

If the electrode resistance is 2 kΩ and we apply a pulse of duration 100 μs and amplitude 40 V then the energy per pulse is 8×10^{-5} J. The frequency at which the pulse is repeated will probably depend upon the acoustic environment but it is unlikely (allowing for periods of no stimulus) to be more than 10 s^{-1}. The mean and peak power requirements will therefore be 0.8 mW and 0.8 W respectively. Even quite small cells can provide a power of ~1 mW for several hundred hours, so battery power supply should not be a problem. For example, batteries used in behind-the-ear hearing aids have a typical capacity of 200 mA h at 1.35 V, giving 0.8 mW for 340 hours.

It was shown above (see Figure 2.4) that there is an optimum pulse duration if the energy in the current pulse is to be minimised. However, this duration will vary with the size and type of nerve fibre which is to be stimulated. In a particular situation it may be possible to minimise power consumption in this way. Most workers have used pulses of around 100 μs duration.

Another way in which power requirements can be minimised is by placing the electrodes as close as possible to the nerve which is to be stimulated and using a large electrode in order to minimise contact impedance. However, there is no point in having an electrode of greater dimension than the underlying nerve as additional current flow will be required, with no effect on the potential developed along the nerve.

The geometrical arrangement of electrode and nerve will also be determined by the need to localise the point of neural stimulation. Electrical currents cannot be focused and hence the only way to localise stimulation is to use small electrodes placed as close as possible to the nerve. However, small electrodes are associated with high spreading resistance and hence poor electrical efficiency. The optimisation of electrode area within these constraints is an important consideration.

Circuitry

It is not possible in this chapter to give any detailed description of circuitry. Many circuits have been used, but designs become rapidly out of date as new components become available. For this reason no circuits for audio signal processing and pulse modulation will be given. However, two areas common to all electrotactile devices will be discussed briefly: the generation of the relatively high voltages required for stimulation, and the low-frequency isolation of the output.

An output transformer can be used to step-up the battery supply voltage to the 60 V which may be required for stimulation. From Figure 2.9 it can be seen that this transformer has to operate efficiently over a wide range of frequencies between about 1 and 50 kHz, and it must handle the peak power of the pulse, which was calculated in the previous section as 0.8 W. It is quite difficult to make a very small transformer to meet this specification. Figure 2.10 shows a circuit which avoids this problem – a switching-regulator design which operates at a single high frequency and is required to generate a high-voltage supply to meet only the average power requirement of a few milliwatts. The high peak powers

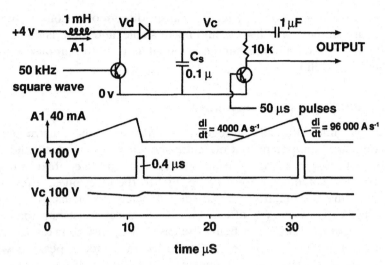

Figure 2.10 A switched inductor design to generate up to 100 V, which can then be used to output a pulse to the electrodes.

of the stimulation pulse are supplied by the storage capacitor C_s. The inductor required in this design has only about one-fifth of the volume of the transformer alternative and the circuit can deliver 40 mW at an efficiency of 70%.

When generating high voltages to stimulate the subject, adequate isolation must be available to prevent a d.c. potential appearing on the electrodes. A d.c. potential directly applied to skin electrodes is not only very painful but also will produce a skin ulcer very rapidly. Even quite small d.c. voltages applied to the skin will produce ulcers so that care must be taken to ensure that this cannot happen. Some form of a.c. coupling is generally used. A transformer cannot pass direct current, so it provides a safe method of generating the high-voltage output pulses required. If the electrodes are directly linked to a high-voltage power supply, adequate capacitative coupling is necessary between the electrodes and the electronics.

A question which often arises in discussion about electrical stimulators is whether a 'constant-current' or 'constant-voltage' design should be used, i.e. whether the output circuitry should produce a specified electrode current or a specified electrode voltage. There are advantages and disadvantages to either type which will not be discussed in detail here. In summary, the threshold of stimulation for a nerve is determined by the current so a constant-current design will give a constant level of stimulation even when the resistance of the electrodes changes. Constant-current stimulation can also, by careful design, be more efficient; however it can give rise to high current densities underneath an electrode if the area of contact becomes reduced, and so cause discomfort. Constant-voltage designs are simpler to construct and make stable, and there is much to be said for keeping circuitry as simple as possible, to both minimise size and maximise reliability.

Safety and output pulse waveform

There are internationally agreed standards for the construction of electromedical equipment, but none are specific to electrotactile aids. The question of safety has already been touched upon in the context of making sure that d.c. potentials cannot be applied to the electrodes. A few more comments may be helpful to avoid specific safety problems.

The balls of the fingers offer a lower electrical resistance than most other parts of the body. That being the case, care must be taken to ensure that the output of the electrotactile device does not appear anywhere which can be touched by the fingers of the wearer. If the case of the device is made of metal then a current might flow between the case and the electrodes attached to the subject. Particular care should be made to ensure that any current that flows across the chest is limited to a safe value. A fitted cardiac pacemaker would be a contraindication.

Probably the most controversial aspect of safety design is that which concerns the waveform of the output pulses. Will the continuous application of electrical pulses cause a biological effect underneath the electrodes, and if so is the shape of the current pulse important? There is no firm evidence that the application of pulses of high-frequency current have any long-term effects. However, very low frequencies might well have an effect as electrolysis can occur and cause electrochemical changes underneath the electrodes. It has been argued that if tissue is electrically non-linear then pulses can give rise to direct current in the tissue. However, measurements made by the authors have not found any evidence for significant tissue non-linearity at the levels of current used in electrotactile aids.

If the production of low-frequency currents and hence electrochemical changes by the stimulation pulses is a serious worry, then an improvement which has been suggested is to use bipolar pulses. It was concluded above (see Figure 2.9) that the low-frequency components in a bipolar pulse are fewer than in a monopolar pulse. The hope is that the two opposite polarity pulses will produce a net electrochemical change of zero. In Figure 2.9 the two phases were shown as consecutive and identical except for the polarity difference; however, many workers use interphase delays or an exponentially decaying second phase (Tillman and Piroth, 1987). Some formats of bipolar pulse are more difficult to produce than monopolar ones and the power requirements may be greater. The choice of (a.c.-coupled) monopolar or bipolar pulses is still controversial and there have been in-depth studies (Donaldson and Donaldson, 1986) which have questioned whether differences in the format of such pulses are significant.

Single- and Multichannel Devices

The main aim of this chapter has been to look at the problems specific to electrotactile devices: aspects such as signal-processing strategies, choice of subjects and the evaluation of devices are covered in later chapters. A comparative review of some vibrotactile devices is given in Chapter 9, but a brief review of electrotactile devices will be given here.

Single-channel devices

It is necessary to draw a line between cochlear implants, which are not being considered here, and electrotactile devices. Only devices which do not involve any surgery will be considered here, so that the extracochlear device of Fourcin et al. (1979) will not be considered as it involves surgical placement of an electrode into the middle ear.

Dodgson et al. (1983) used a pair of metal watch straps on the wrist as electrodes through which 50 µs pulses were applied at frequencies up to 200 s^{-1}. Both amplitude and frequency modulation of the pulses were used, with a zero-crossing detector and divider circuitry to set the pulse frequency. The device was relatively small and worn entirely on the wrist so that trailing wires were avoided.

Bochenek et al. (1989) placed electrodes in the two ear canals and applied a stimulus which was both amplitude and frequency modulated by the incoming sound. Pulses with equal mark/space ratio were used, over a frequency range of 10–100 Hz. Each electrode was a wire projecting into the external auditory meatus from a standard earmould, making contact with the skin of the external meatus by a gauze soaked in saline. Subjects were made aware of environmental sounds and there was some assistance with lip reading. However, it seems most likely that such stimulation induces a primarily auditory sensation via the auditory nerves, any electrotactile sensation being of secondary importance.

Multichannel devices

The use of more than one channel enables different coding strategies to be used. For example, frequency of sound can be encoded as a spatial variable instead of being used to modulate the frequency of the output pulses. Saunders, in 1973, reported on a portable device which presented frequency patterns of sounds to the abdomen via an array of electrodes.

He used bursts of pulses where the number of pulses in each burst determined the perceived intensity of the stimulus. Sparks (1979) also used an array of electrodes on the abdomen: 288 electrodes arranged in a two-dimensional array with frequency as one dimension in 36 steps and amplitude as the other dimension with 8 levels. The method of stimulation was again via packets of pulses with the number of pulses in each packet variable.

If very large numbers of electrodes are to be used then the abdomen is a suitable site as its surface area is large and the electrodes do not interfere too much with body movements. However, other sites have been used. Grant (1980, unpublished Masters thesis, University of Washington) encoded variations in voice fundamental frequency as spatial changes using a ten-electrode linear array on the forearm. Tillman and Piroth (1987) also used an array of electrodes on the forearm: 16 electrodes were used with bipolar constant-current pulses applied sequentially at 100–500 Hz and patterns corresponding to articulatory movements were applied. The fingers are an attractive site for the use of many electrodes; as stated earlier the digital nerves contain almost no efferent fibres and the fingers are well supplied with superficial nerves. A disadvantage in the use of the fingers is that trailing wires are necessary and the electrodes may get in the way when the hands are used for other activities. However, the fingers have been used by Blamey et al. (1988) where the stimulation is presented via eight electrodes positioned over the digital nerve bundles on one hand.

Summary

The use of electrical stimulation of the surface of the skin as an aid to communication has been the subject of a considerable amount of work over the past three decades. Many sites have been tried.

Assuming that a suitable electrode material has been chosen, the most important factors that affect the generation of action potentials in the underlying nerves by stimulation at the skin are first the geometrical arrangement of the electrodes with respect to the nerve and secondly the electrical properties of the tissues surrounding the nerve. The use of too small an electrode to improve localisation leads to problems of high impedance and low stimulation efficiency. In addition stimulation can only occur when the potential gradient between the nodes of Ranvier is large enough to initiate an action potential. Current values of 10 mA are typically required.

The duration of the stimulus is also important. Pulses of about 100 μs width are the most efficient for electrical stimulation. An ideal site is considered to be where the nerve axon comes close to the skin surface and it is possible to stimulate only efferent nerves so as to avoid muscle contraction.

The results of experiments on the number of discriminable levels led to an estimate of 8 bits s^{-1} for the information capacity of an electrotactile channel. Although speech could in theory be transmitted by phonemes at about 50 bits s^{-1}, practical systems require much higher rates. Multichannel systems will have increased information capacity but the potential for speech transmission is limited.

The impedance of the skin decreases with frequency and for 100 µs pulses has a minimum value of about 2 kΩ. Constant-current stimulation is preferred as it is not affected by changes in skin impedance. To prevent skin ulceration it is essential to avoid direct-current stimulation and, to avoid electrochemical changes, pulses with no significant low-frequency components are desirable.

Calculations of power requirements show that it is possible to run a wearable aid for many days on a single miniature battery. Discussion of circuitry for a practical device has been limited to the output circuits particular to electrical stimulators. A carefully designed transformer will provide the two main requirements of high voltage and direct-current isolation but a switched-inductor circuit may be easier to miniaturise in a wearable device.

Devices that have been tried to date have used single-channel stimulation on the wrist and in the ear canal as well as multichannel stimulation on the abdomen, forearm and fingers.

References

BARBER, D.C. and BROWN, B.H. (1984). Applied potential tomography (Review article), *J. Phys. Eng.: Sci. Instrum.* **17**, 723-733.

BISHOP, G.H. (1943). Responses to electrical stimulation of single sensory units of skin. *J. Neurophysiol.* **6**, 361-382.

BOCHENEK, W., CHORZEMPA, A., HAZELL, J.W.P., KICIAK, J. and KUKWA, A. (1989). Non-invasive electrical stimulation of the ear canal as a communication aid in acquired total deafness. *Br. J. Audiol.* **23**, 285-291.

BLAMEY, P.J., COWAN, R.S.C., ALCANTARA, J.I. and CLARK, G.M. (1988). Phonemic information transmitted by a multichannel electrotactile speech processor. *J. Speech Hear. Res.* **31**, 620-629.

BROWN, B.H. and SMALLWOOD, R.H. (1981). *Medical Physics and Physiological Measurement.* Oxford: Blackwell Scientific.

BUTIKOFER, R. and LAWRENCE, P.D. (1978). Electrocutaneous nerve stimulation. *IEE Trans. Biomed. Eng.* **25**(6), 526-531.

DODGSON, G.S. (1982). *An investigation into electrical stimulation at the skin for use in a deaf aid.* PhD thesis, University of Sheffield.

DODGSON, G.S., BROWN, B.H., FREESTON, I.L. and STEVENS, J.C. (1983). Electrical stimulation at the wrist as an aid for the profoundly deaf. *Clin. Phys. Physiol. Meas.* **4**, 403-416.

DONALDSON, N. DE N. and DONALDSON, P.E.K. (1986). When are actively balanced biphasic ('Lilly') stimulating pulses necessary in a neurological prosthesis? II: pH changes: noxious products; electrode corrosion; discussion. *Med. Biol. Eng. Comp.* **24**, 50-56.

FOULKE, E. (1964). The locus dimension as a basis for electrocutaneous communication. *J. Psychol.* **57**, 253-257.

FOURCIN, A.J., ROSEN, S.M., MOORE, B.C.J., DOUEK, E.E., CLARKE, G.P., DODSON, H. and BANNISTER, L.H. (1979). External electrical stimulation of the cochlea: Clinical, psychological, speech-perceptual and histological findings. *Br. J. Audiol.* **13**, 85-107.

GEDDES, L.A. (1972). *Electrodes and the Measurement of Bioelectric Events.* New York: Wiley Interscience.

GEDDES, L.A. and BOURLAND, J.D. (1985). Tissue stimulation: theoretical and practical applications. *Med. Biol. Eng. Comp.* **23**, 131-137.

GESCHEIDER, G.A. (1974). Temporal relations in cutaneous stimulation. In: Geldars, F.A. (ed.), *Conference on vibrotactile communication.* Austin, TX: The Psychonomic Society.

GILMER, B.H. (1961). Toward cutaneous electro-pulse communication. *J. Psychol.* **52**, 211-222.

HAWKES, G.R. (1961). Cutaneous discrimination of electrical intensity. *Am. J. Psychol.* **74**, 45-53.

HOFFMANN, C. (1984). Transmission of speech information for the deaf through electric excitation of the skin. *Audiological Akustok/Acoustics* **23**, 4-21.

KACZMAREK, K.A. (1991). Electrotactile and vibrotactile displays for sensory substitution systems. *IEEE Trans. Biomed. Eng.* **38**, 1-16.

LINDNER, R. (1937). The physiological fundamentals of the electrical speech feeling and their application in the training of deaf mutes. *Z. Sinnesphysiol.* **67**, 114-144.

MCADAMS, E.T. (1987). *A study of electrode-tissue impedances encountered in cardiac pacing.* PhD thesis, University of Leeds.

MCNEAL, D.R. (1976). Analysis of a model for excitation of myelinated nerve. *IEEE Trans. Biomed. Eng.* **23**(4), 329-337.

PETHIG, R. (1979). *Dielectric and Electronic Properties of Biological Materials.* Chichester: John Wiley.

PFEIFFER, E.A. (1968). Electrical stimulation of sensory nerves with skin electrodes for research, diagnosis, communication and behavioural conditioning. A survey. *Med. Biol. Eng.* **6**, 637-651.

PLONSEY, R. and BARR, R.C. (1988). *Bioelectricity: A Quantitative Approach.* New York: Plenum Press.

RABINER, L.R. and SCHAFER, R.W. (1978). *Digital Processing of Speech Signals.* New York: Prentice Hall.

SAUNDERS, F.A. (1973). Electrocutaneous displays. In: Geldard, F.A. (ed.), *Cutaneous Communication Systems and Devices.* Austin, TX: The Psychonomic Society, pp. 20-26.

SAUNDERS, F., HILL, W. and SIMPSON, C. (1980). Speech perception via the tactile mode: Progress report. IEEE Conference on Acoustics, Speech and Signal processing. (Reprinted in: Levitt, H., Pickett, J.M. and Houde, R. (eds), *Sensory aids for the hearing impaired.* New York: IEEE Press, pp. 594-597.

SPARKS, D.W., KUHL, P.K., EDMONDS, A.E. and GRAY, G.P. (1979). Investigating the MESA: The transmission of connected discourse. *J. Acoust. Soc. Am.* **65**(3), 810-815.

TILLMAN, H.G. and PIROTH, H.G. (1986). System for electrocutaneous stimulation. *J. Acoust Soc. Am.* **79** (Suppl. 1).

Chapter 3
The Design of Vibrotactile Transducers

ROGER W. CHOLEWIAK and MICHAEL WOLLOWITZ

Tactile transducers, as defined in this chapter, are those devices that stimulate the skin to provide information to individuals who are limited because of either sensory disability or experience overload in other sensory modalities. Such devices historically have been adapted from other communication systems. An early example of a tactile transducer for deaf persons involved placing a 'speaking tube' against the skin (Gault, 1924). The inevitable failure of this device was owing to several levels of incompatibility: the frequency range of the signal was not matched to that of the skin (which is, practically speaking, 10–400 Hz), the mechanical characteristics of the driving signal did not match the skin's, and the features of the signal were not those that the skin can best appreciate. The success of more recent developments in devices and transducers is a result of their being specifically designed for the skin with an appreciation of such problems and hence with attempts to overcome them. In this chapter some of the characteristics of the skin that are most relevant to the design of tactile transducers will be discussed, as well as some of the physical considerations to be brought to bear in the design of transducers. Transducer designs that are currently used in research and applied areas of tactile communication will also be described.

The Skin as a Transmission Medium

Three of the major areas that have to be considered when designing devices for tactile communication systems are: (1) the overall mechanical properties of the skin; (2) the variation in the skin's characteristics as a function of body site; and (3) the effect of varying stimulus characteristics at a given site. Many of the other important issues involved with the processing of both simple and complex tactile stimuli are discussed in other chapters of this volume, particularly Chapter 1.

The mechanical properties of skin

The skin is a complex multilayered organ (physically, it is 'a boundary of a stratified mechanical continuum' (Langberg, 1987)). Within its layers lie the structures that have been implicated in the sense of touch (see Figure 3.1 and Andres and Düring, 1973). These 'receptors' respond to a variety of environmental events, including mechanical, thermal, chemical and electrical stimuli, some with incredible sensitivity (Khanna and Sherrick, 1981; Cholewiak and Collins, 1991). Two major layers of skin have been defined: the epidermis is the outermost layer, with the dermis below it. Both of these can be subdivided into other layers with unique cellular complements, containing different populations of organelles, and with different degrees of internal cohesiveness (Montagna, 1956; Di Fiore, 1964; Quilliam, 1978). Mechanically stimulating the skin, commonly done with sinusoidal or pulsatile waveforms, produces a complex effect as it is deformed. The skin is a *viscoelastic* material: its viscosity is the property by which, like a thick liquid, it resists deformation and dissipates energy internally. Elasticity, conversely, is the spring-like property of the skin, evidenced by the fact that it returns to its original shape quickly after being deformed. When the skin is deformed it stores some of the energy used to distort it and then releases it in returning to the original shape (see, e.g., Tregear, 1966; Lamoré and Keemink, 1988).

A measure of the degree to which the skin deforms in response to an applied force is its *mechanical impedance*. It depends on the viscoelastic properties and density of the skin as well as characteristics of the stimulus, which include the frequency of stimulation and geometric factors such as the size of the contactor. Impedance (defined in general terms as the quotient of force by velocity) can be determined by simultaneously measuring the velocity of the motion imparted to the skin and the force exerted by the transducer. These measurements are typically and most easily made at the contact site ('driving point impedance'). A more difficult but possibly more useful evaluation of the effect of a stimulus on deep or distant receptors would be made by determining the velocity at a point removed from the contact site, closer to where the receptors might lie (giving a 'transfer impedance').

How the skin is affected by the incident energy of a stimulus depends on how well the impedance of the transducer is matched to that of the skin. To evaluate this, a measure called the *output impedance* is determined for the transducer, corresponding to the transducer's ability to deliver energy to the skin. It is generally advantageous to design for an output impedance of the same order as the mechanical impedance of the skin. In this discussion of transducers, the 'impedance match' will be an important issue: if the transducer output impedance is much greater than the skin impedance, energy transfer to the skin is inefficient since most of the input electrical power is dissipated within the transducer itself; if much less, the transducer motion is strongly affected by the amount of mechanical loading from the skin.

A tactile stimulus can be pictured as producing a wave of displacement travelling deep into the skin. This wavefront produces forces that dissipate with distance from the source according to the inverse square law. Passing through different layers with their unique densities, the form of the displacement wave changes. Obstacles such as blood vessels or bone may distort the front in one way or another by reflecting, refracting or absorbing the energy. As a result, the sensory nerve ending deep in the skin is acted upon by a very different waveform than that presented to the surface.

Energy from mechanical vibration can generate travelling waves on the surface of the skin that may be transmitted for long distances. Travelling waves generated by vibrating the finger, for example, have been observed to extend well up the arm (Franke et al., 1951; von Békésy, 1960; Keidel, 1968). The most superficial of these can be stopped with a static ring

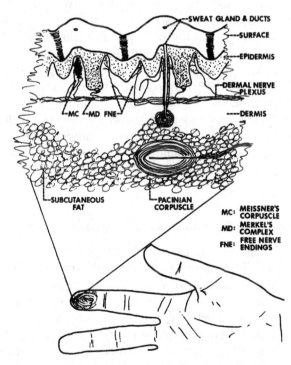

Figure 3.1 A representative cross-section of the skin. The skin of the fingertip is shown with a typical complement of neural end organs asssociated with the sense of touch. The major differences between this sample of glabrous skin and hairy skin are that there are hair follicles, fewer pacinian corpuscles, and overall many fewer receptor structures in hairy skin (adapted from Sherrick and Cholewiak, 1986, by permission of John Wiley & Sons, Inc.).

around the contactor on the skin's surface (Verrillo, 1962; Gescheider et al., 1978), but the deeper waves still tend to spread laterally (Moore and Mundie, 1972; Lamoré and Keemink, 1988).

Variations in the skin as a function of body site

The skin's appearance at one site may differ from that at another: it is flat or furrowed, loose or tight, hairy or smooth (glabrous), thick or thin. On the fingertip there are ridges and valleys, reflecting the random undulations in the papillary layer of the dermis deep below the surface (Quilliam, 1978). Other areas have larger islands of raised tissue, ringed by grooves and pocked with hair follicles and the ducts of sweat glands. These variations in outward appearance reflect more significant subcutaneous differences (see also Chapter 1).

Below the surface, the density of innervation of the neural end organs varies considerably between body sites. The end organs are tightly packed in the fingertips, lips, and genital areas but are rarer at sites closer to the trunk. Many measures of tactile sensitivity are related to the density of innervation. Spatial actuity, as measured by the two-point limen or error of localization, is greatest in regions of high density (Weinstein, 1968). Even estimates of weight and the perception of roughness vary with body site (Stevens, 1979, 1990). Tactile sensitivity as reflected in vibrotactile or pressure thresholds, is also greatest in these regions (Sherrick and Cholewiak, 1986). For 250 Hz vibrotactile stimuli on large (5 mm diameter) contactors, threshold amplitude may be as small as 0.2 µm on the finger or palm. Other sites may require considerably larger displacements. (A common value for a 'comfortable' stimulus amplitude is 12–14 dB (4–5 times threshold), while 'loud' stimuli might be 20–40 dB above threshold. To cover this range, therefore, a tactile transducer has to have a similarly large dynamic range.)

Interactions of stimulus characteristics with body site

In studies involving mechanical stimuli the stiffness and elasticity (i.e. mechanical impedance) of the skin should be matched by that of the mechanical drivers, as described above (Franke, 1951; Alles, 1970; Moore, 1970; Moore and Mundie, 1972; Lamoré and Keemink, 1988). The impedance of the skin varies across body sites and is great enough so that in some places, with stimulators such as piezoceramic benders, the movement of the contactor is readily damped and the waveform presented is not the same as the one desired. For this reason it is common for researchers to use several types of feedback devices on their mechanical stimulators. The most common of these is the accelerometer which allows accurate measurements of displacement for repetitive stimuli such as sinusoids. When the stimulus consists of pulsatile stimuli such as taps, a calibrated strain gauge or an optical sensor system is more useful. In all cases, if these devices are properly mounted at the driving point, they produce electrical signals directly related to the actual displacement of the transducer, and thus the skin.

Another stimulus variable that can interact with choice of body site is the contactor–skin relationship. The static force required on the contactor to produce a given indentation into the skin necessarily varies with the stiffness of the body site chosen for stimulation. As one changes the size of the contactor, either the force with which the contactor presses against the skin or its indentation may be held constant. For example, in order to maintain constant indentation with increasing contactor area the force imposed has to increase because the contactor is pushing against a greater volume of elastic medium. The effects on tactile perception due to the various force/indentation/area factors have been examined (Verrillo, 1962; Craig and Sherrick, 1969; Green and Craig, 1974; Lamoré and Keemink, 1988). The force/indentation parameter is one of the more difficult to control in wearable transducers.

Finally, the punctate nature of tactile sensitivity has to be taken into account in the transducer design. Since the distribution of receptors is not uniform, distinct spots exist where, for example, the sensation of cold can be evoked, in contrast to other points where no thermal sensation may be apparent. Even mechanical stimuli may not produce the most elementary of the skin's sensations, pressure, unless the appropriate points are touched (Geldard, 1972). The observed distribution of such sensitive spots appears to be related to the intensity and area of the stimulus. If the size of the contactor is very small, a sensitive spot could be missed when trying to stimulate the skin and a palpable sensation would not be evoked. The same stimulus at the same intensity level, however, might evoke a suprathreshold sensation if the point of contact were moved slightly (even as small a distance as 1 mm on the fingertip). Because of this, spatial redundancy is commonly included in vibrotactile patterns presented with dense arrays; that is, no single point is expected to be the sole carrier of important information. The optimal stimulator spacing for a given receptor density can be determined by examining the spatial acuity of the skin. Daley and Singer (1975) used the bandwidth of the modulation transfer function (a measure of spatial frequency response) to determine the spatial resolution of an array of vibrators used as a visual prosthesis. This technique can also be applied to other locations on the body's surface.

Tactile Transducer Systems

In this section, several of the major transducer designs currently used in research and in applied cutaneous communication systems will be discussed, limiting the discussion to electromechanical systems. See Chapter 2 for discussions of electrocutaneous systems.

In the laboratory, touch stimuli that produce sensations of pressure, taps, or vibration are delivered to the skin with devices such as von Frey hairs, solenoids, electromagnetic shakers, piezoceramic benders and arrays, or even air puffs. Many of these devices are restricted to the bench top, usually because of power or size requirements. Others cannot be used for wearable aids because they require an external support or reference to work against in order to produce forces upon the skin. These factors have driven many designers to build their systems around the more portable electrocutaneous transducer. Nevertheless, wearable vibrotactile transducers are available.

Design and construction of portable transducers

The design of vibrotactile transducers for wearable tactile aids presents problems distinct from those encountered with bench-top devices. There are obvious concerns with portability and power consumption, but more fundamentally the transducer must be completely self-contained and cannot be supported by any external housing or attachment. (This is in contrast to transducers in which the skin contactor must move relative to a fixed mass, for example the larger shakers). Most portable aids use inertial transducers (e.g. Figure 3.2(b)). In this type of transducer, a mass is suspended by a spring within a rigid case. An alternating force is generated between the internal mass and the case, typically by an electromagnetic coil. Because the case is not rigidly mounted, both it and the internal mass will vibrate. The case is kept in contact with the skin. The advantage of this type of transducer is that the case and contactor are the same. Size and complexity are minimized and complete environmental sealing is possible.

In addition to the requirement that they be self-contained, a number of other parameters such as efficiency, reproduction quality, dynamic range, size, cost, reliability, wearability, and appearance have driven the design and development of transducers for wearable tactile aids. Each involves a range of factors with regard to user population, modes of application, and design of the overall tactile aid system. We will discuss them briefly.

Efficiency

Any wearable tactile aid will be battery powered; the battery is typically the largest and heaviest part of the system. Most of the drain on the battery is in driving the transducer. Consequently, the efficiency of the transducer will determine the size and life of the battery and, in turn, the practicality of the aid as a wearable device. Piezoceramic systems are, in general, more efficient than electromagnetic designs.

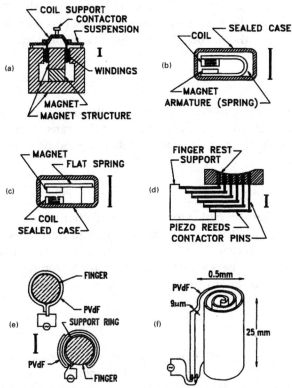

Figure 3.2 Representative cross-section of some vibrotactile transducers. (a) Typical construction of a voice-coil (shaker) transducer; (b) an inertial transducer, similar to that used in the MiniVib-3 and the Tactaid I and II aids (early V1220-V1420 designs); (c) improved inertial transducer similar to the Audiological Engineering M1220 design; (d) cross-section of the Optacon piezoceramic display showing one of 24 rows of contactors; (e) the original and current (split) version of the Leysieffer PVdF ring; (f) the Sensor Electronics PVdF coil. PVdF thickness not to scale in e and f; the bar adjacent to each figure is 1 cm.

Reproduction quality

The ability of a transducer to accurately reproduce a waveform is dependent on its bandwidth, linearity and response time. The need for reproduction accuracy depends on the complexity of the signal produced by the tactile-aid electronics. Linearity is not a major concern since most tactile aids incorporate some type of compression circuitry that causes the drive signal itself to have some non-linear distortion.

Dynamic range

The dynamic range can be important for two reasons. If the tactile aid generates an amplitude-modulated output, the transducer needs to track intensity changes without distortion or buzzing. Also, the optimal perceived intensity for a stimulus varies from user to user, so the output level of the tactile aid must be adjustable to match individual requirements.

Size

From the viewpoint of the user, the smaller the transducer the better. Size limitations depend more on the geometry of the transducer internals than on actual material volume; the cases contain a good deal of empty space.

Cost

The transducers for wearable tactile aids are neither laboratory devices nor clinical instruments. They are consumer products and must be priced accordingly. This becomes more critical as multiple-channel aids requiring many transducers are developed. Too often production quantities of these transducers are too low to provide economies of scale.

Reliability

Tactile transducers may be damaged by impact, environment (e.g. immersion), abuse, or self-induced failure such as metal fatigue. A strong, well-sealed case, tough materials, robust and tamper-resistant assembly methods and careful wiring all contribute to reliability.

Wearability

A wearable aid requires wearable transducers. This means that the transducers should be small, comfortable, lie flat under clothing, and not require excessive pressure against the skin to function. Several single-channel aids have been built with transducers mounted on a watch-like wrist strap. Although convenient, the wrist is a poor location for acuity of perception and the site is not well adapted for multiple-channel aids. The design of harnesses and holders for this and other sites has room for improvement.

Appearance

Although last in the list, the appearance of the transducer is an important factor in its acceptance by child and adult users. People are accustomed to the excellent design and finish of modern consumer products and expect the same in a relatively costly tactile aid.

Electromagnetic designs

The oldest tactile systems are the electromagnetic systems. Historically these have been associated in one way or another with acoustic voice-coil technology. For example, as Levitt (1985, unpublished report at City University of New York) points out, while attempting to develop a speech waveform display for deaf persons, Bell invented the telephone. More recently, however, developments in telephone engineering have preceded advances in sensory aids for the hearing impaired. Gault (1927), for example, used telephone voice coils as the tactile transducers for his vocoder system. However, the transducers used in much of the earliest research on vibrotactile sensitivity were hand held or electromechanically driven tuning forks. Voice-coil or acoustic-speaker systems became more common after Geldard's papers on the perception of mechanical vibration (Geldard, 1940). These systems provided for better control of the frequency, amplitude and waveform of the stimulus than was previously possible, particularly when the systems could be calibrated using piezo-electric crystal displacement transducers combined with optical strobo-scopic measurements. Furthermore, these systems, particularly shakers, are able to deliver a wide range of intensities and their displacement is largely independent of the impedance of the skin. Nevertheless, there have been few advances in the development of devices specifically designed as tactile transducers, despite needs in pure and applied research (Sherrick, 1984).

Voice-coil technology is used in most acoustic drivers (i.e. speakers). A coil is located within a strong radial magnetic field produced by a permanent magnet and a set of pole pieces. A current passing through the coil produces a force that will push the coil along its axis (see Figure 3.2(a)). With proper design, an efficient conversion of energy can be achieved. Voice-coil geometry is commonly used in shakers that have been employed for much of the research on tactile sensitivity. Electromagnetic shakers are useful for presenting vibratory stimuli to the skin over frequencies from 0.1 Hz to 200 or 300 Hz with great efficiency. This design, however, has not generally been used in wearable aids for reasons of weight and cost. A relatively large coil and magnet structure is required to operate the device at low frequencies and high amplitudes; many of the commercial shakers weigh a kilogram or more (the Bruel & Kjaer 4810 commonly used in tactile research weighs 1.1 kg). Although smaller architectures are possible, an efficient voice-coil transducer requires very precise manufacture and alignment, as well as a number of small precision parts, and cost problems may override.

Another type of electromagnetic design that has been investigated for use in tactile aids, and the one that has been chosen for most applications, is the variable-reluctance transducer. Various geometries are possible; typically they employ a permanent magnet, an electromagnetic coil and a spring-loaded armature containing iron or mild steel. The air gap between the magnet and coil must be relatively large compared with an acoustic transducer because of the much larger excursions required. This so greatly reduces the flux in the magnetic circuit that the armature can often be replaced by a non-ferromagnetic suspension with little loss of efficiency. An alternating current applied to the coil creates a magnetic field that alternately reinforces and cancels the field of the permanent magnet, thus causing the armature to vibrate (see Figures 3.2(b),(c)). The variable-reluctance transducer is inherently less efficient than voice-coil devices, but other characteristics have driven its use in wearable tactile aids and development of this type of transducer has led to efficiencies that provide adequately low battery drain. Table 3.1 illustrates some of the characteristics of this type of transducer.

One commercially available device that has been developed specifically for vibratory stimulation is a bone-conduction vibrator (the Radio Ear) that, in turn, has found application in at least one tactile aid for lipreading (Cholewiak and Sherrick, 1986). The molded black case contains a variable-reluctance-type driver that uses a very stiff suspension and an armature loaded with a lead mass to obtain broadband performance above about 300 Hz. Below 300 Hz the transducer is inefficient and its output drops rapidly as frequency decreases. (Note that, as described above and in Chapter 1, the skin is most sensitive to frequencies in the range up to about 400 Hz.) Radio Ear B70 transducers require a high contact force with the skin: this appears to be a result of the large armature mass compared with the 'fixed' case mass; high contact force causes the tissue underlying the skin to be closely coupled to the case, increasing its effective mass. This device lacks the efficiency needed for a wearable tactile aid. The B70 transducers require a signal of 4–5 V peak-to-peak under normal operating conditions, but with a coil impedance of 8 Ω, the current drain is high. They continue to be used in laboratory and clinical work where weight and efficiency are less important than a wide bandwidth, but have been supplanted by newer designs for wearable aids. For example, in one such aid, the Tactaid I, a pack of four 'AA' size Ni–Cd batteries provides sufficient energy to match the power requirements of its transducers.

Another device, the MiniVib-3 (Spens and Plant, 1983) is an aid to lipreading that uses a beam-mounted variable-reluctance design vibrating at a resonant frequency of 250 Hz (similar to that shown in Figure 3.2(b)). The processor/receiver size is only 36 cm³ while the stimulator enclosure, attached to the processor with earphone wire, is only 2.8 cm³, weighing about 55 g. This system simply responds to the intensity of the acoustic waveform, modulating the amplitude of the 250 Hz vibratory signal. Although no frequency information is extracted from the acoustic signal, the prosodic, or rhythmic, information is helpful in understanding speech

Table 3.1 Characteristics of electromagnetic transducers

Configuration	Frequency response (Hz)	Resonance (Hz)	Operating voltage (V)	Operating current (mA)	Displacement amplitude (μm)	Impedance with respect to skin
Audiological Engineering Corporation V1220 (10 × 18 × 25 mm)	200–300	250	<1.2	<25	30	medium
Spens MiniVib-3 (10 × 15 × 20 mm)	230	230	<5	*	25	high
Wake Solenoids (5 × 28.5 mm)	d.c.	*	*	*	2000	low
Queens Aid Solenoids (8 × 23.8 mm)	d.c.–1000	430	5	100	1000	low
RadioEar Bone Conductance Vibs (approx. 15 × 20 × 25 mm)	≥300	1000	<5	*	*	low

* Unknown, not applicable, or unavailable.

(Sherrick, 1991), fulfilling the aim of the designers 'to present an unambiguous representation of the syllabic patterns of speech' (Spens and Plant, 1983). In addition to providing useful information when used in conjunction with lipreading, the device is able to signal important environmental events to the deaf user, such as a telephone or doorbell ringing.

Piezoceramic materials

A number of devices currently use piezoceramic materials as the active element for tactile stimulation. These materials, based on a lead zirconate titanate (PZT) ceramic, are highly efficient transducers of both electrical and mechanical energy; that is, when used as they are in phonographic cartridges, they will generate a current proportional to the applied displacement. On the other hand, when these elements are connected in a driving circuit, they will expand or contract along one or more axis in proportion to the amplitude and polarity of the imposed voltage. Although they are typically used as high-frequency drivers in acoustic systems, they can be constructed with geometry and mass loading to operate with low resonant frequencies. Piezoceramic elements appear in a circuit as capacitors with extremely small losses at the low frequencies used for tactile stimulation.

In a typical design, two thin metalized plates of piezoelectric material are bonded to a conductive shim. The sandwich can then be cut into a variety of shapes depending on the application. When an electric field is applied across the plates, one shrinks and the other expands, and the assembly bends. Many modes of vibration can occur, depending on how the assembly is clamped. For example, disks of this material are used in almost every smoke detector to generate intense high-frequency alarm beeps with a relatively low current draw. When cut into rectangular plates piezoceramics can be readily adapted for use as tactile transducers, typically in a 'beam' configuration (one end rigidly clamped and the other allowed to move in response to the applied voltage). The force produced by the free end as it bends is proportional to the width of the plate, and inversely proportional to its length. The amplitude of the displacement is proportional to the plate's length. In this configuration, the resonant frequency of the bender is inversely proportional to the unclamped length squared. Rubin (Rubin, S.I., 1979, unpublished Masters Thesis, Massachusetts Institute of Technology) surveyed piezoceramic benders for potential use in an experimental vibrotactile array, and describes the test arrangement and frequency responses of several sizes of bender when driving the skin of the finger in a tangential (stroking) mode. Displacement amplitudes were measured with solid-state strain gauges mounted directly on the benders. Rubin found that the strongest sensation for a given input signal, when using a static normal contact force of 10 g, was provided when a bender of 32 × 13 mm was used.

Unfortunately, when used on sites other than the fingertip, piezoceramic elements require input voltages in the range of 100 V or higher to achieve reasonable vibration amplitudes, although current levels are of the order of one or two milliamps. These voltages are typically achieved by passing the output signal through a step-up transformer, thus increasing the mass and volume of the package and reducing electrical efficiency. A connecting cord may be broken or bitten through, exposing the user to an unpleasant, although probably not dangerous, electric shock.

The Optacon (Telesensory Systems, Inc., 455 N. Bernardo Avenue, Mountain View, CA 94039, USA), a reading machine for the blind, is a commercial tactile aid that uses piezoceramic bimorph benders as its transducer elements (Linvill and Bliss, 1966; Bliss et al., 1970). The Optacon employs a self-contained matrix of elements to provide two-dimensional spatial information to the skin of the fingertip. The device has a camera with a 6-column, 24-row array of phototransistors that are used to sense the black/white information on a printed sheet. The dark/light state of these sensors determine the on/off state of an isomorphic set of vibrotactile transducers. In order to be able to pack 144 contactors in such a small space, the benders are stacked in six layers of 24-bender combs. Each comb is offset slightly from the one below it, so that the tips of all 144 elements are visible from above. Attached at right angles to each tip is a steel pin that protrudes into a supporting fingerplate above the array (see Figure 3.2(d)). When driven, the bender first moves downward, pulling the pin away from the fingerplate and building up momentum. On the upward swing it taps the skin then retracts to begin the next cycle. The bender is driven at 230 Hz, its resonant frequency, resulting in a period of 4.35 ms. However, because it is driven at resonance, the stimulus is highly damped by the skin; furthermore, the actual duration of skin contact is only about 0.8 ms (Bliss et al., 1970). It would be better, perhaps, to characterize this stimulus as a 500-Hz haversine presented at a rate of 230 pulses s^{-1}. The intensive dynamic range of the system is relatively small. From threshold to the highest intensity possible without modification, less than 20 dB of psychophysical 'loudness' variation is available (Cholewiak and Collins, 1990). Because its mechanical design prevents the experimeter from having precise control of stimulus amplitudes and waveform, the Optacon is not always an appropriate device for research applications.

Van Doren has developed an alternative arrangement for tactile stimulation using piezoceramic elements that stimulate the skin when they elongate instead of bending (Van Doren, 1987, 1989). This system, originally designed to examine the spatial frequency characteristics of the skin, involves an array of 88 piezoceramic plates stacked like a deck of cards separated by insulating material. The top driving surface of the stack is 19 × 33 mm, with an insulated plate thickness of 0.38 mm (resulting in a

minimum usable spatial bandwidth of 0.76 mm). The user places their
finger or palm on the surface, and, under computer control, the edges of
the individual plates are driven up and down. By synchronizing the action,
traveling waves can be generated that move over the surface of the array.
Although the frequency response of the system is quite good (0–1000 Hz),
the maximum stimulus amplitude is small (at most about 11 μm), which
is an intrinsic limitation of the piezoelectric ceramic technology (Van
Doren, 1987). This displacement is sufficient to study some of the most
sensitive tactile receptors, but for others a greater intensitive dynamic
range is required.

The final configuration of piezoceramic benders discussed here involves
arrays in which the benders are mounted vertically with contactors on
their edges so that the skin is stimulated by tangential or lateral motion.
The lateral mode of stimulation is as effective as indentation (von Békésy,
1960; Alles, 1970). In fact, this may be the most effective mode for
optimally stimulating those receptors most responsible for vibrotactile
pattern perception (Gardner and Palmer, 1989). One of the earliest such
systems was a large 8 × 8 element array using benders 32 mm long and
13 mm wide on 15 mm centers (Rubin, 1979; Cholewiak and Sherrick,
1981), which was used to examine vibrotactile pattern perception on large
areas of the skin, such as the thigh, which require higher stimulus amplitudes and cannot resolve arrays of any greater spatial density (e.g.
Cholewiak, 1979). The size of these elements is such that their resonant
frequency is within the dynamic range of the skin, with the consequence
that they tend to be readily damped. A newer ultra-dense array uses the
same bender configuration, but its elements have a much higher resonant
frequency because they are shorter. This results in a flatter frequency
response over the useful range of 10–400 Hz. The new system is called
the Multipoint TACtile array (MTAC) (Sensor Electronics, Inc., 105 Fairway
Terrace, Mt Laurel, NJ 08054, USA), and includes 256 benders in a 16 × 16
element configuration. The array is small enough for all of the elements
to fit under the fingertip: 16 elements in a row on 0.63 mm centers and
16 rows on 1.27 mm centers. These actuators sweep the skin laterally,
rather than indenting the skin as the Optacon does.

Table 3.2 lists some of the characteristics of piezoceramic transducers.

Polyvinylidene fluoride

One of the newest materials to be used for tactile stimulation is a piezopolymer film called polyvinylidene fluoride (PVdF), or Kynar (Pennwalt
Corporation, 950 Forge Avenue, Valley Forge, PA 19482, USA). This
electromechanical-mechanoelectrical material is a flexible plastic, similar
to ordinary kitchen wrap (e.g. polyvinylidene chloride) in form and thickness. PVdF is available in thicknesses of 9–52 μm. If the sheet is metalized

Table 3.2 Characteristics of piezoceramic transducers

Configuration	Frequency response (Hz)	Resonance (Hz)	Operating voltage (V)	Operating current (mA)	Displacement amplitude (μm)	Impedance with respect to skin
Telesensory Optacon (1.258 × 33 mm horizontal bender + 5–20 mm vertical pin)	d.c. >400	230	<50	<1	<65 indentation	high
Van Doren Plate (25 × 124 mm vertical plates)	d.c. 1000	10 000	<150	<167	<17 indentation	low
Sensor Elect MTAC beam (short vertical bender)	d.c. >400	>800	<350	<5	<200 transverse	low

Table 3.3 Characteristics of piezopolymer transducers

Configuration	Frequency response (Hz)	Resonance (Hz)	Operating voltage (V)	Operating current (mA)	Displacement amplitude (μm)	Impedance with respect to skin
Leysieffer Ring (12 × 10 mm, 9 μm film)	d.c. 1000	800	<160	<10	<10 compression	low
Sensor Elect MTAC Column (1.2 × 26 mm, 9 μm film)	d.c. >2500	5000	<270	<5	<30 indentation	low

front and back, a voltage can be applied across it and it will bend, like other piezoceramic materials. The material has been used commercially in several items, including an internal fan for Macintosh computers driven by line voltage (110 V a.c.). In the fan, the material is held in a beam configuration. However, because it is a thin flexible sheet, its impedance is much less than that of the skin so in this mode it cannot produce a displacement great enough to serve as a tactile stimulus; in applications requiring the production of high forces, unique configurations of PVdF must be used. In one arrangement Leysieffer (1985) wrapped several layers of 9 μm thick PVdF over a split ring 10 mm wide to be slipped over the finger (Figure 3.2(e)). Vibrotactile thresholds of the order of 0.14 μm at 200 Hz were recorded for a 12-layer arrangement, with a power dissipation of about 100 μW (1.6 V). At 20 dB SL, the power required (10 mW) compares favorably with that for electrocutaneous stimulation (6 mW). A sufficient compressive force could be generated in this manner to use several of these in a vocoder design (Leysieffer, 1986).

Another configuration of PVdF that can produce forces sufficient to stimulate the skin is one developed by Sensor Electroncs, Inc. (105 Fairway Terrace, Mt Laurel, NJ 08054, USA), which was an improvement of a concept developed by Linvill (Linvill, 1980; Dameron and Linvill, 1981). In the latest arrangement, 10 turns of 9 μm film are rolled in a bifilar fashion (Patent 4 879 698, E. Langberg at Sensor Electronics), into a long, thin, tube (25 mm × 0.5 mm) that elongates when voltages are applied (Figure 3.2(f)). The multiturn columns can be packed in a tight configuration to produce a relatively dense array. By winding the pliable film into a column it gains sufficient strength to operate in a compressive mode when finger pressure is applied to one end. The force produced by this arrangement is considerable and is sufficient to resist damping by any reasonable loading with skin contact. Specifically, it is calculated that a light touch of 2 psi (14 kPa) interacts with such a column to produce a static actuator deflection of only 0.16 μm (Langberg, 1987). With a maximum of 270 V d.c. the peak amplitude approaches 18 μm, with a maximum peak force of about 0.3 N. If an a.c. power supply is used, peak-to-peak displacement can be doubled; alternatively the length of the column can be increased to increase the displacement.

For stimuli well above threshold over a wide frequency range, these configurations can require high voltages (hundreds of volts, but at milliamps of current). If a dielectric fault occurred these levels could cause material breakdown. A serious drawback of PVdF is that it produces hydrogen fluoride gas when it burns: if this occurs, this highly corrosive and reactive gas must be neutralized locally or dissipated. The design of a system using this material should take into account this potential hazard to the user and to the system. Some characteristics of PVdF devices are shown in Table 3.3.

Development of the Tactaid Transducer – A Case History

As an example of how these considerations might be implemented, the development of the transducer for the Tactaid Vibrotactile Aid will be described. The processor section of the Tactaid was completed before the transducer, so Radio Ear B70 series transducers, which were used during development of the Tactaid, were sold with the processor until custom-designed transducers were developed.

The first type of transducer to be investigated used piezoelectric bimorph benders in a beam configuration. One end of the bimorph was fixed to the case while a small lead mass was attached to the other. The bimorph transducers built in the laboratory proved efficient, requiring only about 100 mW at peak drive levels, but they also tended to have a very peaked frequency response. Work was suspended on this transducer because of two obstacles: the high voltages needed by the transducer would make it necessary to build a step-up transformer into the electronics, also the bimorph geometry tends to be long and wide. The intention was to design a transducer that would work with multiple-channel tactile aids. Multiple transformers would add much to the weight, and large transducer size would not allow the development of a closely packed transducer array.

Parenthetically, a commercial bimorph-based tactile aid (the TAM) has been produced by Summit in the UK (Summit C.P., B irmingham, UK). It is a single-channel unit with the transducer built into a wrist band. A pulse transformer in the electronics case raises the voltage on the connecting cord to about 100 V. The bandwidth of this unit is equivalent to transducers built by Audiological Engineering Corporation (AEC) and Spens, to be described below.

The transducer built by Karl-Erik Spens in Sweden for the MiniVib-3 tactile aid was carefully studied (Spens and Plant, 1983). This variable-reluctance design is similar in concept to the Radio Ear devices but uses a different spring geometry. Instead of a flat stiff spring, a stamped steel plate was bent into a 'U' with the coil and magnet facing each other on the inside surfaces. One side of this armature was then cemented to the small molded case (similar to Figure 3.2(b)). The result was a less stiff suspension that allowed greater travel. Because of the low stiffness, no additional mass was needed to lower the resonant frequency and the transducer was small and light and did not require high contact force. The coil impedance was 100 Ω so the current drain was quite low.

This transducer design was seen as the best developed to date, but it still suffered several significant flaws: the bandwidth was narrow and the resonant frequency varied from one unit to another; the output frequency was adjusted to partially compensate for this variation. Several construction details proved unreliable; for example, the suspension was unhardened, leading to alignment problems. Furthermore, as with the Radio Ear devices, the electrical connector consisted of several small parts assembled into the case. These were difficult to assemble, could be damaged in use, and did not provide a good environmental seal.

The first transducer series developed by Audiological Engineering (in 1986) was designed using a simple model of analysis of inertial transducers (see Appendix 3.1) and based in part on the Spens design. The most basic improvement was the use of hardened steel and a modified geometry for the cantilever spring, providing better control of stiffness, frequency response, and unit-to-unit reproducibility, as well as improving resistance to impact damage. A one-piece molded connector was also incorporated. This simplified the assembly and allowed the molded case to be completely sealed. Cyanoacrylate adhesives were chosen to cement the armature to the case and to seal the case; this has proven to be a very reliable method of assembly. The final design also included an external steel spring clip to make it easier to mount the transducer on clothes or an elastic band.

The coil impedance on these transducers was 22 Ω and was matched to a drive circuit that supplied amplitude-modulated output. Two versions were produced: the V1220 with a 250 Hz resonant frequency and the V1420 with a 375 Hz resonant frequency, matched to two versions of the Tactaid II, a two-channel wearable tactile aid. The higher frequency was found to provide better voicing discrimination but certain users, particularly older people, had poor sensitivity at this frequency, especially in cold weather. The lower frequency device is more efficient and is preferred by some teachers. The skin has a greater dynamic range at lower frequencies so less compression of the signal is required.

In 1988 the design was modified to improve reliability. The bent steel armature of the original design was difficult to adjust; because of manufacturing variations or impact, it would occasionally bend too far, allowing the magnet and steel core of the coil to stick together. In addition, in the original version the magnet was attached to the case, with the coil acting as the suspended mass in order to achieve the most efficient ratio of case to internal mass (Figure 3.2(b)). Unfortunately, the wires leading to the coil were continuously flexing and would occasionally break. The new version replaced the bent armature with a flat strip of tempered steel cantilevered from one end of the case (Figure 3.2(c)). This was easier to build and proved more reliable: it also changed the mass ratio and, in combination with a redesigned coil, allowed the coil and magnet locations to be reversed, virtually eliminating failure of the coil lead wires.

A 7-channel wearable tactile aid is being developed. In conjunction with this processor a new, smaller, transducer has been developed (the M1120). This transducer has a longer cantilever spring and a redistributed case mass to achieve a wide dynamic range and short response time without significant loss of efficiency.

Design for limited production

Wearable tactile aids are limited-production devices but must have a high-quality appearance and feel if they are to be commercially successful. Every molded, stamped or formed component carries tooling and set-up charges that may be difficult to amortize in a small production run, especially if rework or redesign is required. Mold making and set-up charges for a typical plastic part might run to $10 000. For a tactile transducer, the part might be made in a quantity of 1000 at an incremental cost of $0.50 each. By comparison, commercial hearing aid parts would be made 10 000 pieces at a time, at an incremental cost of $0.35 each. The total cost per item is thus $10.50 for the tactile transducer part but only $1.35 for the hearing aid part.

The way to manage this type of cost is to keep the design simple and to try to anticipate production pitfalls, for example selecting variable-reluctance over voice-coil designs. The voice coil has certain advantages that lead it to be chosen in audio speakers and shakers, however it requires the careful assembly of precision parts which keeps costs high. The variable-reluctance design is inherently simpler and, by adopting it, expensive manufacturing operations can be eliminated.

It is almost always advantageous to use off-the-shelf components and preassembled components whenever possible, even if compromises must be made in the overall design. For example, a preassembled electrical connector on a transducer can reduce parts and assembly cost as well as improving reliability.

Other Sources

Other sources that might be helpful in developing vibrotactile systems are: Bliss Tactile Displays Conference (Bliss, 1970), Geldard's conference on Cutaneous Communication System and Devices (Geldard, 1974), the chapter by Craig and Sherrick on dynamic tactile displays (Craig and Sherrick, 1982), Sherrick's article on displays and devices (Sherrick, 1984), and Boring's compendium on the senses (Boring, 1942).

Appendix 3.1: Analysis of Inertial Transducers

A simple model, based on that developed by Franklin and Franklin (1983), can be developed to analyse the motion of an inertial transducer. The model is used to estimate the vibration amplitude for a given input signal amplitude and frequency. The model is generalized to show the ratio of vibration amplitude to applied force; thus it is independent of the parameters determining the conversion of electrical power to applied force. This model has proven useful for determining reasonable values for the

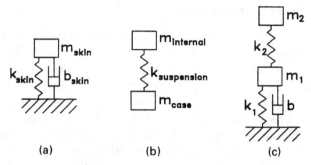

Figure 3.3 Dynamic models of the skin. (a) Simplified model of the skin; (b) simple dynamic model for an inertial transducer; (c) the combined dynamic model of skin and transducer.

case and internal masses and for the spring stiffness. It is assumed that, all other things being equal, greater vibration amplitude results in greater sensation. Effects on sensation due to contactor area and contact force are not considered in this model.

A simple linearized model for the physical response of the skin is used here. The skin is modeled with single mass, stiffness, and resistance elements as shown in Figure 3.3(a). The skin is treated as a single mass connected to a fixed base by a linear spring and a linear damper. The actual mass, elasticity, and resistance parameters are considered to be dependent on the contact area.

The transducer is modeled as shown in Figure 3.3(b). It consists simply of a case mass and an internal mass connected by a spring. Within the transducer the damping is assumed to be much less than that of the skin and is ignored. The force, whether electromagnetic or piezoelectric, acts equally on both masses but in opposite directions.

The combined model is shown in Figure 3.3(c), and the parameters are defined as:

m_1 = combined case and skin mass
m_2 = internal mass
k_1 = spring constant for the skin
k_2 = spring constant for the internal mass suspension
b = damping factor for the skin
F = applied force
x_1 = displacement of the case (and skin surface)
x_2 = displacement of the internal mass

The equations of motion for m_1 and m_2 are:

$$m_1 s^2 x_1 = F + k_2 x_2 - bs x_1 - (k_1 + k_2)x_1 \qquad (3.1a)$$
$$m_2 s^2 x_2 = -F + k_2 x_1 - k_2 x_2 \qquad (3.1b)$$

where s is the operator d/dx.

The equations can be combined and reorganized as

$$[(m_2s^2 + k_2)(m_1s^2 + bs + (k_1 + k_2)) - k_2^2]x_1 = m_2s^2F \qquad (3.2)$$

This can be expanded and written in transfer equation form as

$$\frac{x_1}{F} = \frac{m_2s^2}{m_1m_2s^4 + m_2bs^3 + ((k_1 + k_2)m_2 + k_2m_1)s^2 + k_2bs + k_1k_2} \qquad (3.3)$$

For the next step, it is assumed that the input F will have the form of a constant amplitude sinusoid. This is equivalent to driving the transducer with a sinewave generator, as would often be done in threshold response testing. In this case, the replacement $s = j\omega$ can be made, where j is the square root of -1 and ω is the angular frequency in rad s^{-1}.

Making this substitution in (3.3) and combining real and imaginary terms, gives us

$$\frac{x_1}{F} = \frac{A}{B + jC} = \frac{AB - jAC}{B^2 + C^2} \qquad (3.4)$$

where

$$A = m_2\omega^2$$
$$B = m_1m_2\omega^4 - ((k_1 + k_2)m_2 + k_2m_1)\omega^2 + k_1k_2$$
$$C = -m_2b\omega^3 + k_2b\omega$$

To eliminate the complex term from the equation it is necessary to find the absolute value of equation:

$$\frac{|x_2|}{|F|} = \frac{[(AB)^2 + (AC)^2]^{1/2}}{B^2 + C^2} = \frac{|A|}{(B^2 + C^2)^{1/2}} \qquad (3.5)$$

This equation can be used to generate plots of $|x_1/F|$ as a function of driving frequency. It is convenient to substitute frequency f in cycles per second (Hz) for angular frequency ω in using the relation $\omega = 2\pi f$.

This derivation is used to calculate the amplitude of the case vibrations. A similar process sequence gives $|x_2|$, the amplitude of vibration of the internal mass. The resulting equation is:

$$\frac{|x_2|}{|F|} = \frac{[(A_rB + A_iC)^2 + (A_iB + A_rC)^2]^{1/2}}{B^2 + C^2} \qquad (3.6)$$

where

$$A_r = (-m_1\omega^2 + k_1)$$
$$A_i = b\omega$$

Equation 3.6 is particularly useful in the design of transducers in which the internal mass is significantly less than the case mass. In this case the internal mass has a greater vibration amplitude than the case and care must be taken to provide sufficient clearance for this motion.

Values for the mass, stiffness, and damping of the skin can be taken from equations and parameters determined by Franke (1951)

$$m_{skin} = \pi a^3 r/3 \tag{3.7a}$$
$$k_1 \equiv k_{skin} = 3\pi a n_1 \tag{3.7b}$$
$$b \equiv b_{skin} = 3\pi a^2 r[(n_1/r)^{1/2} + n_2/ar] \tag{3.7c}$$

where a is effective contactor radius, r is 1.1 g cm^{-3} (= 1.1 × 10^3 kg m^{-3}), n_1 is 2 × 10^4 dyne cm^{-2} (= 2 × 10^3 Pa) and n_2 is 150 dyne s cm^{-2} (= 15 Pa s).

Figure 3.4 shows the results calculated using equation 3.7 with different ratios of m_1 to m_2 with the contact area held constant. The value of k_2 was adjusted to maintain an approximately constant peak or resonant frequency. The response varies between a relatively broad band curve when the internal mass is relatively large to a highly peaked but more efficient curve when the internal mass is small. Even if a tactile aid operates at a constant frequency, making the transducer bandwidth too narrow can cause problems: firstly, changes in transducer placement and variations between transducers can shift the resonant frequency so that it no longer matches the output signal, resulting in even lower efficiency than might be achieved with a more broad band design.

A second concern has become more important as the design of the tactile aid electronics has improved: a resonant transducer cannot instantly

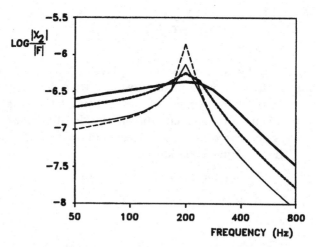

Figure 3.4 The calculated response curves for an inertial vibrotactile transducer. Corresponding parameters: K$_1$ = 1.51 × 10^5 dyne cm^{-1}; b = 2020 dyne s cm^{-1}, m_{skin} = 0.58 g; a = 0.8 cm; (– – – –) m_1 5.0 g, m_2 1.25 g, k_2 1.7 × 10^6 dyne cm^{-1}; (——) m_1 5.0 g, m_2 5.0 g, k_2 4.2 × 10^6 dyne cm^{-1}; (- - - -) m_1 2.5 g, m_2 5.0 g, k_2 3.2 × 10^6 dyne cm^{-1}; (—) m_1 1.25 g, m_2 5.0 g, k_2 2.8 × 10^6 dyne cm^{-1}.

Table 3.4 Resonant frequency and Q (tuning) of representative transducers

Transducer	f_o (Hz)	Q‡
M1220 (AEC)*	250	3.6
V1420 (AEC)	375	8.7
B70 (Radio Ear)	1108	4.1
B72 (Radio Ear)	868	10.0
P2 (AEC)†	260	16.0

*The M1220 is a prototype design, not yet in production.
†The P2 is an experimental Bimorph-type inertial transducer developed by Audiological Engineering Corp. (AEC).
‡The Q-factor was determined by the 3-dB drop-off method.
All transducers were tested in contact against the forearm.

start or stop vibrating; it may take 5–20 ms for the transducer to follow the input signal. As more information is transmitted through the transducer this time lag may cause 'blurring' that degrades the signal.

Table 3.4 shows results obtained by Rabinowitz* in a study of frequency response of several tactile transducers. The wide range of bandwidths and resonant frequencies is obvious. The M1220 transducer is noteworthy in that it combines a low resonant frequency with low Q-factor.

Acknowledgments

The authors would like to express their sincere appreciation to Amy A. Collins, David A. Franklin and Carl E. Sherrick for their advice and helpful criticisms during the preparation of this manuscript. The preparation was supported by Grant DC 00076-27 from the National Institutes of Health, US Department of Health and Human Services, to Princeton University. The second author is a consultant to Audiological Engineering Corporation, which also supported preparation of this manuscript.

References

ALLES, DAVID, S. (1970). Information transmission by phantom sensations. *IEEE Trans. Man–Machine Systems* **11**, 85–91.

ANDRES, K.H. and DÜRING, M. VON (1973). Morphology of cutaneous receptors. In: Iggo, A. (ed.), *Handbook of Sensory Physiology: Somatosensory system*, Vol. 2. New York: Springer, pp. 3–28.

---

*Unpublished observations by Dr William Rabinowitz, communicated to Audiological Engineering Corporation in April 1990.

BÉKÉSY, G. VON (1960). *Experiments in Hearing.* New York: McGraw-Hill.

BLISS, J.C. (1970). Tactile Displays Conference. *IEEE Trans. Man–Machine Systems* 11, 1–125.

BLISS, J.C., KATCHER, M.H., ROGERS, C.H. and SHEPARD, R.P. (1970). Optical-to-tactile image conversion for the blind. *IEEE Trans. Man–Machine Systems* 11, 58–64.

BORING, E.G. (1942). *Sensation and Perception in the History of Experimental Psychology.* New York: Appleton-Century.

CHOLEWIAK, R.W. (1979). Spatial factors in the perceived intensity of vibrotactile patterns. *Sens. Proc.* 3, 141–156.

CHOLEWIAK, R.W. and COLLINS, A.A. (1990). The effects of a plastic-film covering on vibrotactile pattern perception with the Optacon. *Behav. Res. Meth. Instrum. Comp.* 22, 21–26.

CHOLEWIAK, R.W. and COLLINS, A.A. (1991). Sensory and physiological bases of touch. In: Heller, M.A. and Schiff, W.R. (eds), *The Psychology of Touch.* Hillsdale, NJ: Lawrence Erlbaum Associates, pp. 23–60.

CHOLEWIAK, R.W. and SHERRICK, C.E. (1981). A computer-controlled matrix system for presentation to the skin of comaplex spatiotemporal patterns. *Behav. Res. Meth. Instrum.* 13, 667–673.

CHOLEWIAK, R.W. and SHERRICK, C.E. (1986). Tracking skill of a deaf person with long-term tactile aid experience. *J. Rehab. Res. Dev.* 23, 20–26.

CRAIG, J.C. and SHERRICK, C.E. (1969). The role of skin coupling in the determination of vibrotactile spatial summation. *Percept. Psychophys.* 6, 97–101.

CRAIG, J.C. and SHERRICK, C.E. (1982). Dynamic tactile displays. In: Schiff, W. and Foulke, E. (eds), *Tactual Perception: A Sourcebook.* Cambridge: Cambridge University Press. pp. 209–233.

DI FIORE, M.S.H. (1964). *An Atlas of Human Histology.* Philadelphia: Lea & Febiger.

DALEY, M.L. and SINGER, M. (1975). A spatial resolution measure of cutaneous vision. *IEEE Trans. Systems, Man, Cybernet.* 16, 124–125.

DAMERON, D.H. and LINVILL, J.G. (1981). Cylindrical PVF$_2$ electromechanical transducers. *Sensor & Actuators* 2, 73–84.

FRANKE, E.K. (1951). *Mechanical impedance measurements of the human body surface.* Air Force Technical Report No. 6469, Wright Air Development Center.

FRANKE, E.K., GIERKE, H.E. VON, OESTREICHER, H.L. and WITTERN, W.W. VON (1951). *The propagation of surface waves over the human body.* (USAF Technical Report 6464.) United States Air Force, Aero Medical Laboratory, Wright-Patterson Air Force Base.

FRANKLIN, D. and FRANKLIN, L. (1983). *Bimorph skin transducers: A preliminary study.* Report to the Research Laboratory of Electronics, Massachusetts Institute of Technology.

GARDNER, E.P. and PALMER, C.I. (1989). Simulation of motion on the skin: I. Receptive fields and temporal frequency coding by cutaneous mechanoreceptors of OPTACON pulses delivered to the hand. *J. Neurophysiol.* 62, 1410–1436.

GAULT, R.H. (1924). Progress in experiments on tactual interpretation of oral speech. *Soc. Psychol.* 14, 155–159.

GAULT, R.H. (1927). 'Hearing' through the sense organs of touch and vibration. *J. Franklin Inst.* 204, 329–358.

GELDARD, F.A. (1940). The perception of mechanical vibration I–IV. *J. Gen. Psychol.* 22, 243–308.

GELDARD, F.A. (1972). *The Human Senses.* New York: Wiley.

GELDARD, F.A. (ED.) (1974). *Cutaneous communication systems and devices.* Austin, TX: The Psychonomic Society.

GESCHEIDER, G.A., CAPRARO, A.J., FRISINA, R.D., HAMER, R.D. and VERRILLO, R.T. (1978). The effects of a surround on vibrotactile thresholds. *Sens. Proc.* **2**(2), 99-115.

GREEN, B.G. and CRAIG, J.C. (1974). The role of vibration amplitude and static force in vibrotactile spatial summation. *Percept. Psychophys.* **16**, 503-507.

KEIDEL, W.D. (1968). Electrophysiology of vibratory perception. In: Neff, W.D. (ed.), *Contributions to Sensory Physiology*, Vol. 3. New York: Academic Press, pp. 1-79.

KHANNA, S.M. and SHERRICK, C.E. (1981). The comparative sensitivity of selected receptor systems. In Gualtierotti, T. (ed.), *The Vestibular System: Function and Morphology*. New York: Springer, pp. 337-348.

LAMORÉ, P.J.J. and KEEMINK, C.J. (1988). Evidence for different types of mechanorecep-tors from measurements of the psychophysical threshold for vibrations under differ-ent stimulation conditions. *J. Acoust. Soc. Am.* **83**, 2339-2351.

LANGBERG, E. (1987). *Magnetic Tactile Array, Contract N43-NS-7-2394*. Final Report submitted to National Institute of Neurological and Communicative Disorders and Stroke. National Institutes of Health, Bethesda, Maryland.

LEYSIEFFER, H. (1985). Vibrotaktile Reizgeber mit PVDF (Polyvinylidenfluorid) als Elektromechanischen Wandler. *Fortschr. der Akustik – DAGA* **6**, 863-866.

LEYSIEFFER, H. (1986). A wearable multi-channel auditory prosthesis with vibrotactile skin stimulation. *Audiol. Acoust.* **25**, 230-251.

LINVILL, J.G. and BLISS, J.C. (1966). A direct translation reading aid for the blind. *Proc. IEEE* **54**, 40-51.

LINVILL, J.G. (1980). PVdF models, measurements, and devices. *Ferroelectrics* **28**, 291-296.

MILLER, J.M. and TOWE, A.L. (1979). Audition: Structural and acoustical properties. In: Ruch, T. and Patton, H.D. (eds), *Physiology and Biophysics*. Philadelphia: Saunders, pp. 376-434.

MONTAGNA, W. (1956). *The Structure and Function of Skin*. New York: Academic Press.

MOORE, T.J. (1970). A survey of the mechanical characteristics of skin and tissue in response to vibratory stimulation. *IEEE Trans. Man-Machine Systems* **11**, 79-84.

MOORE, T.J. and MUNDIE, J.R. (1972). Measurement of specific mechanical impedance of the skin: Effects of static force, site of stimulation, area of probe, and presence of a surround. *J. Acoust. Soc. Am.* **52**, 577-584.

QUILLIAM, T.A. (1978). The structure of finger print skin. In: Gordon, G. (ed.), *Active Touch. The Mechanism of Recognition of Objects by Manipulation: A Multidisciplinary Approach*. Oxford: Pergamon, pp. 1-18.

SHERRICK, C.E. (1984). Basic and applied research on tactile aids for deaf people: Progress and prospects. *J. Acoust. Soc. Am.* **75**, 1325-1342.

SHERRICK, C.E. (1991). Tactual sound- and speech-analyzing aids for deaf persons. In: Christman, C.L. and Albert, E.N. (eds), *Cochlear Implants: A Model for the Regulation of Emerging Medical Device Technologies*. Norwell, MA: Kluwer Academic Publishers, pp. 189-219.

SHERRICK, C.E. and CHOLEWIAK, R.W. (1986). Cutaneous Sensitivity. In: Boff, K., Kaufman, L. and Thomas, J.L. (eds), *Handbook of Perception and Human Performance*. New York: Wiley, pp. 12-1-12-58.

SPENS, K.-E. and PLANT, G. (1983). *A tactual 'Hearing' aid for the deaf*. Paper presented at the 10th International Congress of Phonetic Sciences, Utrecht, 1-6 August.

STEVENS, J.C. (1979). Thermo-tactile interactions: Some influences of temperature on touch. In: Kenshalo, D.R. (ed.), *Sensory Functions of the Skin of Humans*. New York: Plenum Press, pp. 207-222.

STEVENS, J.C. (1990). Perceived roughness as a function of body locus. *Percept. Psychophys.* 47(3), 298-304.

TREGEAR, R.T. (1966). *Physical Functions of the Skin*. New York: Academic Press.

VAN DOREN, C.L. (1987). A device for measuring spatiotemporal sensitivity. *J. Acoust. Soc. Am.* 81, 1906-1916.

VAN DOREN, C.L. (1989). A model of spatiotemporal tactile sensitivity linking psychophysics to tissue mechanics. *J. Acoust. Soc. Am.* 85, 2065-2080.

VERRILLO, R.T. (1962). Investigation of some parameters of the cutaneous threshold for vibration. *J. Acoust. Soc. Am.* 34, 1768-1773.

WEINSTEIN, S. (1968). Intensive and extensive aspects of tactile sensitivity as a function of body part, sex, and laterality. In: Kenshalo, D.R. (ed.), *The Skin Senses*. Springfield, Illinois: Thomas, pp. 195-222.

Chapter 4
Communication of the Acoustic Environment via Tactile Stimuli

JANET M. WEISENBERGER

Impressive demonstrations of communication ability by deaf-blind individuals using so-called 'natural' means of tactile speech reception, together with data from psychophysical and perceptual studies of the spatial and temporal resolution abilities of the tactile system, argue that the tactile channel is a viable option for communication of information about the acoustic environment. Recent results from laboratory studies of devices that convert acoustic signals into vibrotactile or electrotactile signals offer further support for this argument. In this chapter, results from evaluations of a number of commercially available and laboratory prototype tactile aids will be discussed in terms of what aspects of the acoustic environment can successfully be communicated tactually, and how future designs for tactile devices might improve such communication.

Reed and colleagues (Reed et al., 1978, 1985, 1989; Delhorne, Reed and Durlach, 1988) have reported on the abilities of several highly trained deaf-blind users of 'natural' methods of tactile speech reception. In the Tadoma method (Norton et al., 1977), the hand of the receiver is placed on the face and neck of the talker. Information is obtained through the hand about facial and neck activity during speech (lip and jaw movements, oral cavity airflow, laryngeal vibration). These cues are sufficient for surprisingly good reception of connected speech (Reed et al., 1989). Work with users of tactile fingerspelling and tactile signing, in which letter shapes or signs are presented into the hand of the receiver, has also shown highly accurate reception of speech information (Delhorne, Reed and Durlach, 1985, 1988). The performance of users of these natural methods attests to the capabilities of the tactile sense for processing very complex inputs from the acoustic environment; their primary limitation is that they require physical contact between talker and receiver, prohibiting the reception of acoustic signals from more distant sources. However, these methods involve only the tactile and kinesthetic modalities, and do not require additional input from another sensory channel, such as vision.

Psychophysical studies of the ability of the tactile system to resolve vibratory and electrical stimulation suggest certain dimensions that would be suitable for transduction of information about the acoustic environment. A more comprehensive discussion of tactile abilities can be found in Chapter 1, and only a few pertinent findings are reviewed here. For example, the Weber fraction for discrimination of the intensity of a vibratory stimulus has been measured at approximately 0.20 across a wide range of reference intensities (Craig, 1972). Sherrick (1991) notes that this value is not appreciably larger than the Weber fraction of 0.12–0.18 for auditory stimuli measured at conversational sound levels by Jesteadt, Weir and Green (1977). However, frequency or temporal resolution acuities are not comparable between auditory and tactile modalities: temporal resolution of 3–5 ms has been found for vibratory stimuli (Gescheider, 1974; Weisenberger, 1986), which, although not equal to auditory abilities, is sufficient for transmission of fine-structure temporal aspects of acoustic waveforms, such as syllabic rate or phonemic rate. While frequency discrimination in the tactile system is poor relative to that for the auditory system (Weber fractions in the vicinity of 0.25 as measured by Rothenberg et al., 1977), measures of spatial acuity at different locations on the body surface (Weinstein, 1968) suggest that a spatial transformation of acoustic frequency into location on the skin is feasible. Indeed, this transformation has been investigated repeatedly, beginning with Gault (1927), and recent implementations have shown promise for tactile reception of acoustic stimuli.

Several steps are involved in the realization of a tactile device for conveying acoustic information, including:

1. determination of the aspects of the acoustic environment that are to be transmitted;
2. generation of appropriate coding and presentation strategies for transmission of the selected acoustic information;
3. design and construction of a device that incorporates the coding and presentation strategies in a power-efficient, wearable, and cosmetically acceptable fashion;
4. design and implementation of appropriate training and evaluation procedures.

A more detailed discussion of points 2 and 3 can be found in Chapters 5 and 6, point 4 is the subject of Chapter 8; accordingly, the main focus of this chapter will be on the first point.

Communication of the Acoustic Environment

Background acoustic stimulation

Giolas (1982) states, 'the primary consequence of a hearing impairment is the possible loss of verbal communication efficiency'. While an

interference in verbal communication is clearly the most serious consequence, hearing is typically used for functions other than verbal communication. A cogent discussion of awareness of auditory aspects of the
world around us is provided by Ramsdell (1978), who argues that
hearing gives us a sense of relatedness to the world, on a very primitive
level. Without conscious attention by the listener, auditory stimulation
in the background serves to connect the normally hearing person with
the world in a way not provided by a more conscious, deliberate level
of hearing.

The loss of a sense of 'connectedness' encountered by a hearing-
impaired person can lead to confusion or depression. Ramsdell argues that
an unconscious awareness of background events provides an 'affective
tone' that is an important component of a sense of security and well-being.
Further, changes in background auditory stimulation typically evoke a
conscious response in the listener, and lead to appropriate responses.
Hearing-impaired persons who cannot hear these changes in background
stimulation often react with annoyance at their failure to understand what
is happening around them.

Changes in the level or nature of background acoustic stimulation serve
as a signal to the listener, providing information or warning of potential
harm and allowing the listener to take appropriate countermeasures.
Ramsdell describes the conscious attendance by a listener to these stimuli
as a second level of sound awareness, referred to as the signal or warning
level. The ability to respond quickly to such warnings provides a sense of
security and safety that may not be available to a hearing-impaired person.
This level of awareness involves not only identification of the signal but
also the ability to determine its source.

Simple tactile aids, even those employing only a single channel and
presenting only temporal envelope information about acoustic events,
could provide sufficient background stimulation to restore a feeling of
connectedness to the world. While this aspect of auditory ability can be
provided by hearing aids to those with less severe hearing impairments,
tactile aids or other sensory devices might be more successful for those
with profound impairment.

In considering 'higher' levels of hearing, a variety of listener tasks can
be described, which vary in the degree of analysis of the acoustic stimulus and complexity of the communicative response required. A hierarchy
of listening tasks requiring finer and finer analysis of the input stimulus is
described by Weisenberger and Miller (1987), and is shown in Table 4.1.

Detection

Perhaps the simplest task performed by a listener who is consciously
attending is the detection of a stimulus. Studies reported in the auditory

Table 4.1 Levels of processing of acoustic stimuli

Task	Analysis of waveform
Detection	Presence or absence of energy
Discrimination	Differentiation of two or more waveforms on some basis
Identification	Selection of salient aspects of waveform
Environmental sounds	Amplitude envelope
Syllable stress pattern	Amplitude envelope
Phonemes	Spectral/temporal fine structure
Words	Spectral/temporal fine structure and amplitude envelope
Sentences	Spectral/temporal fine structure and amplitude envelope
Connected speech	Spectral/temporal fine structure and amplitude envelope
Comprehension	Waveform aspects above plus cognitive factors, such as context cues

literature notwithstanding (e.g. Lindner, 1968), it can be argued that a stimulus must be detectable before it can be processed further. In addition, minimal analysis of the waveform is necessary for detection. Thus, the first requirement of a sensory device such as a tactile aid is that it render acoustic stimuli detectable to the wearer.

The normal auditory system can detect a vast range of sound, covering some 120 dB. With its excellent frequency, temporal, and intensity discrimination abilities, the auditory channel determines what input constitutes relevant targets and rejects irrelevant input as 'noise'. Given that most tactile aids provide at best a crude approximation of the processing performed by the normal auditory system, it may not be desirable to render all acoustic stimuli detected by the normal ear detectable through the aid. A more useful strategy may be to focus on stimuli that are likely to be relevant to the individual (i.e. falling in the range of speech and environmental sounds at relatively close range). This strategy may help to mitigate the difficulty of isolating target signals from background noise, a problem encountered by sensory aids of all kinds but particularly important with tactile aids. An adjustable microphone gain may give sufficient flexibility for detection in different envionments. In any event, the degree of processing of the input acoustic stimulus required for the detection task is minimal; a simple determination of the presence or absence of energy will suffice.

Localization

A more complex task is that of locating the source of an acoustic stimulus. Although recent data suggest some individual variability in sound localization performance (e.g. Wightman and Kistler, 1989a,b), the normal listener can localize quite effectively in the horizontal plane. Localization is primarily binaural; low-frequency acoustic signals are localized primarily on the basis of phase differences occurring between the two ears (including arrival time and ongoing phase differences), and high-frequency signals are localized primarily on the basis of intensity differences between the two ears as a result of head-shadow effects. The ideal localization device would therefore involve a comparison of two or more inputs, and would require more than one transducer (or at least more than one 'mode' of stimulation).

However, a tactile aid might not operate exactly like the normal auditory system in this respect, particularly if real-time inputs were used. The normal binaural auditory system can detect phase/time differences in the microsecond range, but the temporal resolution abilities of the tactile system do not approach these values. Richardson (1982) notes that the tactile system is largely insensitive to phase differences in vibratory stimuli, consistent with the system's temporal properties. Empirical studies provide some support for these ideas.

High-frequency sounds, for which inter-aural intensity differences mediate localization, pose a lesser problem. Intensity discrimination is fair in the tactile system, and a device that provides inter-locus intensity differences to two or more loci might have some success in cueing source location. The simplest means of accomplishing this would involve mounting microphones on both sides of the head or body, to take advantage of shadow effects, and transmitting input signals to tactile transducers at two locations (possibly, but not necessarily, one on each side). Other, more complicated, strategies for stimulus input could be conceived, along with strategies for transforming input phase differences of low-frequency stimuli into a form more usable by the tactile system.

A tactile device that could yield accurate information about the location of a sound source based on the tactile cues alone may be desirable, but the importance of providing such information may be subject to debate. Because of the limited processing ability of the tactile system, it may be better to focus on providing information necessary for more complex auditory tasks. This is worth considering on two levels: first, a rough approximation of the location of a source can be accomplished by movement of the observer, even with a single-channel device which does not explicitly code localization cues, so if movement is practical specific coding of location may not be as necessary; second, in many situations the detection of a stimulus produces an alerting response that involves looking around to locate the most likely source of the sound. Thus the primary utility of a tactile device designed to provide information about sound location would be in situations where no visual cues were available. Laboratory devices designed to present such information are described later.

Discrimination and identification

An arguably more complex task, in terms of the necessary level of analysis of the acoustic waveform, is that of discrimination or identification of stimuli. *Discrimination* is typically described as the task of determining whether stimulus A is different from stimulus B along any of a number of dimensions. *Identification* is typically described as the task of isolating the unique features of a stimulus leading to the ability to name that stimulus. It is beyond the scope of this chapter to discuss in depth the question of whether stimulus A must be identified in order to discriminate it from stimulus B, and the two tasks are described together.

The kind of analysis of the acoustic waveform can be similar for the two tasks. The types of acoustic stimuli that typically need to be identified or discriminated in everyday situations cover a wide range, from environmental sounds (ringing telephones, barking dogs) to connected conversation. Aspects of waveform analysis for a number of tasks involving stimuli falling in this range are described below.

Amplitude envelope

Some identification and discrimination tasks can be performed using information available in the waveform envelope of the acoustic stimulus: having detected the presence of an acoustic waveform, the listener can extract further information about the stimulus from temporal and intensity variations in the waveform envelope.

This level of waveform analysis may be appropriate when attempting to distinguish classes of sounds with wide variation in their envelope characteristics. Environmental sounds (car horns, door-bells) fit this criterion and many environmental sounds can be identified or discriminated on the basis of distinctive temporal envelope characteristics. Even a relatively simple tactile device employing a single tactile transducer might be able to present waveform envelope information with sufficient fidelity for environmental sound identification. The usefulness of such an ability to increase understanding and awareness of events occurring around them is noted in anecdotal reports of hearing-impaired persons.

Amplitude envelope cues also distinguish among speech sounds, providing information about syllable number, syllable stress, and speech rhythm (segmentation). Studies of auditory coding strategies for speech perception have shown that even a simple amplitude-modulated tonal signal that reproduces the temporal waveform of speech can provide significant information to listeners who can simultaneously lipread (e.g. Grant et al., 1985).

Although single-channel aids may be quite effective at preserving amplitude envelope cues, multichannel devices, with transducers in different locations along the skin surface, might break up the integrity of the envelope and actually impair this aspect of speech recognition (Carney and Beachler, 1986; Bernstein, Eberhardt and Demorest, 1990). This issue will be addressed later in the chapter.

Fine structure temporal features

While overall amplitude envelope cues can yield surprising benefits in identifying acoustic signals, many signals, particularly speech sounds, are difficult or impossible to distinguish based on envelope cues alone. For these a more in-depth analysis of the acoustic waveform is necessary. In speech, discrimination at the phoneme level is accomplished by using fine-structure information, which can be either spectral or temporal.

One example of the use of temporal fine-structure information in the normal auditory system is the perception of consonant voicing based on differences in voice onset time (VOT). The differences between voiced and voiceless stop consonants are typically measured in tens of milliseconds, a range potentially detectable by the tactile system under optimal conditions. It is not clear whether temporal gaps corresponding to VOT can be perceived in running speech, but reasonable performance might be anticipated for isolated syllables.

Duration cues can also be useful for other aspects of phoneme identification, for example in identifying medial vowels. For short words or syllables, vowel duration may correspond well with total word duration, and a tactile aid which preserved only temporal envelope cues might be effective in vowel discriminations based on duration. Other distinctions involving durational cues may be facilitated, such as distinguishing stop consonants from fricatives.

The preservation of the temporal fine structure of the acoustic signal in a tactile aid may prove beneficial to the wearer, although some attempt to match the information presented to the temporal resolution properties of the tactile system would be required for optimal results.

Fine structure spectral features

For the purposes of understanding speech, the ability to analyze the spectral fine structure of the acoustic stimulus is crucial. The normal auditory system has excellent abilities in this regard, possibly well beyond what is necessary for phoneme identification. The converse is true for the tactile system, which demonstrates very poor frequency resolution, particularly for frequencies in the range in which absolute detection is best. Thus, for a tactile aid to be successful in conveying spectral information about an acoustic stimulus an encoding strategy must be designed that either takes into account or bypasses entirely the question of tactile frequency resolution.

One form of spectral cue that has been shown to be effective in auditory studies as a supplement to lipreading is *voice fundamental frequency*, F0. Grant et al. (1985) found that presentation of a frequency-modulated fixed-amplitude tonal signal (FM), an amplitude-modulated fixed-frequency signal (AM), or a frequency- and amplitude-modulated signal (AM–FM), all led to improvements when combined with lipreading over scores for lipreading alone. When amplitude information was added to the FM signal in the AM–FM condition, the highest levels of performance were observed. Findings such as these argue that F0 cues can provide important information, and these may be useful in the design of a tactile aid.

For phoneme identification and discrimination, it is clear that spectral information is of great importance. Many sounds can be distinguished on the basis of relatively steady formant (a characteristic energy peak in the spectrum of a speech signal) frequencies (F1, F2 or F3), and others on the basis of formant transitions, or changes in formant frequency in an ascending or descending direction.

There is some disagreement as to which formant is most informative in signalling the uniqueness of a phoneme, or whether a contrast of several formant values may be necessary. While this issue may be more or less academic for the normal auditory system, it becomes important in considering the design of a tactile aid; given limited processing ability, it may be desirable to concentrate on displaying information in a frequency range most likely to yield optimal identifiability of speech sounds, based on results from auditory studies. On the other hand, one might decide to present only information not already available in the lipreading signal, to minimize redundancy. The issue of redundant versus complementary information is discussed below.

'Higher level' processing

The ability to identify individual phonemes in speech may be necessary for understanding everyday conversation, but proficiency at identifying phonemes in isolated syllables does not ensure proficiency in understanding running speech. The continuous stimulation of connected speech signals creates a situation in which individual phonemic targets are 'masked', with both forward and backward masking effects playing a role. It is also unlikely that a tactile aid could process connected speech in real time if the observer were attempting to identify strings of individual phonemes. The 'higher order' aspects of such processing include cross-modal integration of the information from lipreading with that supplied by the tactile aid and more 'cognitive' or 'top-down' operations, such as use of contextual cues of a syntactic or semantic nature. These higher order processes are not specific to the processing of tactile inputs, but may be complicated by the need to transform tactile signals into lexical form.

In attempting to integrate visual and tactile inputs in processing speech signals, the question arises whether the two inputs should be complementary. The optimal balance of redundant versus complementary information in the signals provided by the two modalities has not been empirically demonstrated; however, cues to place of articulation are readily available from lipreading, whereas cues to manner of articulation or consonant voicing are less available (e.g. Summerfield, 1987). Most multichannel tactile devices tested to date are relatively poor transmitters of place information, but have in many cases provided information about manner and voicing. This complementarity of cues may contribute to high levels of performance in identifying speech signals.

The ability to use context cues to predict topic and syntax is an important determinant of the success a user will have in understanding speech. This is true for tactile devices, cochlear implants and hearing aids. The substantial inter-subject differences observed in connected speech tasks may be attributable to differences in this ability, which is dependent to a large degree on facility with language, and which may be reduced for some hearing-impaired persons. In testing the ability of a tactile aid to transmit connected speech, test materials should be chosen that are suited to the language level of the subject, to avoid possible confounding effects. In a task where performance with connected speech is tested using lipreading alone and lipreading with tactile aid, an individual subject may be assumed able to use context cues equally under both testing conditions. A within-subject comparison of performance is valid, but differences in the ability to use context may make between-subject comparisons difficult. For this reason, data from connected speech tasks are often reported for individual subjects rather than pooled across groups.

In testing a tactile aid or other sensory device, most researchers are interested in determining the degree to which it will benefit the hearing-impaired in everyday situations. Because most such situations involve the processing of connected speech, usually in conversation, tasks have been developed that attempt to approximate to these everyday situations; one such is *connected discourse tracking*, originally developed by DeFilippo and Scott (1978). Tracking involves the presentation of connected text by a talker to a listener, and the verbatim repetition of this text by the listener. A time-based measure, the number of words per minute transmitted from talker to listener, is used to determine performance. Text is presented a word, a phrase, or a sentence at a time, and correction strategies are employed to assist the listener. Although this task does not exactly mimic normal conversation, the use of prepared text allows some degree of control over the input. When performed in a live-voice setting, a number of sources of variability arise, including local variation in text difficulty, lipreadability of the talker and facility of the talker and listener with correction strategies. These, and others, have been noted in the literature (e.g. DeFilippo, 1988; Tye-Murray and Tyler, 1988), and strategies for modification of the tracking task have been proposed (e.g. Matthies and Carney, 1988). Despite its problems, tracking remains one of the tests most often used in evaluating a sensory aid's ability to transmit connected speech.

Tactile Aid Designs for Transmission of Acoustic Stimuli

Tactile aids can be classified according to several schemes, including number of channels (number of tactile transducers), modality of stimulation (vibrotactile or electrotactile), location of transducer array on body surface, type of processing strategy. A thorough discussion of tactile aid classification schemes is found in Reed, Durlach and Braida (1982). Study of the options indicated by these classifications may yield important insights about the transmission of acoustic stimuli via the tactile system. Results from tactile-aid evaluations conducted in the author's and other laboratories address the effect of a number of design variables on communication of acoustic information.

Single-channel tactile aids

Single-channel tactile aids, so designated because only a single tactile transducer, or 'channel', is utilized, are relatively simple in design. This simplicity has facilitated the commercial introduction of wearable versions. In deciding what information to convey through a single transducer, a number of possibilities can be considered. Perhaps the simplest approach can be found in the Fonator and Minifonator (Siemens Hearing Instruments), which detect incoming acoustic stimulation and present a band-limited version of this input on the transducer, using the transducer as a sort of loudspeaker. Relatively little signal processing is performed by the device, and much of the quality of the original input is maintained: in fact, holding the transducer of one of these devices next to the ear results in a percept akin to that heard through a low-fidelity loudspeaker.

The utility of this input to the tactile system has been studied by several investigators. Carney and Beachler (1986) and Carney (1988) found that the Fonator was quite effective in conveying syllable number and stress pattern. Similar results for the Minifonator were reported by Weisenberger (1989a), the device performing well in sound detection, identification of environmental sounds and syllable rhythm and stress. However, these tasks are dependent on preservation of amplitude envelope information, and do not necessarily require fine-structure temporal or spectral cues; in fact, the limited range of frequencies to which the tactile system is responsive and the relatively poor ability to resolve frequency might argue that the fine-structure cues that are present in the signal presented by a device such as the Minifonator are not perceived by the tactile system. This argument was supported by Weisenberger and Russell (1989), who compared the Minifonator and the Minivib3 (AB Special Instrument), a single-channel device that extracts the envelope of the incoming acoustic signal and uses it to modulate the amplitude of a fixed frequency vibratory carrier, thus presenting only envelope information to the wearer. (Other commercial tactile aids employing a similar strategy include the Summit TAM and Audiological Engineering Tactaid I.) Both devices performed well in tasks in which envelope information should be sufficient, such as sound detection, limited-set environmental sound identification, and syllable rhythm and stress identification (see Figure 4.1(a–c)). However, neither was effective in providing the fine-structure information necessary for phoneme identification, even in very limited sets (4 items), as shown in Figure 4.1(d). These data suggest that only envelope cues were used by wearers of the Minifonator, and that any additional information present in the tactile signal was not available. Thus, at least for the single-channel tactile aids available to date, only information about the waveform envelope of the acoustic signal is transmitted.

Although waveform envelope cues are not effective for differentiating phonemes presented solely to the tactile aid, this information may be useful when combined with lipreading: Miyamoto, Myres and Punch (1987), Skinner et al. (1988), and Weisenberger et al. (1991) all reported gains with single-channel devices in connected speech tracking over rates for lipreading alone. The benefit is modest, however, in the range of five words per minute. Improvements provided by single-channel devices in connected speech are likely to result from cues to segmentation and phrasing which are present in the amplitude envelope.

Use of single-channel tactile aids in educational settings appears to benefit language acquisition of profoundly hearing-impaired children. Two case studies (Proctor and Goldstein, 1983; Geers, 1986) showed that the vocabulary of young children fitted with a single-channel tactile aid increased rapidly. For these children, the primary function of the device seemed to be in alerting them to the presence of acoustic stimulation and focusing attention on the talker's mouth. The tactile aid also served to cue envelope structure and provided feedback about the quality of the child's vocalizations.

Although the information presented by single-channel tactile aids does not permit perception of acoustic stimulation comparable to that possible with the normal auditory system, single-channel devices do allow some communication of features of the acoustic environment. They are useful for sound detection, and for the identification of sounds that can be differentiated on the basis of envelope cues. Anecdotal reports suggest that

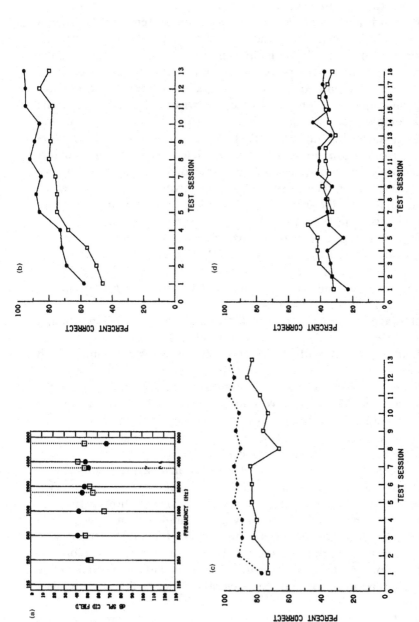

Figure 4.1 Performance of subjects in four tasks with two single-channel vibrotactile aids, the Minifonator (□) and Minivib (●). (a) Performance in a sound-field detection audiometric task, averaged across three subjects; (b) performance of subject PB in identifying recorded environmental sounds with the Minifonator and Minivib. A set of 20 items was used, presented in a five-item multiple choice response format, so that chance performance was 20%; (c) performance of subject CB in identifying the syllable number and stress of 15 recorded words consisting of monosyllabic, trochaic, and spondaic items. Chance performance for this task was 33%; (d) averaged performance for three subjects in a four-item task consisting of words differing only in initial consonant, using the initial consonants /t,d,s,z/. Chance performance for this task was 25%.

these devices are also beneficial in providing a sense of 'connectedness' with the world by conveying background acoustic stimulation.

Two-channel tactile aids

The localization of sound sources is normally mediated by the binaural auditory system, and would be a desirable attribute of a sensory substitution device. A few attempts to provide information about stimulus location in a tactile aid have been described, with most of the work being carried out by Richardson (Richardson, 1982; Richardson and Frost, 1977, 1979; Richardson, Wullemin and Saunders, 1978). Following earlier work by von Békésy (1959) and Gescheider (1965, 1970), Richardson argued that tactile sound localization must depend solely on intensity differences, since the tactile system is not responsible to small phase differences. In Richardson's device, square wave pulse trains were delivered to the tip of the index finger of both hands, and input microphones were placed at both ears. When subjects were permitted to move their heads to localize sound sources, performance with this tactile device was comparable to auditory localization of the same sounds. Further, subjects improved considerably with practice, suggesting that long-term use of the device might result in accurate tactile localization.

In Richardson's data, the best localization performance was found when the stimulus was located at an azimuth angle of 60°, a location that generated intensity differences of 10 dB between the two tactile stimulators. At other angles the intensity differences fell to as low as 2 dB. Richardson concluded that the good performance observed when head movement was permitted involved subjects turning to place the stimulus at a 60° angle.

Weisenberger et al. (1987) constructed a two-channel tactile device that utilized microphones and transducers mounted on hard Lucite earmolds, one inserted into each ear canal. In testing this device our acoustic signals were used: narrow-band noises centered at 500 Hz, 1000 Hz or 2000 Hz, and a broad-band noise. Stimuli were delivered to one of five loudspeakers placed in a 180° array in front of the subject. Results (summarized in Figure 4.2(a)) indicated that the 2000 Hz signals were most accurately localized, while the other signals proved more difficult. The 2000 Hz signals were probably easiest to localize because they generated the largest intensity differences at the vibrators, other signals creating only small intensity differences (phase differences created by the low-frequency signals were probably not perceptible through the device). The authors concluded that a more successful tactile localization aid could be devised that transformed any differences in input at the two ears into an intensity difference at the vibratory stimulators.

In attempting to convey spectral features of acoustic stimuli to facilitate

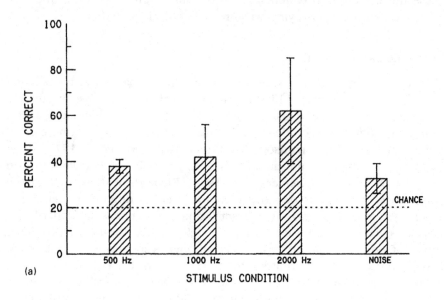

(a)

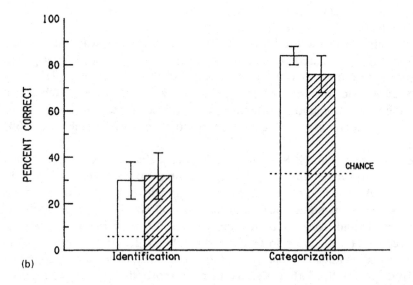

(b)

Figure 4.2 Performance of subjects with two-channel tactile aids. (a) Mean and standard error of sound localization performance with a two-channel earmold vibrator, averaged across five subjects for stimuli presented to one of five possible loudspeakers arranged in 180° semicircle in front of the subject. Stimuli were narrow-band noises centered at 500, 1000 or 2000 Hz, or a broad-band noise; (b) performance of three subjects with the Tactaid II (▨) and the single-channel Minivib (▢) on a syllable number and stress task. A 15-item stimulus set consisting of monosyllabic, trochaic, and spondaic items was presented live-voice. Subjects were scored on whether the correct stimulus item was identified from the list of 15 (identification), as well as on whether the response was an item with the correct syllable number and stress (categorization).

more complex auditory tasks than detection or localization, the abilities of the tactile system itself must be taken into account. Given its poor frequency resolution and the resultant difficulties in conveying spectral features of acoustic stimuli as tactile frequency, one reasonable approach to the design of tactile devices is to transform input frequency into a dimension along which the tactile system shows good resolution (e.g. space). An early suggestion for such a strategy was suggested by von Békésy (1959). The simplest implementation of this strategy involves dividing the input spectrum in two, directing the output of the low-frequency half to one transducer and the high-frequency half to another transducer in a different location on the skin surface. A number of two-channel tactile aids have been devised, including the KS 3/2 (Telex) and the Tactaid II (Audiological Engineering), which have been marketed commercially.

The addition of a second channel could be expected to increase the amount of spectral information available in the signal, and so performance with such a device could be significantly better than that with a single-channel tactile aid. This might hold true for even relatively simple two-channel devices, but the addition of a second envelope stimulus could interfere with overall envelope cues provided by a single channel, and thus it is possible that performance might be impaired relative to that with a single-channel device.

In an empirical comparison of single- and two-channel devices, Broadstone and co-workers compared performance in a variety of tasks using either the single-channel Minivib3 or the two-channel Tactaid II (Broadstone, Weisenberger and Kozma-Spytek, 1989, unpublished data). Overall, results showed that the addition of the second channel did *not* impair the ability to make identifications based on envelope cues, such as syllable rhythm and stress. Averaged data for this task are shown in Figure 4.2(b). However, the only task for which a reliable improvement for all subjects was seen using the two-channel device was an 's-detection' task, in which subjects were asked to determine which of a pair of words differing only in the inclusion of an initial or final /s/ had been presented. One subject also performed better in a sentence identification task using the Tactaid II. But in general, the addition of a second channel, while it did produce improved detection of fricatives, did not lead to higher scores in word identification tasks.

Work by Lynch et al. (1989), using connected speech tracking with hearing-impaired subjects, found small benefits (less than 10 words per minute) over lipreading alone when the Tactaid II was used, suggesting a small but reliable degree of benefit provided by the device. Other investigators (e.g. Geers and Moog, 1991) have noted improvements in isolated aspects of speech perception and production for children wearing the Tactaid II. More impressive benefits were reported by Cholewiak and Sherrick (1986), in a case study of one adult subject wearing the two-channel Telex KS 3/2 device. In this study, substantial improvements over lipreading alone were found when lipreading was combined with the tactile aid in the connected discourse tracking task. They suggested that the long-term experience of the subject with the tactile aid (over a number of years) may have contributed to the high performance. Because of the relatively recent introduction of tactile aids into commercial use, long-term experience is rare; results such as those reported by Cholewiak and Sherrick suggest that a true assessment of the potential benefit of a tactile device may not be provided in short-term laboratory studies.

Multichannel tactile aids

A further extension of the strategy of transforming input acoustic frequency into place on the skin surface is found in multichannel tactile aids, which employ multiple tactile transducers to convey spectral information about the acoustic stimulus. Such devices can use any of a number of coding strategies in selecting the features of the stimulus to be communicated; several of these are briefly mentioned later in this chapter, and a more in-depth discussion is provided in Chapter 6. Perhaps the most common approach has been the channel vocoder, in which the envelope outputs from a bank of bandpass filters are used to drive a set of fixed-frequency tactile transducers. While early tactile vocoders showed only mild promise (Wiener et al., 1951; Engelmann and Rosov, 1975), recent implementations have indicated more substantive benefits.

Brooks and her colleagues (Brooks et al., 1986a,b; Scilley, P.L., 1980, unpublished data) reported impressive performance of one adult subject in a variety of speech perception tasks using the Queen's University tactile vocoder, a 16-channel device with an array of magnetic solenoid transducers arranged linearly along the forearm. This subject acquired a 250-word vocabulary of items recognized through the tactile aid alone, and identified a large percentage of open-set sentence material when the aid was combined with lipreading. After a short period of connected speech tracking, benefits in excess of 20 words per minute over lipreading alone were observed. This subject's performance provided encouraging evidence that tactile aids could be a viable route for conveying acoustic information to hearing-impaired persons.

Number of channels

In attempting to produce small, power-efficient and wearable versions of tactile aids, one important consideration is the number of tactile transducers to be used. In modern designs, the transducers represent a significant portion of the total power consumption of the device, and a successful tactile aid would incorporate the smallest number of channels that could still transmit sufficient speech information to the wearer.

Direct comparisons of devices with different numbers of channels, but in which all other device features are held constant, are rare. Some initial insights may be gained from a study by Weisenberger (1988, 1989b), in which the performance of the Tactaid V, a 5-channel prototype tactile aid, was compared with the 16-channel Queen's vocoder. In very simple tasks, such as minimal-pairs phoneme identification, the two devices performed comparably. When larger closed-set tasks were employed in conjunction with lipreading, however, the Queen's aid was superior. But the picture was not entirely straightforward: when connected speech tracking was tested, one of the three subjects performed much better with the Queen's aid, the second only slightly better with the Queen's aid, and for the third subject performance with the two devices was comparable. These results are illustrated in Figure 4.3. Taken as a whole, these data do not provide a simple answer to the question of the optimal number of channels, but they do offer some encouragement for the use of fewer channels for wearable implementations. The data also point to a frequently encountered phenomenon in evaluating a tactile device: performance of a tactile aid on simple closed-set tasks is not always indicative of the benefit that will be seen in connected speech tasks.

Pilot work comparing 16-channel and 8-channel versions of the Queen's vocoder suggests that, at least for some subjects, eight channels may yield equivalent levels of speech perception performance. Overall, the results suggest that substantial amounts of speech information are conveyed by multichannel devices, even by those employing fewer channels.

Modality of stimulation

Another approach is to avoid the use of vibratory stimulation altogether. Several devices have been investigated that utilize electrotactile stimulation, a stimulus mode that raises some difficulties of its own. The major problem in coding acoustic inputs for electrotactile presentation is the extremely limited dynamic range of the tactile system for electrical stimulation, typically not exceeding 10 dB. Thus, in electrotactile devices that attempt to provide information about sound intensity over a range greater than about 10 dB, it is necessary to transform the input in some way, possibly by compressing the amplitude range of the acoustic stimulus, or by coding input intensity in some other form, such as pulse rate or pulse width.

Early promise was shown by the MESA (multipoint electrotactile stimulator array) in studies by Sparks et al. (1978, 1979). The MESA employed a two-dimensional abdomen array coding intensity vertically and frequency horizontally. Subjects tested with this device performed well in closed-set

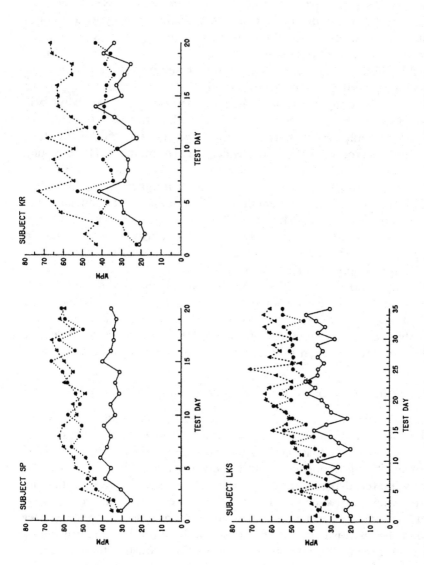

Figure 4.3 Connected discourse tracking performance of three subjects under lipreading plus Tactaid V (●) and lipreading plus Queen's vocoder (▲) conditions, compared with lipreading alone (○). Data are plotted as words per minute tracking performance across 1-h test sessions. Each data point reflects the average of two 5-min tests under each tactile aided condition, and one 5-min test of lipreading alone.

word and phoneme identification, and experienced some benefits over lipreading alone when connected speech was presented.

The first wearable and commercially marketed multichannel tactile aid was an electrotactile device: the Tacticon TC-1600, a 16-channel electro-tactile vocoder with a linear array of electrical stimulators worn on the abdomen. Input intensity was mapped as pulse rate changes. Saunders, Hill and Simpson (1976) found good identification of closed-set items with a precursor of the Tacticon; in a comparison of the Tacticon with the Queen's aid, Weisenberger, Broadstone and Saunders (1989) found that both devices performed well in minimal pairs phoneme identification and other closed-set tasks, with and without lipreading. However, when connected speech tracking was tested, the Queen's aid yielded final levels of improvement over lipreading alone of 40–50 words per minute, but the improvement provided by the Tacticon was in the order of 5–10 words per minute. These results are shown in Figure 4.4. In view of the compa-rable levels of performance found on single-item tasks, these differences in performance for connected speech were puzzling. The authors concluded that performance of a tactile aid on single-item tasks was not predictive of the success of that device with connected speech, suggest-ing that the wearer of a tactile aid may use different processing strategies, and possibly different stimulus information, in the two types of task.

Weisenberger's group were able to eliminate two possible reasons for the differences in connected speech performance. First, the influence of a noise-suppression circuit in the Tacticon, which may have adversely affected the perception of ongoing speech, was eliminated, by training subjects with versions of the Tacticon with and without the circuit: no differences in performance were observed. Second, a version of the Queen's aid that could be worn on either the abdomen or the forearm was constructed to determine whether location of stimulator array had affected the results: no differences were found for the two array locations. One further possibility is that the vibratory mode of stimulation is better at conveying speech information via the tactile system than the electrical mode. Corroborating results were obtained by Rakowski, Brenner and Weisenberger (1989), who evaluated a 32-channel electrotactile vocoder, the Audiotact (Sevrain-Tech), also worn on the abdomen. They obtained a pattern of results similar to that observed for the Tacticon (good perfor-mance with single-item tasks, but little or no benefits in connected speech tracking with the device).

However, promising results with an electrotactile device have been reported for the Tickle-Talker (Cowan et al., 1988, 1990), an eight-channel electrotactile device which stimulates the digital nerves on the fingers of one hand. Recent reports from this group indicate improvements in connected speech tracking of up to 30 words per minute over lipreading alone for subjects engaged in long-term work with the device. That these

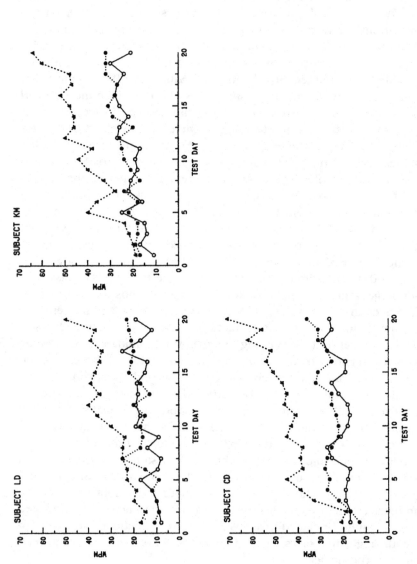

Figure 4.4 Connected discourse tracking performance of three subjects under lipreading plus Tacticon (●), lipreading plus Queen's vocoder (▲), or lip reading alone (○). Data are plotted as words per minute tracking performance across 1 h test sessions. Each data point reflects the average of two 5-min tests under each tactile-aided condition, and one 5-min test of lipreading alone.

results suggest that electrotactile stimulation is inferior to vibrotactile stimulation is an over-simplification; because the coding strategy used by the Tickle-Talker involves feature extraction rather than a spectral vocoder approach, the comparison is not completely straightforward. However, the Tickle-Talker data suggest that there is as yet no final word on the relative effectiveness of electrical or vibratory modes of stimulation for tactile aids.

Coding strategies

The aspects of the acoustic environment to be conveyed through a tactile aid can also be selected by implementing a particular coding strategy. Most devices discussed above have been channel vocoders, but other coding strategies may be equally or more effective. One strategy that requires more sophistication is the extraction of particular features from the speech signal. Boothroyd and colleagues (e.g. Boothroyd and Hnath-Chisholm, 1988) have investigated tactile devices that display voice fundamental frequency (F0) in a single-channel or multichannel design, and have found them to have some promise as an assistive device for the hearing impaired. These 'pitch' displays have shown benefits in single-item tasks and in connected speech, and are of particular interest in that they provide a signal to the wearer that is not typically provided by vocoder designs.

A feature-extraction strategy has also been incorporated into two recent designs. Once device that has shown good results in laboratory and limited field testing is the previously mentioned Tickle-Talker. The location of the electrode receiving stimulation indicates the value of the second formant (F2) of the speech sound, while pulse rate is used to code F0. Evaluation of this device (Cowan et al., 1988, 1990) indicates that substantial benefits are obtainable after training, in both single-item and connected speech tasks. As mentioned above, recent data from Cowan's laboratory show significant improvements in connected speech tracking when the Tickle-Talker is used. Pilot work with this device (Brenner and Weisenberger, 1990) supports these findings. A vibrotactile formant extraction aid has also been developed, the Tactaid VII (Audiological Engineering), which uses seven vibrators in a flexible array that can be worn on any of a number of body sites. This device displays F2 as location on the stimulator array. Initial work in the author's and other laboratories (Osberger, 1991) suggests potential benefit from this device, in both single-item and connected-speech tasks.

Yet another coding strategy that has been investigated is the use of principal component analysis, a speech-analysis technique designed to reduce the redundancy in most speech sounds. Principal component analysis uses across frequency correlations in spectral energy in a waveform to produce a small set of independent parameters, which contain information about the overall spectral shape of the waveform, rather than only its spectral peaks. One such device, investigated by Weisenberger, Craig and

Abbott (1991), consisted of a 30-element, two-dimensional array worn on the forearm, and displayed the value of the first two principal components of the input waveform in an x,y format. The algorithm used was designed to maximize the separability of vowels, and indeed this device yielded excellent identification performance for stimuli differing in medial vowel. Consonant features of manner and voicing were also transmitted effectively by the device, and impressive benefits to lipreading were demonstrated. For three trained subjects, tracking performance was 30–40 words per minute better than for lipreading alone; several subjects reached tracking rates of 80 words per minute when the device was used in conjunction with lipreading, with occasional scores in excess of 90. Given the 'normal-hearing' tracking rates of 100 words per minute typically reported in the literature, aided values in the 80–90 range are extremely promising. This device, as a laboratory prototype, was not wearable, but further investigations in a wearable application are warranted.

Conclusions and Implications for Further Research

Several points mentioned in the preceding sections merit further discussion.

In general, research supports the notion that considerably more information about the acoustic environment can be communicated by a multichannel tactile aid than by a single-channel aid. In addition, adding multiple channels does not necessarily impair the quality of information successfully communicated by a single-channel device, such as syllable number, stress pattern, and other envelope-dependent cues. This is not to say that single-channel and two-channel tactile devices have no value; the ability to detect acoustic stimuli, the feeling of 'connectedness' with the environment and the ability to identify stimuli based on envelope cues (as in environmental sounds) represent significant everyday abilities denied to the profoundly hearing-impaired who cannot be aided by conventional devices.

The relative comparability of tactile aids and cochlear implants has been difficult to evaluate empirically in the past, due to the lack of commercially available, wearable multichannel tactile devices. As multichannel tactile aids become commercially viable, such comparisons can be tested. This issue is discussed in Chapter 9.

An important issue is that performance of a tactile device in single-item, analytical training tasks is not indicative of performance of the same device in connected speech tasks. This lack of predictability is problematic on several levels. First, single-item testing is relatively simple to perform and relatively simple to standardize. Connected speech testing, particularly connected discourse tracking, on the other hand, is much more difficult, requiring considerable training of the talker and the listener, so that (to some degree) improvements seen early in training may reflect task learning and improvements in talker–listener interaction as much as improvements provided by the tactile aid itself. Further, tracking is quite difficult to standardize, although some efforts to produce laser-disk versions of connected discourse tracking are under way (e.g. Levitt, 1988). The correction strategies employed by the talker, text variability, talker lip readability, and other variables introduce considerable fluctuation in tracking scores. Second, the fact that some tactile devices might be beneficial in single-item tasks but not in connected speech tasks may reflect characteristics of the wearer as much as of the device itself. The subject may attend to different aspects of the tactile signal when processing connected speech, or employ different cognitive strategies with the same aspects of the tactile signal. Changes in the design of tactile devices might be effected to facilitate the changing cognitive strategies of the subject. This aspect of tactile aid use has received relatively little attention, and seems a potentially fruitful area for further exploration.

Finally, the whole issue of how to train a patient or subject to be an effective tactile aid user needs extensive investigation. It has never been verified whether the methods that are most effective for training in the use of hearing aids are also the most appropriate for tactile aids. Because the signal is quite different in the two cases, involving not only different modalities, but also different codings, it is quite likely that different training paradigms would be most effective. Similarly, training programs might differ depending on which aspects of the acoustic environment are to be communicated. Some evidence supporting this can be found in the analysis of confusion matrices obtained in single-item tasks with tactile aids. Typically, the pattern of confusions that occur with a tactile device are quite different from those that occur in auditory presentations, whether to the normal auditory system or to hearing-aided patients. At the very least, this finding suggests that the specific speech features selected for training with a tactile device might be different from those selected for training with a hearing aid, but it may also be that the tasks selected, the kind of instruction given, and the methods for testing and error correction might be different for tactile inputs, particularly regarding how to integrate tactile and visual inputs. These questions have received relatively little attention in the literature.

One area of research that has not been discussed in detail in this chapter is the possibility of using tactile devices to supplement both visual and auditory inputs or using a tactile aid and a hearing aid together. Preliminary efforts in this direction can be found in work by Lynch et al. (1989), who show the relative benefits provided in various combinations of tactile, auditory, and visual stimulation for the hearing-impaired. Further investigations might produce a clearer picture of which aspects of the acoustic stimulus are best communicated by which sensory modality, and may shed light on the whole question of multimodal processing of stimuli.

Two conclusions can be drawn from the data discussed in this chapter: first, that tactile aids can be used successfully to communicate a variety of features of the acoustic environment; second, that considerable further research is necessary in the design and evaluation of tactile aids to determine the benefits potentially available from the tactile sensory channel.

Acknowledgments

The author wishes to thank Susan M. Broadstone, Linda Kozma-Spytek, Christine Brenner and Deanna Buehlhorn for their contributions to this research and to the preparation of this chapter. Support for this work was provided by grant DC00306 from the National Institutes of Health, Bethesda, MD, USA.

References

BÉKÉSY, G. VON (1959). Similarities between hearing and skin sensations. *Psycholog. Rev.* **66**, 1-22.

BERNSTEIN, L.E., EBERHARDT, S.P. and DEMOREST, M.E. (1989). Single-channel vibrotactile supplements to visual perception of intonation and stress. *J. Acoust. Soc. Am.* **85**, 397-405.

BOOTHROYD, A. and HNATH-CHISHOLM, T. (1988). Spatial, tactile presentation of voice fundamental frequency as a supplement to lipreading: Results of extended training with a single subject. *J. Rehab. Res. Dev.* **25**, 51-56.

BRENNER, C. and WEISENBERGER, J.M. (1990). Evaluation of a wearable multichannel tactile aid. *J. Acoust. Soc. Am.* **88**, s192(A).

BROOKS, P.L., FROST, B.J., MASON, J.L. and GIBSON, D.M. (1986a). Continuing evaluation of the Queen's University tactile vocoder I: Identification of open-set words. *J. Rehab. Res. Dev.* **23**, 119-128.

BROOKS, P.L., FROST, B.J., MASON, J.L. and GIBSON, D.M. (1986b). Continuing evaluation of the Queen's University tactile vocoder II: Identification of open-set sentences and tracking narrative. *J. Rehab. Res. Dev.* **23**, 129-138.

CARNEY, A.E. (1988). Vibrotactile perception of segmental features of speech: A comparison of single- and multichannel aids. *J. Speech Hear. Res.* **31**, 438-448.

CARNEY, A.E. and BEACHLER, C.R. (1986). Vibrotactile perception of suprasegmental features of speech: A comparison of single-channel and multichannel instruments. *J. Acoust. Soc. Am.* **79**, 131-140.

CHOLEWIAK, R.W. and SHERRICK, C.E. (1986). Tracking skill of a deaf person with long-term tactile aid experience: A case study. *J. Rehab. Res. Dev.* **23**, 20-26.

COWAN, R.S.C., ALCANTARA, J.I., BLAMEY, P.J. and CLARK, G.M. (1988). Preliminary evaluation of a multichannel electrotactile speech processor. *J. Acoust. Soc. Am.* **83**, 2328-2338.

COWAN, R.S.C., BLAMEY, P.J., GALVIN, K.L., SARANT, J.Z., ALCANTARA, J.I. and CLARK, G.M. (1990). Perception of sentences, words, and speech features by profoundly hearing-impaired children using a multichannel electrotactile speech processor. *J. Acoust. Soc. Am.* **88**, 1374-1384.

CRAIG, J.C. (1972). Difference threshold for intensity of tactile stimuli. *Percept. Psychophys.* **11**, 150-152.

DEFILIPPO, C.L. (1988). Tracking for speechreading training. *Volta Rev.* **90**, 215-239.

DEFILIPPO, C.L. and SCOTT, B.L. (1978). A method for training and evaluating the reception of ongoing speech. *J. Acoust. Soc. Am.* **63**, 1186-1192.

DELHORNE, L.A., REED, C.M. and DURLACH, N.I. (1985). A study of the reception of tactile fingerspelling. *Am. Speech Lang. Hear. Assoc.* **27**, 81(A).

DELHORNE, L.A., REED, C.M. and DURLACH, N.I. (1988). The reception of sign language through the tactile sense. *Am. Speech Lang. Hear. Assoc.* **30**, 136(A).

ENGELMANN, S. and ROSOV, R. (1975). Tactual hearing experiment with deaf and hearing subjects. *Exceptional Children* **41**, 243-253.

GAULT, R.H. (1927). 'Hearing' through the sense organs of touch and vibration. *J. Franklin Inst.* **204**, 329-358.

GEERS, A.E. (1986). Vibrotactile stimulation: Case study with a profoundly deaf child. *J. Rehab. Res. Dev.* **23**, 111-117.

GEERS, A.E. and MOOG, J.S. (1991). Evaluating the benefits of cochlear implants in an educational setting. *Am. J. Otol.* **126**(Suppl. 1), 116-125.

GESCHEIDER, G.A. (1965). Cutaneous sound localization. *J. Exp. Psychol.* **70**, 617-625.

GESCHEIDER, G.A. (1970). Some comparisons between touch and hearing. *IEEE Trans. Man-Machine Systems* **11**, 28-35.

GESCHEIDER, G.A. (1974). Temporal relations in cutaneous stimulation. In: Geldard, F.A. (ed.), *Cutaneous Communication Systems and Devices.* Austin, TX: The Psychonomic Society, pp. 33-37.

GIOLAS, T.G. (1982). *Hearing-handicapped adults.* Englewood Cliffs, NJ: Prentice-Hall.

GRANT, K.W., ARDELL, L.H., KUHL, P.K. and SPARKS, D.W. (1985). The contribution of fundamental frequency, amplitude envelope, and voicing duration cues to speechreading in normal-hearing subjects. *J. Acoust. Soc. Am.* **77**, 6710-677.

JESTEADT, W., WEIR, C.C. and GREEN, D.M. (1977). Intensity discrimination as a function of frequency and sensation level. *J. Acoust. Soc. Am.* **61**, 169-177.

LEVITT, H. (1988). Videophonetics. *J. Acoust. Soc. Am.* **84**, S46(A).

LINDNER, W.A. (1968). Recognition performance as a function of detection criterion in a simultaneous detection-recognition task. *J. Acoust. Soc. Am.* **44**, 204-211.

LYNCH, M.P., EILERS, R.E., OLLER, D.K., URBANO, R.C. and PERO, P.J. (1989). Multisensory narrative tracking by a profoundly deaf subject using an electrocutaneous vocoder and a vibrotactile aid. *J. Speech Hear. Res.* **32**, 331-338.

MATTHIES, M.L. and CARNEY, A.E. (1988). A modified speech tracking procedure as a communicative performance measure. *J. Speech Hear. Res.* **31**, 394-404.

MIYAMOTO, R.T., MYRES, W.A. and PUNCH, J.L. (1987). Tactile aids in the evaluation procedure for cochlear implant candidacy. *Hear. Instr.* **38**, 33-37.

NORTON, S.J., SCHULTZ, M.C., REED, C.M., BRAIDA, L.D., DURLACH, N.I., RABINOWITZ, W.M. and CHOMSKY, C. (1977). Analytic study of the Tadoma method: Background and preliminary results. *J. Speech Hear. Res.* **20**, 574-595.

OSBERGER, M.J., ROBBINS, A.M., TODD, S.L. and BROWN, C.J. (1991). Initial findings with a wearable multichannel vibrotactile aid. *Am. J. Otol.* **12**(Suppl.1), 179-182.

PROCTOR, A. and GOLDSTEIN, M.H. JR (1983). Development of lexical comprehension in a profoundly deaf child using a wearable vibrotactile communication aid. *Language Speech Hear. Serv. Schools* **14**, 138-149.

RAKOWSKI, K., BRENNER, C. and WEISENBERGER, J.M. (1989). Evaluation of a 32-channel electrotactile vocoder. *J. Acoust. Soc. Am.* **86**, S83(A).

RAMSDELL, S.A. (1978). The psychology of the hard-of-hearing and the deafened adult. In: Davis, H. and Silverman, S.R. (eds), *Hearing and Deafness*. New York: Holt, Rinehart and Winston, pp. 435-446.

REED, C.M., RUBIN, S.I., BRAIDA, L.D. and DURLACH, N.I. (1978). Analytic study of the Tadoma method: Discrimination ability of untrained observers. *J. Speech Hear. Res.* 21, 625-637.

REED, C.M., DURLACH, N.I. and BRAIDA, L.D. (1982). Research on Tactile Communication of Speech: A Review. *ASHA Monographs No. 20*. Rockville, MD: American Speech-Language-Hearing Association.

REED, C.M., RABINOWITZ, W.M., DURLACH, N.I., BRAIDA, L.D., CONWAY-FITHIAN, S. and SCHULTZ, M.C. (1985). Research on the Tadoma method of speech communication. *J. Acoust. Soc. Am.* 77, 247-257.

REED, C.M., DURLACH, N.I., DELHORNE, L.A., RABINOWITZ, W.M. and GRANT, K.W. (1989). Research on tactual communication of speech: Ideas, issues, and findings. *Volta Rev.* 91, 65-78.

RICHARDSON, B. (1982). Using the skin for the purpose of sound localization. In: Gatehouse, R.W. (ed.), *Localization of Sound: Theory and Applications*. Groton, CT: Amphora Press, pp. 155-168.

RICHARDSON, B.L. and FROST, B.J. (1977). Sensory substitution and the design of an artificial ear. *J. Psychol.* 96, 259-285.

RICHARDSON, B.L. and FROST, B.J. (1979). Tactile localization of the direction and distance of sounds. *Percept. Psychophys.* 25, 336-344.

RICHARDSON, B.L., WULLEMIN, D.B. and SAUNDERS, F.J. (1978). Tactile discrimination of competing sounds. *Percept. Psychophys.* 24, 546-550.

ROTHENBERG, M., VERRILLO, R.T., ZAHORIAN, S.A., BRACHMAN, M.L. and BOLANOWSKI, S.J. JR (1977). Vibrotactile frequency for encoding a speech parameter. *J. Acoust. Soc. Am.* 62, 1003-1012.

SAUNDERS, F.A., HILL, W.A. and SIMPSON, C.A. (1976). Speech perception via the tactile mode: A progress report. *Proceedings of the IEEE International Conference on Acoustics, Speech and Signal Processing* 54, 594-597. (Reprinted in: Levitt, H.F., Pickett, J.M. and Houde, R.A. (eds), *Sensory Aids for the Hearing Impaired*. New York: IEEE Press, 1980.)

SHERRICK, C.E. (1991). Tactual sound- and speech-analyzing aids for deaf persons. In: Christman, C.L. and Albert, E.N. (eds), *Cochlear Implants: A Model for the Regulation of Emerging Medical Device Technologies* (in press).

SKINNER, M.W., BINZER, S.M., FREDERICKSON, J.M., SMITH, P.G., HOLDEN, T.A., HOLDEN, L.K., JUELICH, M.F. and TURNER, B.A. (1988). Comparison of benefit from vibrotactile aid and cochlear implant for postlingually deaf adults. *Laryngoscope* 98, 1092-1099.

SPARKS, D.W., KUHL, P.K., EDMONDS, A.A. and GRAY, G.P. (1978). Investigating the MESA (Multipoint Electrotactile Speech Aid): The transmission of segmental features. *J. Acoust. Soc. Am.* 63, 246-257.

SPARKS, D.W., ARDELL, L.A., BOURGEOUIS, M.R., WIEDERMAN, B. and KUHL, P.K. (1979). Investigating the MESA (multipoint electrotactile speech aid): The transmission of connected discourse. *J. Acoust. Soc. Am.* 65, 810-815.

SUMMERFIELD, Q. (1987). Some preliminaries to a comprehensive account of audio-visual speech perception. In: Dodd, B. and Campbell, R. (eds), *Hearing by Eye: The Psychology of Lip-reading*. Hillsdale, NJ: Erlbaum, pp. 3-51.

TYE-MURRAY, N. and TYLER, R.S. (1988). A critique of continuous discourse tracking as a test procedure. *J. Speech Hear. Dis.* 53, 226-231.

WEINSTEIN, S. (1968). Intensive and extensive aspects of tactile sensitivity as a function of body part, sex, and laterality. In: Kenshalo, D.R. (ed.), *The Skin Senses*. Springfield, IL: Thomas, pp. 195–222.

WEISENBERGER, J.M. (1986). Sensitivity to amplitude-modulated vibrotactile signals. *J. Acoust. Soc. Am.* **80**, 1707–1715.

WEISENBERGER, J.M. (1988). Effects of number of channels on speech perception with tactile aids. *J. Acoust. Soc. Am.* **84**, s45(A).

WEISENBERGER, J.M. (1989a). Evaluation of the Siemens Minifonator vibrotactile aid. *J. Speech Hear. Res.* **32**, 24–32.

WEISENBERGER, J.M. (1989b). Tactile aids for speech perception and production by the hearing-impaired. *Volta Rev.* (Monograph) **91**(5), 79–100.

WEISENBERGER, J.M. and MILLER, J.D. (1987). The role of tactile aids in providing information about acoustic stimuli. *J. Acoust. Soc. Am.* **82**, 902–916.

WEISENBERGER, J.M. and RUSSELL, A.F. (1989). Comparison of two single-channel tactile aids for the hearing-impaired. *J. Speech Hear. Res.* **32**, 83–92.

WEISENBERGER, J.M., BROADSTONE, S.M. and KOZMA-SPYTEK, L. (1991). Relative performance of single-channel and multichannel tactile aids for the hearing-impaired. *J. Rehab. Res. Dev.* **28**, 45–56.

WEISENBERGER, J.M., BROADSTONE, S.M. and SAUNDERS, F.A. (1989). Evaluation of two multi-channel tactile aids for the hearing-impaired. *J. Acoust. Soc. Am.* **89**, 1764–1775.

WEISENBERGER, J.M., CRAIG, J.C. and ABBOTT, G.D. (1991). Evolution and evaluation of a principal-components tactile aid for the hearing-impaired. *J. Acoust. Soc. Am.* **90**, 1944–1957.

WEISENBERGER, J.M., HEIDBREDER, A.F. and MILLER J.D. (1987). Development and preliminary evaluation of an earmold sound-to-tactile aid for the hearing-impaired. *J. Rehab. Res. Dev.* **24**, 51–66

WIENER, N., WIESNER, J.B., DAVID, E.E. and LEVINE, L. (1951). Felix (Sensory Replacement Project). *Quarterly Progress Reports*, Research Laboratory of Electronics, MIT.

WIGHTMAN, F.L. and KISTLER, D.J. (1989a). Headphone simulation of free-field listening. I: Stimulus synthesis. *J. Acoust. Soc. Am.* **85**, 858–867.

WIGHTMAN, F.L. and KISTLER, D.J. (1989b). Headphone simulation of free-field listening. II: Psychophysical validation. *J. Acoust. Soc. Am.* **85**, 868–878.

Chapter 5
Signal Processing Strategies for Single-channel Systems

IAN R. SUMMERS

The development of single-channel tactile aids was pioneered by Gault in the 1920s (Gault, 1924, 1926) – improvised devices such as a tin can held in the fingers no doubt have a much longer history. (For an early insight, see Rousseau, 1762.) Several single-channel aids have been commercially distributed in relatively large numbers over the past ten years, but there is little evidence to suggest that the optimum design for this type of device has been established.

For the purposes of this chapter, single-channel aids are defined as those which convey information via a single vibrator or single pair of electrodes on the skin. However, the line between single-channel and multichannel is not easily drawn, and the discussion will also touch on aids in which a single acoustic feature (e.g. voice pitch) is transmitted via an array of transducers or electrodes, and on some two- or three-channel devices.

Questions that must be answered when specifying the design of a single-channel tactile aid include:

1. *What capacity* has the tactile channel?
2. *What information* is most usefully transmitted?
3. *What coding strategy* is best?

Possible answers are discussed below. It should be noted that there is no a priori reason to suppose that the vibrotactile and electrotactile cases are equivalent: on the contrary, some elements of vibrotactile perception relate to the response of receptors in the skin which are not involved when electrical stimulation is applied directly to the sensory nerves; some elements of electrotactile perception are particular to electrical stimulation since they relate to the response characteristics of electrode/nerve transduction.

What Capacity?

Perception by the sense of touch and via electrotactile stimulation have been discussed at length in Chapters 1 and 2, respectively. The skin can recognise spatial and spatiotemporal patterns as well as temporal patterns of tactile sensation and is thus not used to its best advantage when stimulation is at a single site. The capacity of a single tactile channel is limited to the extent that tactually transmitted information cannot substitute for any more than a small part of normal hearing.

With vibrotactile stimulation, performance may be further limited by the response of the output transducer (see Chapter 3). In laboratory experiments it may be possible to use vibrators with near-ideal response (see, for example, Rothenberg et al., 1977) but requirements of cosmetic acceptability and low power consumption for the output transducer in an acceptable body-worn aid have led to the use of vibrators with very restricted performance (see, for example, Summers and Farr, 1989a,b). Cosmetic considerations may affect performance in another way, at least in the vibrotactile case, since they favour stimulation sites such as the forearm rather than sites such as the fingertip where tactual acuity may be greater.

It is almost certainly unrealistic to hope that a single-channel device will be able to convey sufficient information to allow speech reception at normal rates via the tactile channel alone, and so in practice we must consider the tactile transmission of speech-related information as a supplement to lipreading. In the non-speech context, however, the single-channel capacity is such that significant benefit (e.g. in terms of environmental awareness) may be derived from a stand-alone tactile signal.

What Information?

Those features of the acoustic environment which might usefully be made available to a hearing-impaired person are discussed in Chapter 4. Perhaps the most restricted application of the tactile channel is for transmission of one particular environmental feature, such as the sounding of a doorbell. This is easily achieved if the 'target' device is hard-wired into the tactile stimulator, but may require sophisticated pattern-recognition techniques if a microphone signal is used as input (Uvacek and Moschytz, 1988). For general environmental awareness – for detection of significant sources of sound, for some discrimination between sources and for estimation of background noise level in order to determine an appropriate voice level – the tactile channel must convey information as to the intensity, temporal pattern and/or gross spectral content of sounds (see, for example, Dodgson et al., 1983). Most aids, however, are primarily designed to give information which improves the speech perception of the user.

Single-channel aids to speech reception will generally be used to supplement lipreading. The potential of a relatively small amount of supplementary information to improve lipreading performance has been shown in experiments using acoustic presentation (Risberg, 1974; Rosen, Fourcin and Moore, 1981; Breeuwer and Plomp, 1984; Plant, Macrae and Dillon, 1984; Grant et al., 1985) and electrical stimulation of the cochlea (Rosen et al., 1989). Given that a single tactile channel cannot transmit all the information in a speech signal, one obvious strategy is to identify some significant part of this information which is not available visually and present this via the sense of touch.* Speech features which are denied to the lipreader include most of those which indicate suprasegmental information (i.e. stress, intonation and inflection) and, at the segmental level, the features necessary to differentiate between visually similar phonemes, i.e. phonemes falling within the various 'viseme' groups (Bement et al., 1988; Owens and Blazek, 1985). (Blamey and Cowan (Chapter 9) suggest that the majority of likely tactile aid users will have some residual hearing, in which case the appropriate speech features may be restricted to those not available visually or by audition.) Relevant acoustic parameters of the speech waveform include:

1. the amplitude envelope,† which indicates sentence stress and also contains some phonemic information (Van Tassell et al., 1987);
2. voice fundamental frequency (corresponding to the subjective parameter of voice pitch), which indicates stress and intonation and can give phonemic and suprasegmental information by signalling presence or absence of voicing (Klatt, 1976; Faulkner and Fourcin, 1989);
3. gross spectral features (e.g. balance between high and low frequencies, spectral centre of gravity) which carry phonemic information such as the distinction between voiced, unvoiced and mixed excitation (Traunmuller, 1980; Breeuwer and Plomp, 1984) – zero crossing frequency is a related parameter (Dodgson et al., 1983). For vowel sounds, the zero-crossing frequency of an appropriately bandpass-filtered speech signal can give an estimate of formant frequency, that is, it can indicate the position of one of the characteristic peaks in the vowel spectrum (Scott and De Filippo, 1977; Blamey et al., 1987).

---

*It is at least arguable, however, that this is not always the best tactic. Under adverse conditions, such as poor illumination of the speaker, it may be better to use the tactile channel to reinforce or duplicate information which might ideally be available through vision alone.

†The amplitude envelope is conveniently obtained by rectification and smoothing. Details of the amplitude envelope of a speech signal depend on the effective time constant of the smoothing process - a relatively long time constant (say, 20 ms) gives an envelope whose features correspond to the time-variation of speech intensity; a short time constant (say, 1 ms) gives an envelope whose fluctuations retain some information as to spectral features, such as voice fundamental frequency.

The benefit from aids which extract a particular speech feature for tactile presentation is often limited by the poor performance of feature-extraction circuitry under everyday conditions of background noise, reverberation, etc. Pitch-extractor circuits, which measure voice fundamental frequency, are particularly vulnerable in this respect – the analogue circuits which have typically been used in body-worn devices (Boothroyd, 1985; Howard, 1990) only perform well on 'clean' signals. However, recent developments in pattern-recognition techniques may provide a solution to these problems (Howard and Huckvale, 1988).

When developing a system intended primarily for the tactile transmission of speech features, an important secondary consideration must be the output produced in response to non-speech inputs. Acoustic parameters such as intensity and spectral distribution may be as informative in relation to environmental sounds as they are in relation to speech; however, a parameter such as voice fundamental frequency may be of little significance when inappropriately extracted from the general acoustic background.

What Coding Strategy?

There are two distinct approaches to the question of tactile coding. The first, here referred to as 'direct', essentially involves no coding at all. An amplified microphone signal is applied to a vibrator on the skin with the minimum of preprocessing. (The equivalent electrotactile operation has only rarely been used (Nelson, 1959), as some signal processing is generally considered necessary to produce current pulses suitable for nerve stimulation.) In the second strategy – the 'processing' approach – a limited number of features extracted from the acoustic input are used to modulate a tactile stimulus whose varying parameters are intended to match the perception available via the skin. (A suitable stimulus might, for example, be a pulse train with amplitude and frequency modulation.)

The direct approach

This is based on the conviction that, given sufficient access to an acoustic signal, the skin will be able to extract useful information (Gault, 1924, 1926; Schulte, 1972). In practice there may be problems: some important features may not be in a form that is easily perceived by the sense of touch; significant components in the tactile stimulus may be masked by less significant components (Gescheider, Bolanowski and Verrillo, 1989).

Another obvious disadvantage of this scheme is that, because of the poor response of the skin to high frequencies, most information above 500 Hz in the original acoustic signal will be lost. Such information can be brought into the perceptual range of the skin by using vocoder methods to compress the speech bandwidth (Brown, B.H., 1989, personal communication) or by means of transposition techniques which convert from high to low frequency, the transposed signal being combined with direct low-frequency information (as in the Siemens Minifonator, see below). Such attempts to increase the frequency range in the original acoustic signal that is available via the tactile channel may sometimes be counter-productive, since one advantage of the direct approach – that some gross frequency discrimination is guaranteed because low frequencies are detected and high frequencies are not – is lost. A similar point can be made in relation to the use of filtering to compensate for the high-frequency fall off of tactile response.

The direct approach might seem outdated. It was first developed by Gault in 1924, at a time when little information was available about the differences between auditory and tactile perception, and when the available technology provided few alternatives. However, there are many unanswered questions regarding the more sophisticated coding strategies which might now appear more appropriate (see below), and the direct approach still offers some attractions for the aspiring manufacturer of an inexpensive, reliable body-worn aid.

An example of a single-channel aid of the 'direct' type currently in widespread use is the Siemens Minifonator (Weisenberger, 1989). This consists of a body-worn electronics unit linked to a wrist-worn electromechanical vibrator. The amplified microphone signal, after low-pass filtering at 1 kHz, is applied directly to the output transducer. High-frequency information (4 kHz and above), transposed to frequencies below 500 Hz by non-linear circuitry, can be added to the direct signal if required. This aid can give significant benefit to the user, in terms of environmental awareness and as a support to lipreading (see Chapter 11). However, its performance is limited by some additional factors unrelated to its direct coding strategy: the vibratory output is insufficiently strong for some users and the electronics unit is perhaps too bulky at $85 \times 85 \times 28$ mm.

The processing approach – choice of tactile output

In systems which are based on this approach, the quantity of information presented to the skin is generally less than with the 'direct' schemes. However, the selected acoustic features are chosen as being particularly significant and are coded so that they should be easily perceived, the intention being to convey a greater amount of useful information in this way.

The capacity of a single tactile channel is such that it can successfully transmit information derived from only one or two acoustic features which vary on a timescale of, say, 100 ms or longer (Sherrick, 1985; Kokjer, 1987; Rabinowitz et al., 1987; Gescheider et al., 1990). It is convenient to picture the information transfer down such a channel in terms of temporal patterns in the tactile stimulus:

> The tactile sense gathers information about sound signals by recognising such features as how long an excitation lasts; whether an excitation consists of a constant or a changing amplitude; ... what are the rhythms, relative intensities and so forth... Tactile information about frequency components ... is perceived only indirectly as changes in those temporal properties.
>
> (Franklin, 1984)

The type of frequency analysis found in the ear, by which several simultaneous acoustic stimuli can be independently characterised in terms of intensity and frequency, is not available from a single site on the skin, and so the best tactic may be to altogether avoid competing stimuli in the tactile channel. Hence the widespread use of periodic stimuli with amplitude and/or frequency modulation (see below).

An interesting alternative is the amplitude-modulated-dual-fixed-frequency system (Bernstein, Eberhardt and Demorest, 1989) which uses stimulation with a mixture of 40 and 400 Hz signals. A subjective effect akin to continuously variable stimulus frequency is produced by changing the relative proportion of the two components. (For a similar scheme, see Weisenberger, Heidbreder and Miller, 1987.)

Another variant (Boston, 1975; Scott and De Filippo, 1977) involves coding in terms of stimulus 'quality' – periodic or random. There are some problems with this: the limitations of the tactile modality are such that the periodic/random distinction is difficult to discriminate for short-duration stimuli; if the stimulus also carries information via amplitude modulation, perception of this is worse for noise carriers than for sinusoidal carriers (Weisenberger, 1986).

The processing approach – some examples

Since it is much easier to design an electromechanical output transducer that operates over a narrow frequency range than a wide-band system, the use of an amplitude-modulated single-frequency system is attractive in the case of vibrotactile aids. The output frequency is generally fixed in the range 200–400 Hz, to which the skin is most sensitive in terms of displacement threshold.

A simple example of this type of device is the TAM aid (Summit, Birmingham, UK) which has been distributed in large numbers since its commercial release in 1986. This device (an earlier version is described by Summers and Martin, 1980) has an output at 200 Hz which is keyed on and off according to whether the amplitude of the microphone signal is above or below a user-set threshold. This 'on/off' coding has the advantage of making few demands on the tactile perception of the user, but the limited information which it can transmit means that the TAM is essentially an environmental aid only (Summers, Peake and Martin, 1981). Ling and Sofin (1975) have used a similar coding strategy to signal the presence of high-frequency consonants.

A more sophisticated version of this approach can be found in the Minivib (Special Instrument AB, Stockholm, Sweden), whose fixed-frequency output is amplitude modulated by a signal derived from the amplitude envelope of the low-pass filtered acoustic input, this envelope being to some extent high-pass filtered so as to accentuate changes of input level (Spens and Plant, 1983). A similar device is described by I.M. Beguesse (1976, unpublished data) (see also Proctor and Goldstein, 1983).

The converse coding scheme – variable stimulus frequency and fixed amplitude – lends itself to the coding of voice fundamental frequency (Rothenberg and Molitor, 1979; Bernstein, Eberhardt and Demorest, 1989). In practice the output amplitude is generally switched between a fixed level and zero since there are periods when no significant information is available for coding. With vibrotactile stimulation it is possible to use either pulse trains or sinusoids in this connection, the former having the advantage that the skin's sensitivity to pulses varies with stimulus frequency to a lesser degree than does its sensitivity to sine waves (Rothenberg et al., 1977; Bernstein, Schecter and Goldstein, 1986). An acoustic version of this system has been applied with some success to patients with some residual hearing (Rosen et al., 1987).

Use of a periodic stimulus with both frequency and amplitude modulation has obvious attractions in terms of increased information transfer (Sherrick, 1985; Rabinowitz et al., 1987). Grant et al. (1985) found that a frequency/amplitude-modulated sine wave gave significant benefit when presented acoustically to normally hearing subjects as a supplement to lip-reading. A tactile equivalent can be found in the aid developed by Plant (Teck Enn Loi and Plant, 1986) which uses the novel rotary transducer described by Traunmuller (1980). In one configuration of this device, voiced speech sounds are coded as a periodic signal whose amplitude corresponds to the speech intensity in the frequency range 500–1000 Hz and whose frequency corresponds to the voice fundamental frequency, transposed into the range 40–140 Hz. This signal is combined for output with a fixed-frequency (300 Hz) signal whose amplitude corresponds to the speech intensity in the frequency range >5 kHz.

In one of the few comparable electrotactile studies, Dodgson et al. (1983) coded the zero-crossing frequency and intensity of the acoustic input as the frequency and amplitude, respectively, of current pulses applied through an electrode pair on the wrist.

If stimulus amplitude and frequency are varied to code two independent acoustic parameters, it is necessary to ensure that changes in frequency do not result in apparent changes in stimulus intensity. This is essentially a question of working along appropriate equal-sensation

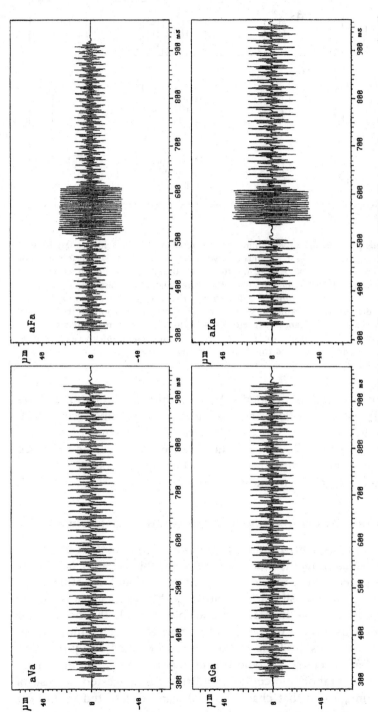

Figure 5.1 Vibratory output from a device which gives voiced/unvoiced information (Summers and Farr, 1989b). The examples shown correspond to the nonsense syllables aVa, aFa, aGa and aKa. Unvoiced sounds are indicated by a strong high-frequency stimulus. Voiced sounds (including those with mixed excitation) are indicated by a weaker low-frequency stimulus. Additional information is available from gaps in the output which correspond to silences in the original speech. In a study using computer-synthesized stimuli, Farr has shown that subjects can easily discriminate (86% success) between tactually presented patterns similar to those shown in the figure (Farr, J., 1989, unpublished data). The piezoelectric output transducer used in this device has a sharp mechanical resonance at 220 Hz. For the 'unvoiced' output it is driven with a 220 Hz square wave. In the 'voiced' case it is driven with a 36 Hz square wave, giving an output which appears as a series of tonebursts.

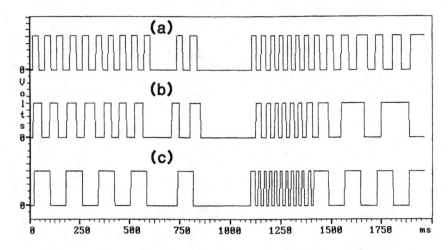

Figure 5.2 Various presentations of voice fundamental frequency for the sentence 'My horse has *three* white legs' (male speaker). (a) Square wave at F0; (b) after a linear transformation of the (nominal) frequency range 100–200 Hz into the range 40–220 Hz; (c) after an extreme non-linear transformation to a 'low/high' (50/300 Hz) representation (see also Figure 5.3). In each case the stress on the word '*three*' is indicated by a rise in frequency. (The gaps in voicing correspond to the fricatives in 'hor*se*' and '*three*'). The transformations in (b) and (c) are intended to accenuate significant F0 changes so as to faciliate their tactual perception (Summers and Farr, 1989a). Note that for greater clarity of reproduction, square-wave frequencies in the figure are one-eighth of the true frequencies quoted above.

contours. The problem is avoided when amplitude and frequency are simultaneously varied to code a single acoustic feature (Edmondson, 1974; Summers and Farr, 1989a,b; see also Sherrick, 1985). Figure 5.1 shows a variant of this scheme applied to the transmission of the voiced/unvoiced distinction – just one example from the wide range of coding strategies based on amplitude and/or frequency modulation.

The processing approach – some general coding considerations

There are probably as many proposed solutions to the question of coding as there are designs of tactile aid. One reason for this diversity lies in the constraints imposed by the tactile modality. On one hand, for stimulation parameters such as intensity and frequency, dynamic ranges available through the skin are less than those available through the normal ear (Keidel, 1974). This has led to the use of compression techniques so that the full range of sounds available to the ear can be detected by the skin. On the other hand, acuity of tactile perception at a single site is limited in comparison to auditory perception, and this has suggested the use of expansion techniques so that changes which can be detected by the ear are also tactually discriminable.

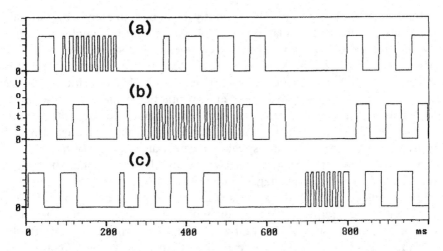

Figure 5.3 Variation of F0 for differently stressed versions of the sentence 'Look on the chair', presented as square-wave frequency after reduction to a 'low/high' representation in which only gross F0 changes are preserved. The 'low/high' assignment was determined by comparing the instantaneous value of F0 in the original speech to a threshold value, automatically set at 20% above the F0 value at the start of the sentence (Summers, 1986). This transformation is intended to facilitate the tactual perception of significant F0 changes (Summers and Farr, 1989a). The stress in (a), (b) and (c) falls on the first, second and fourth words, respectively. In each case the stressed word is indicated by a rise in frequency, also by a lengthening of the syllable in comparison to the unstressed equivalent. (The gaps in voicing correspond to the unvoiced sounds in 'Loo*k*' and '*ch*air'.) For greater clarity of reproduction, the 'low' and 'high' outputs are represented by square-wave frequencies of 12.5 and 75 Hz – higher frequencies such as 40/400 Hz are more suitable for tactile presentation.

When implementing signal-processing strategies of the type described above, the necessary electronic hardware commonly has two sections: the first operates on the input signal and produces an output or outputs corresponding to the acoustic feature(s) which are to be tactually transmitted; the second produces a tactile stimulus whose parameters are determined by these features. Such a system allows a great deal of flexibility at the interface between the two sections. For example consider a pitch extractor, whose output voltage varies linearly with voice fundamental frequency F0, coupled to a voltage-controlled oscillator which drives a vibrotactile output transducer. Such a system is essentially frequency-to-voltage followed by voltage-to-frequency, and may be configured so that the frequency of the tactile output is equal to F0. However, many other configurations are possible: the frequency range of the output can be offset and/or expanded with respect to that of the input, or derived via a non-linear transformation (Rothenberg and Molitor, 1979; Bernstein, Eberhardt and Demorest, 1989; Summers and Farr, 1989a) – the investigator is probably spoilt for choice. Similar considerations apply to the coding of other acoustic features. Figures 5.2 and 5.3 show variously processed presentations of F0 from a male speaker.

In designing aids for use by recently deafened persons (or normally hearing test subjects!) it may be desirable to attempt to match the subjective magnitude of tactually perceived changes to the subjective magnitude of changes in the corresponding acoustic feature when perceived aurally (Marks, 1987; Petrosino et al., 1988). However, this consideration may have little relevance to most users and in practice a more suitable aim is to maximise the dynamic range of significant changes in the tactile output in order to facilitate their perception. It may be easier to achieve this aim in the speech context if inter-speaker normalisation is employed.

Normalisation of tactile stimuli derived from different speakers has potential advantages and disadvantages. Taking voice pitch as example, the range of F0 produced by typical speakers (men, women and children) coincides well with the frequency range in which the skin is most sensitive (50–500 Hz). This suggests a coding scheme in which the tactile stimulus has a frequency equal to F0. However, a particular speaker will occupy only approximately one octave of the overall F0 range of more than three octaves (Hess, 1983). This may cause problems when training tactile aid users to recognise characteristic intonation patterns, since a typical male voice will produce a stimulus at the lower end of the F0 range but a typical female voice will lie at the upper end of the range, where the tactile sensation is quite different and frequency discrimination is poorer (Rothenberg et al., 1977; Sherrick, 1985). These problems may be solved by normalising the various pitch ranges so that the tactile stimulus moves over approximately the same frequency range, irrespective of speaker (see, for example, Bernstein, Eberhardt and Demorest, 1989). This scheme has an added advantage that the dynamic range of the output can be expanded so that intonation patterns move over the full frequency range available on the skin and should thus be more easily perceived (Rothenberg and Molitor, 1979). However, practical implementation of this normalisation is difficult (for one possibility, see Figure 5.3 and Summers, 1986) and it can be argued that the consequent loss of information about the pitch range of the speaker is undesirable. A similar discussion can be applied to the tactile transmission of the speech amplitude envelope: compression techniques may be used so that peak levels of tactile stimulation are invariant over a wide range of input voice levels and the amplitude envelope of whatever speaker can then be coded over a wide dynamic range. This may facilitate the identification of significant features in the amplitude envelope, but potentially useful information (such as the speaker's mood or the distance from which he or she is speaking) is lost. It is the author's opinion that normalisation techniques are worth pursuing: improved speech reception is of primary importance to potential tactile aid users and the capacity of a single-channel device – at least under every-day conditions when the user's attention may not be fully directed towards the tactile stimulus – is such that the information presented should be as little and as clear as possible.

Extensions of Single-channel Strategies

Some aids with more than one output channel can be considered as extended versions of a single-channel device rather than multichannel aids in the true sense.

Two-channel and three-channel devices

Given the ability of the skin to process spatial information, stimulation at more than one site is an attractive possibility. A small step in this direction is the use of two or three channels.

The Tactaid II (Audiological Engineering Corporation, Somerville, MA, USA) has two vibrotactile transducers which can be worn side by side on the wrist. Each produces a fixed-frequency stimulus at 375 Hz (250 Hz in an alternative version; and 400 Hz in early examples), one channel being amplitude modulated by the amplitude envelope of input signals in the range 100 Hz to 1.8 kHz, and the other by the amplitude envelope of input signals in the range 1.5–10 kHz. This device incorporates noise suppression circuitry: the tactile output is produced only in response to transient signals such as speech; steady input signals are interpreted as general background noise and produce no output. The Kanievski aid (Cholewiak and Sherrick, 1986), now marketed as the Telex KS 3/2 (Telex Communications Inc., Rochester, MN, USA), is also a two-channel vibrotactile device, with an output transducer on each wrist.

The Scott SRA-10 vibrotactile aid (Friel-Patti and Roeser, 1983) derives from an interesting earlier device which had a combination of both vibrotactile and electrotactile outputs (Scott and De Filippo, 1977). The SRA-10 codes low-frequency information as an amplitude- and frequency-modulated sine wave. Mid and high frequencies are coded as amplitude-modulated random noise, and are intended to be distinguished by quality of tactile sensation. In addition, the various frequency regions of the input signal are spatially encoded along a linear array of three vibrators – high frequencies on the centre, mid frequencies on the two outer vibrators and low frequencies on all three. This coding in terms of area of stimulation, rather than the more obvious coding as linear position, seems an attractive possibility but has attracted little further interest.

An electrotactile example of a two-channel device can be found in the Signalon (Uvacek and Moschytz, 1988). Two different stimulus intensities at two different locations on the wrist are used to signal four types of alarm signal.

The extent to which it is possible to make use of the information potentially available from two-channel systems has been investigated. Broadstone, Weisenberger and Kozma-Spytek (1989, unpublished manuscript) (see also Chapter 4) compared the single-channel Minivib with the Tactaid

II and concluded that the addition of a second channel produced little benefit. Eberhardt et al. (1990) reported a negative effect on lipreading performance from the addition of a second high-frequency channel to a system transmitting voice fundamental frequency.

The use of two channels to give directional 'stereotactile' information and hence allow separation of competing sources is an interesting possibility which has received relatively little attention (Weisenberger, Heidbreder and Miller, 1987; Weisenberger and Miller, 1987; Richardson, 1990). Gescheider (1965, 1968, 1970) describes laboratory investigations of tactile localisation and reports:

> ...after a few sessions of practice, cutaneous sound localisation was about as accurate as auditory sound localisation. Cutaneous sound localisation, therefore, seems to hold promise as a possible supplement to or substitution for auditory sound localisation.

Devices with multi-stimulator arrays

The Portapitch (Yeung, Boothroyd and Redmond, 1988) has a linear array of 16 vibrotactile transducers which are ranged along the user's forearm at 6-mm intervals. Voice pitch is coded as stimulus position (in terms of which one of the transducers is activated) and also as stimulus frequency. A recent study has indicated that this device is not particularly successful in transmitting pitch information (Kishon-Rabin, Hanin and Boothroyd, 1990) but this may be due to failings in its feature extraction circuitry rather than problems inherent to the coding scheme. A similar electro-tactile device, with ten electrode pairs at 2-cm spacing along the forearm, is described by Grant et al. (1986).

Comparison of Coding Strategies

There have been relatively few comparative evaluations of different coding strategies and/or different tactile aids. In studying reports on those investigations which have taken place, it is often difficult to discover whether the relative success or failure of a particular device is attributable to the choice of acoustic feature(s) to be coded, to the reliability or otherwise of the feature extractors that may have been used, or to the choice of coding strategy. In order to look separately at these problem areas, more studies are needed of the benefit from aural presentation of various acoustic features (Blamey, Martin and Clark, 1985; Grant et al., 1985; Boothroyd, 1988), in which case problems of coding are minimised; also more studies on the discrimination of synthesised 'speech-like' signals under various types of tactile coding (Farr, J., 1989, unpublished data; Eilers et al., 1990), in which case problems which relate to choice and extraction of acoustic features are circumvented.

In Chapter 11 of this volume, Thornton describes a comparative trial of four commercially available aids with significantly different coding strategies: the TAM, Minivib, Minifonator and Tactaid II. His results are not easily interpreted as an indication in favour of one particular coding scheme or other. The TAM scores well overall, despite its relatively crude signal processing.

The same four aids were compared in a study by Plant (1989) which also included the Tacticon TC-1600 – a multichannel electrotactile device. The results from Plant's test battery '... show a clear overall superiority for the Minivib', and this aid was also the most popular among his subjects. Weisenberger and Russell (1989) compared the Minivib and Minifonator and found that subjects did not make use of the additional spectral information present in the Minifonator output, concluding that '... performance with the Minifonator was not superior to that with the Minivib on any task. In fact, in many of the tasks, the Minivib yielded higher levels of performance.' Both these observations contrast with the relatively poor showing of the Minivib in Thornton's study, presumably due to differences in test materials and subject training. The latter factor is a potential source of many problems in comparative trials since it may be very difficult to match the effectiveness of training for devices with different coding schemes.

Several investigators (e.g. Rothenberg and Molitor, 1979; Bernstein, Eberhardt and Demorest, 1989; Summers and Farr, 1989a) have looked in some detail at variants of one particular coding strategy – in the examples quoted, the coding of voice fundamental frequency as vibrotactile frequency. For questions of tactile coding to be answered with any confidence more studies of this type (whose aim is to optimise a particular strategy), as opposed to studies which evaluate devices whose design has been pre-ordained, are needed.

Comparison of Single-channel and Multichannel Systems

At first sight it seems obvious that multichannel systems offer more potential benefit than single-channel devices. However effective a single-channel aid might be, a more effective device should result from application of the same coding strategy to the stimulus from a multichannel device, with additional information coded onto the spatial dimension (Bernstein, Eberhardt and Demorest, 1989). It is less obvious, however, that any advantage offered by existing multichannel aids (Saunders, 1985; Brooks et al., 1986; Blamey et al., 1988) over existing single-channel devices outweighs the engineering, cosmetic and ergonomic disadvantages which are associated with multichannel designs. The picture is further confused by the results of studies (Carney and Beachler, 1986; Carney, 1988; Plant, 1989;

Kishon-Rabin, Hanin and Boothroyd, 1990) which show that single-channel aids perform no worse than some multichannel devices in comparative trials. It seems likely that there is potential for both types of aid; perhaps with multichannel devices for the more committed user and single-channel devices for those (perhaps the majority) who will only accept an aid with minimal practical disadvantages.

Conclusion

There have been many studies which relate to the question of tactile coding. Systems using a variety of coding schemes have been shown to transmit useful information, and several aids are currently in every-day use in considerable numbers. However, the design of such devices is some way from being optimised. With further investigations to provide the necessary data, it is realistic to hope that better single-channel tactile aids will become available in the next 5-10 years.

References

BEMENT, L., WALLBER, J., DE FILIPPO, C.L., BOCHNER, J. and GARRISON, W. (1988). A new proto-col for assessing viseme perception in sentence context: the lipreading discrimina-tion test. *Ear. Hear.* **9**, 33-40.

BERNSTEIN, L.E., EBERHARDT, S.P. and DEMOREST, M.E. (1989). Single-channel vibrotactile supplements to visual perception of intonation and stress. *J. Acoust. Soc. Am.* **85**, 397-405.

BERNSTEIN, L.E., SCHECTER, M.B. and GOLDSTEIN, M.H. (1986). Child and adult vibrotactile thresholds for sinusoidal and pulsatile stimuli. *J. Acoust. Soc. Am.* **80**, 118-123.

BLAMEY, P.J., MARTIN, L.F.A. and CLARK, G.M. (1985). A comparison of three speech coding strategies using an acoustic model of a cochlear implant. *J. Acoust. Soc. Am.* **77**, 209-217.

BLAMEY, P.J., DOWELL, R.C., CLARK, G.M. and SELIGMAN, P.M. (1987). Acoustic parameters measured by a formant-estimating speech processor for a multiple-channel cochlear implant. *J. Acoust. Soc. Am.* **82**, 38-47.

BLAMEY, P.J., COWAN, R.S.C., ALCANTARA, J.I. and CLARK, G.M. (1988). Phonemic information transmitted by a multichannel electrotactile speech processor. *J. Speech Hear. Res.* **31**, 620-629.

BOOTHROYD, A. (1985). A wearable tactile intonation display for the deaf. *IEEE Trans. Acoust. Speech Signal Process.* **33**, 111-117.

BOOTHROYD, A. (1988). Perception of speech pattern contrasts from auditory presenta-tion of voice fundamental frequency. *Ear. Hear.* **9**, 313-321.

BOSTON, D.W. (1975). An instrument facilitating the perception and discrimination of voiced sounds and fricatives using a single vibrotactile cue. *Br. J. Audiol.* **9**, 84, 89.

BREEUWER, M. and PLOMP, R. (1984). Speechreading supplemented with frequency-selec-tive sound-pressure information. *J. Acoust. Soc. Am.* **76**, 686-691.

BROOKS, P.L., FROST, B.J., MASON, J.L. and GIBSON, D.M. (1986). Continuing evaluation of the Queen's University tactile vocoder. *J. Rehab. Res. Dev.* **23**, 119-128, 129-138.

CARNEY, A.E. (1988). Vibrotactile perception of segmental features of speech: A comparison of single-channel and multi-channel instruments. *J. Speech Hear. Res.* **31**, 438-448.

CARNEY, A.E. and BEACHLER, C.R. (1986). Vibrotactile perception of suprasegmental features of speech: A comparison of single-channel and multichannel instruments. *J. Acoust. Soc. Am.* **79**, 131-140.

CHOLEWIAK, R.W. and SHERRICK, C.E. (1986). Tracking skill of a deaf person with long-term tactile experience: A case study. *J. Rehab. Res. Dev.* **23**, 20-26.

DODGSON, G.S., BROWN, B.H., FREESTON, I.L. and STEVENS, J.C. (1983). Electrical stimulation at the wrist as an aid for the profoundly deaf. *Clin. Phys. Physiol. Meas.* **4**, 403-416.

EBERHARDT, S.P., BERNSTEIN, L.E., DEMOREST, M.E. and GOLDSTEIN, M.H. (1990). Speechreading sentences with single-channel vibrotactile presentation of voice fundamental frequency. *J. Acoust. Soc. Am.* **88**, 1274-1285.

EDMONDSON, W.H. (1974). Preliminary experiments with a new vibrotactile speech training aid for the deaf. *Proceedings of the Speech Communication Seminar*, Stockholm, **4**, 41-48.

EILERS, R., LYNCH, M., OLLER, D.K. and VERGARA, K. (1990). Mechanisms of multi-modal processing of speech information. Paper presented at the International Conference on Tactile Aids, Hearing Aids and Cochlear Implants, Sydney.

FAULKNER, A. and FOURCIN, A.J. (1989). Speech-pattern presentation to the deaf: Speech perception and production. In: Tubach, J.P. and Mariani, J.J., eds, *Proceedings of Eurospeech '89, Paris.* **2**. Edinburgh: CEP Consultants Ltd, pp. 718-721.

FRANKLIN, D. (1984). Tactile aids: new help for the profoundly deaf. *Hear. J.* **37**, 20-24.

FRIEL-PATTI, S. and ROESER, R.J. (1983). Evaluating changes in the communication skills of deaf children using vibrotactile stimulation. *Ear Hear.* **4**, 31-39.

GAULT, R.H. (1924). Progress in experiments on tactual interpretation of oral speech. *J. Abnorm. Soc. Psychol.* **19**, 155-159.

GAULT, R.H. (1926). Touch as a substitute for hearing in the interpretation and control of speech. *Arch. Otolaryngol.* **3**, 121-135.

GESCHEIDER, G.A. (1965). Cutaneous sound localization. *J. Exp. Psychol.* **70**, 617-625.

GESCHEIDER, G.A. (1968). Role of phase-difference cues in the cutaneous analog of auditory sound localization. *J. Acoust. Soc. Am.* **43**, 1249-1254.

GESCHEIDER, G.A. (1970). Some comparisons between touch and hearing. *IEEE Trans. Man–Machine Systems* **11**, 28-35.

GESCHEIDER, G.A., BOLANOWSKI, S.J. and VERRILLO, R.T. (1989). Vibrotactile masking: Effects of stimulus onset asynchrony and stimulus frequency. *J. Acoust. Soc. Am.* **85**, 2059-2064.

GESCHEIDER, G.A., BOLANOWSKI, S.J., VERRILLO, R.T., ARPAJIAN, D.J. and RYAN, T.F. (1990). Vibrotactile intensity discrimination measured by three methods. *J. Acoust. Soc. Am.* **87**, 330-338.

GRANT, K.W., ARDELL, L.H., KUHL, P.K. and SPARKS, D.W. (1985). The contribution of fundamental frequency, amplitude envelope, and voicing duration cues to speech reading in normal-hearing subjects. *J. Acoust. Soc. Am.* **77**, 671-677.

GRANT, K.W., ARDELL, L.H., KUHL, P.K. and SPARKS, D.W. (1986). The transmission of prosodic information via an electrotactile speechreading aid. *Ear Hear.* **7**, 328-335.

HESS, W. (1983). *Pitch Determination of Speech Signals: Algorithms and Devices.* Berlin: Springer.

HOWARD, D.M. (1990). Peak-picking fundamental period estimation for hearing prostheses. *J. Acoust. Soc. Am.* **86**, 902-910.

HOWARD, I.S. and HUCKVALE, M.A. (1988). Speech fundamental period estimation using a trainable pattern classifier. In: Ainsworth, W.A. and Holmer, J.N., eds, *Proceedings of the Seventh FASE Symposium, Speech '88*. Edinburgh: Institute of Acoustics, pp. 129-136.

KEIDEL, W.D. (1974). The cochlear model in skin stimulation. In: Geldard, F.A. (ed.), *Cutaneous Communication Devices and Systems*. Austin, TX: The Psychonomic Society, pp. 27-32.

KISHON-RABIN, L., HANIN, L. and BOOTHROYD, A. (1990). Lipreading enhancement by a spatial tactile display of fundamental frequency. Paper presented at the International Conference on Tactile Aids, Hearing Aids and Cochlear Implants, Sydney.

KLATT, D.H. (1976). Linguistic uses of segmental duration in English: acoustic and perceptual evidence. *J. Acoust. Soc. Am.* **59**, 1208-1221.

KOKJER, K.J. (1987). The information capacity of the human fingertip. *IEEE Trans. Syst. Man Cybernet.* **17**, 100-102.

LING, D. and SOFIN, B. (1975). Discrimination of fricatives by hearing-impaired children using a vibrotactile cue. *Br. J. Audiol.* **9**, 14-18.

MARKS, L.E. (1987). On cross-modal similarity: Perceiving temporal patterns by hearing, touch, and vision. *Percept. Psychophys.* **42**, 250-256.

NELSON, M. (1959). Electrocutaneous perception of speech sounds. *Arch. Otolaryngol.* **69**, 445-448.

OWENS, E. and BLAZEK, B. (1985). Visemes observed by hearing-impaired and normal-hearing adult viewers. *J. Speech Hear. Res.* **28**, 381-393.

PETROSINO, L., FUCCI, D., HARRIS, D. and RANDOLPH-TYLER, E. (1988). Lingual vibrotactile/auditory magnitude estimation and cross-modal matching: Comparison of suprathreshold responses in men and women. *Percept. Mot. Skills* **67**, 291-300.

PLANT, G. (1989). A comparison of five commercially available tactile aids. *Aust. J. Audiol.* **11**, 11-19.

PLANT, G., MACRAE, J. and DILLON, H. (1984). Lipreading with minimal auditory cues. *Aust. J. Audiol.* **6**, 65-72.

PROCTOR, A. and GOLDSTEIN, M.H. (1983). Development of lexical comprehension in a profoundly deaf child using a wearable, vibrotactile communication aid. *Lang. Speech Hear. Serv. Schools* **14**, 138-149.

RABINOWITZ, W.M., HOUTSMA, A.J.M., DURLACH, N.I. and DELHORNE, L.A. (1987). Multidimensional tactile displays: Identification of vibratory intensity, frequency, and contactor area. *J. Acoust. Soc. Am.* **82**, 1243-1252.

RICHARDSON, B.L. (1990). Separating signal and noise in vibrotactile devices for the deaf. *Br. J. Audiol.* **24**, 105-109.

RISBERG, A. (1974). The importance of prosodic speech elements for the lipreader. *Scand. Audiol. Suppl.* **4**, 153-164.

ROSEN, S.M., FOURCIN, A.J. and MOORE, B.C.J. (1981). Voice pitch as an aid to lipreading. *Nature (Lond.)* **291**, 150-152.

ROSEN, S.M., WALLIKER, J.R., FOURCIN, A.J. and BALL, V. (1987). A microprocessor-based acoustic hearing aid for the profoundly impaired listener. *J. Rehab. Res. Dev.* **24**, 239-260.

ROSEN, S.M., WALLIKER, J., BRIMACOMBE, J.A. and EDGERTON, B.J. (1989). Prosodic and segmental aspects of speech perception with the House/3M single-channel implant. *J. Speech Hear. Res.* **32**, 93-111.

ROTHENBERG, M. and MOLITOR, R.D. (1979). Encoding voice fundamental frequency into vibrotactile frequency. *J. Acoust. Soc. Am.* **66**, 1029-1038.

ROTHENBERG, M., VERRILLO, R.T., ZAHORIAN, S.A., BRACHMAN, M.L. and BOLANOWSKI, S.J. (1977), Vibrotactile frequency for encoding a speech parameter. *J. Acoust. Soc. Am.* **62**, 1003-1012.

ROUSSEAU, J.J. (1762). Emile. *Oeuvres de Jean Jaques Rousseau*, volume 7. Amsterdam: Neaulme, pp. 237-238. (For an English translation of the relevant passage, see Geldard, F.A. (1966). Cutaneous coding of optical signals: the optohapt. *Percept. Psychophys.* **1**, 377-381.)

SAUNDERS, F. (1985). *Tacticon 1600 Electrocutaneous Vocoder.* Tacticon Corporation, USA.

SCHULTE, K. (1972). Fonator system: Speech stimulation and speech feedback by technically amplified one-channel vibrations. In: Fant, G., ed., *International Symposium on Speech Communication Ability and Profound Deafness*. Washington: A.G. Bell Association, paper no. 36.

SCOTT, B.L. and DE FILIPPO, C.L. (1977). Progress in the development of a tactile aid for the deaf. Paper presented at the 94th meeting of the Acoustical Society of America, Miami Beach, FA, December.

SHERRICK, C.E. (1985). A scale rate for tactual vibration. *J. Acoust. Soc. Am.* **78**, 78-83.

SPENS, K-E. and PLANT, G. (1983). A tactual 'hearing' aid for the deaf. *Speech Trans. Lab. Q. Prog. Stat. Rep. 1*. Stockholm, Royal Institute of Technology, pp. 52-56.

SUMMERS, I.R. (1986). An improved tactile aid for the deaf. *IEE (UK) Conference Publication 258*, pp. 184-188.

SUMMERS, I.R. and FARR, J. (1989a). Coding strategies for a single-channel tactile aid. *Br. J. Audiol.* **23**, 299-304.

SUMMERS, I.R. and FARR, J. (1989b). Development of a single-channel tactile aid for the profoundly deaf. In: Tubach, J.P. and Mariani, J.J., eds, *Proceedings of Eurospeech '89, Paris*. **2**. Edinburgh: CEP Consultants Ltd, pp. 706-709.

SUMMERS, I.R. and MARTIN, M.C. (1980). A tactile sound level monitor for the profoundly deaf. *Br. J. Audiol.* **14**, 30-33.

SUMMERS, I.R., PEAKE, M.A. and MARTIN, M.C. (1981). Field trials of a tactile acoustic monitor for the profoundly deaf. *Br. J. Audiol.* **15**, 195-199.

TECK ENN LOI and PLANT, G. (1986). A single-transducer vibrotactile aid to lipreading. *Proceedings of the First Asian-Pacific Regional Conference on Deafness*, Hong Kong, pp. 435-446.

TRAUNMULLER, H. (1980). The Sentiphone: A tactual speech communication aid. *J. Comm. Dis.* **13**, 183-193.

UVACEK, B. and MOSCHYTZ, G.S. (1988). Sound alerting aids for the profoundly deaf. *Proceedings of the IEEE International Symposium on Circuits and Systems*, ISCAS-88. New York: IEEE.

VAN TASELL, D.J., SOLI, S.D., KIRBY, V.M. and WIDIN, G.P. (1987). Speech waveform envelope cues for consonant recognition. *J. Acoust. Soc. Am.* **82**, 1152-1161.

WEISENBERGER, J.M. (1986). Sensitivity to amplitude-modulated vibrotactile signals. *J. Acoust. Soc. Am.* **80**, 1701-1715.

WEISENBERGER, J.M. (1989). Evaluation of the Siemens Minifonator vibrotactile aid. *J. Speech Hear. Res.* **32**, 24-32.

WEISENBERGER, J.M. and MILLER, J.D. (1987). The role of tactile aids in providing information about acoustic stimuli. *J. Acoust. Soc. Am.* **82**, 906-916.

WEISENBERGER, J.M. and RUSSELL, A.F. (1989). Comparison of two single-channel vibrotactile aids for the hearing-impaired. *J. Speech Hear. Res.* **32**, 83-92.

WEISENBERGER, J.M., HEIDBREDER, A.F. and MILLER, J.D. (1987). Development and preliminary evaluation of an earmold sound-to-tactile aid for the hearing-impaired. *J. Rehab. Res. Dev.* **24**, 51-66.

YEUNG, E., BOOTHROYD, A. and REDMOND, C. (1988). A wearable multichannel tactile display of voice fundamental frequency. *Ear Hear.* **9**, 342-350.

Chapter 6
Signal Processing Strategies for Multichannel Systems

JAMES L. MASON and BARRIE J. FROST

In his pioneering studies, Gault (1924) made the first systematic attempts to use the tactile sense as a substitute channel for presenting acoustic information to the skin. Although his first experiments simply involved having artificially deafened subjects learn to discriminate words by placing their palms against the end of a long tube down which words were transmitted, he later used electronically amplified sounds presented to the skin through vibrators. After extensive learning, Gault's subjects were able to discriminate vowel sounds, individual words from a moderately sized set, and sentences from a fixed set. However, the limitations of the skin to resolve frequency information above about 300 Hz impeded further progress, and ultimately gave rise to multichannel devices (which Gault himself pioneered), which were specifically designed to circumvent the bandwidth limitations of the skin.

Before examining the signal processing strategies that have been employed by a number of groups working in this field a caution is in order. The design and evaluation of any sensory substitution device involves an incredibly complex array of variables, all of which may contribute substantively to the final performance of the device. Sometimes features of the signal processor will contribute most to variance in the final performance, in other instances the interfacing with the human receiver will impose considerable constraints, in yet others the characteristics of the receivers themselves will predominate. Because these devices all involve a new form of perceptual learning, the training and evaluation procedure may critically determine performance. Consequently, the author's group is of the opinion that many fine devices have been developed that might have produced substantially better performances if they had been fine tuned on the basis of performance data, and, most importantly, if subjects had been more extensively trained and tested with more complex and discriminable real-world stimuli (Kirman, 1974; Richardson and Frost, 1977). In the acquisition of speech through a normally functioning auditory system, a very considerable amount of time is involved, and performance proceeds from the discrimination of a few holistic Gestalt patterns first, to a gradually expanding universe of 'objects' where finer and more analytic discriminations are possible later. We do not insist that children first learn to discriminate all of the 40 or more basic phonemes of their native tongue before combinations in syllables are presented, which in turn must be mastered before words are introduced. Yet evaluation of the utility of many devices has often involved no more than a few hours' experience, and the tests have often required immediate, fine, analytical discriminations of the sort usually demanded only of well-practised observers. Readers should keep this caveat in mind, because ultimate performance attainable with any tactile vocoder system will depend on these factors and their complex interactions, and the development of realistic, reasonable, and standardised sets of training and evaluation procedures.

Over the past two decades there have been many excellent reviews and comparative evaluations of the various forms of tactile vocoder, and it is not the intention to repeat that material here (Kirman, 1973; Reed, Durlach and Braida, 1982; Sherrick, 1984; Pickett and McFarland, 1985). Rather the different general principles that have been incorporated into the various vocoders that have been built and tested will first be outlined, and on the basis of this analysis they will be divided into a number of classes, and then the various strategies that have been used to implement their operating characteristics will be compared.

Multichannel Devices

One of the fundamental ways in which tactile hearing devices differ is in the degree to which the acoustic signal is processed before it is presented to the skin. Many scientists and engineers chose to present the acoustic signal to the skin in as 'direct' or 'raw' a form as possible because they believe that the invariant features of speech will eventually be learned and automatically extracted by the central somatosensory system. This view has received support in recent years because of the clearly demonstrated plasticity, even into adulthood, of the somatosensory system (Merzenich et al., 1983a,b, 1984; Roe et al., 1990). These studies suggest that although the somatosensory cortex may not initially possess feature extractors to handle some of the basic dynamic patterns in the manner required for skilled recognition of the speech stream presented through the skin, they may well build the appropriate units with repeated experience of the

---

*The multichannel devices described in this chapter are, for the most part, based on a vocoder-type design (Dudley, 1939) in which the distribution of output signal across the different channels corresponds to the distribution of energy with frequency in the speech input (or to some frequency-related parameter).

invariant patterns specifying the phonemic structure. Others believe that tactile perception of speech may be facilitated by feature extraction, i.e. by preprocessing the acoustic signal to recognise some features of the speech pattern electronically. This predigested information can then be presented to the skin in a condensed form. The basic rationale behind this approach is that it ensures that information critical for any generic speech recognition device is presented to the receiver, and in the process may reduce the redundancy in the information flow through the somatosensory system.

Direct devices

Perhaps the most direct system is the single-channel device that transduces the acoustic information directly into vibrotactile information presented to one locus on the skin. Chapter 5 deals specifically with these devices so they will not be discussed further in this chapter.

Given the multidimensional nature of the acoustic signal and the multidimensional nature of normal auditory perception, it was an obvious and simple step to realise that multichannel arrays of some form might be required to provide sufficiently rich and systematic information via the somatosensory system for speech to be processed in the central nervous system. Although some speech theorists argue that there are unique processors of speech in the human brain, it is also clear through the acquisition of skills such as reading that this information can be accessed through sensory systems other than the auditory system. Considering the acoustic signal itself, the frequency, intensity and time domains need to be translated into an equivalent three-space involving the skin before 'hearing through touch' is feasible. There are several ways in which this could be accomplished and some of these have been incorporated into tactile vocoders: Table 6.1 shows some of these possibilities. In this section some prototype devices that have used certain of these configurations will be identified.

Since the major problem with early single-channel devices centred around the wearer's inability to discriminate frequency information provided in the transduced acoustic signal, the obvious solution was to provide a 'frequency-to-place' transform on the skin, similar to the place principle that operates along the basilar membrane (Moore, 1982). Gault, after realising the inherent limitations of the skin to extract frequency information developed the 'Teletactor', the first multichannel vocoder system (Gault and Crane, 1928). This system bandpass filtered the speech signal into five channels and then presented the information to the fingers of one hand through five independently activated vibrators. The five bands were: below 250 Hz, 250–500 Hz, 500–1000 Hz, 1000–2000 Hz and above 2000 Hz, and were systematically arranged with the low-frequency infor-

Table 6.1 Direct devices

Type	Name	Pre-empha-sis	Chan-nels	Input frequency range	Post-proces-sing	Display Type	Display Location
Frequency to place	Englemann and Rosov	No	24	85 Hz–10 kHz	No	Linear, vibrotactile	Thighs
	Saunders	Yes	20	190 Hz–6.2 kHz	No	Linear, electro-cutaneous	Abdomen
	Queen's	Yes	16	160 Hz–8 kHz	Logarithmic compression	Linear, vibrotactile	Forearm
Frequency + ampli-tude to place	Goldstein	Yes	18	250 Hz–7.7 kHz	No	Optacon	Fingertip
	Sparks	No	36	85 Hz–10.5 kHz	Logarithmic processing	36 × 8 Array, electro-cutaneous	Abdomen
	Snyder	Yes	24	100 Hz–5 kHz	Logarithmic processing	Optacon	Fingertip
Time-swept	Clements	Yes	24	100 Hz–5 kHz	Logarithmic compression	Optacon	Fingertip
	Ifukube	Yes	16	200 Hz–4.4 kHz	Lateral inhibition	16 × 3 Array, vibrotactile	Fingertip
Duplex frequency to place	Guilke	No	160	410 Hz–2.9 kHz	No	Linear, vibrotactile	Fingers

mation sent to the thumb and information from successively higher filters to the remaining digits in order so that the high-frequency output went to the little finger. Although this device appeared to be a substantial improvement on single-channel systems, subjects still apparently had difficulty in discriminating phonemes with higher frequency information, because there was no attempt to match the output signal to the frequency range in which the skin is sensitive.

Subsequently, a number of similar devices have been built that all employ essentially the same processing strategy – that is, a 'frequency-to-place' tactile system, with time and intensity directly coded. The next prototype built using this basic principle was the 'Felix', developed at MIT by Wiener and Wiesner from 1949-51 (see Kirman, 1973), which was originally constructed as a five-channel vocoder, but was later expanded to a seven-channel device. Different filter characteristics from Gault's Teletactor were chosen: 0-400, 400-800, 800-1400, 1400-2400 and 2400-15000 Hz in the original five-channel 'Felix', and 0-200, 200-400, 400-670, 670-1000, 1000-1400, 1400-2400 and 2400-15000 Hz in the modified version. Perhaps the most important development introduced in the Felix was a clear attempt to match the output of the vibrators to the skin sensitivity by using a carrier frequency of 300 Hz. It is now known that this frequency is close to the optimum for stimulating the pacinian corpuscles, and therefore this innovation overcame one of the basic problems of the Teletactor, which lost a lot of high-frequency information through preserving frequency in the output signal to the skin. Wiener and Wiesner also experimented with electrical stimulation of the skin in place of vibrotactile stimulation. One of the puzzling things about this enterprise is the reason it was abandoned, since it seems to have most of the important features of the more recently developed 'frequency-to-place' vocoder systems that have been demonstrated to work reasonably well. It is worth noting here that Wiener and Wiesner were primarily concerned with whether the device carried enough information to uniquely specify all the phonemes in English and, as Richardson and Frost (1977) have pointed out, such an analytical task presented at the outset of complex perceptual learning may have overtaxed the system. What results might have been obtained had more extensive training been given on material that was initially more discriminable?

Other 'frequency-to-place' tactile systems that have been developed include the 160-channel device built by Guelke and Huyssen (1959), which also used tuned reed oscillators to stimulate the fingers, thereby providing a 'duplex frequency to (frequency and) place' coding system; a 10-channel device built in Sweden by Rösler (1957) and evaluated by Lövgren and Nykvist (1959) and Pickett and Pickett (1963); a 23-channel vocoder built and evaluated by Engelmann and Rosov (1975); a 20-channel electrotactile vocoder constructed and evaluated by Saunders et al. (1980); and a 16-channel device built by the authors' group and evaluated by P.L. Scilley (1980, unpublished data), Mason, Scilley and Frost (1981), Brooks and Frost (1983, 1986), Brooks et al. (1985, 1986a,b, 1987), and Weisenberger and Miller (1987).

Given that the skin is a two-dimensional surface, it is possible to represent one of the acoustic dimensions along the second skin dimension. This processing strategy has been employed in some tactile vocoder systems, where a 'frequency-to-place' transform is represented along one skin dimension, and intensity (or rather energy or amplitude within frequency bands) on the other. This class of vocoder device is shown as 'frequency and amplitude to place' in Table 6.1. The vocoders developed and tested by Yeni-Komshian and Goldstein (1977), Mook (D. 1978, unpublished thesis), Sparks et al. (1978) and Snyder et al. (1982) have all used this strategy, with a 'bar-graph' type of display (where additional stimulators in the intensity dimension were turned on as energy in that band increased).

Some vocoder developers have used the second spatial dimension of the skin to present time-sequence information, and have left intensity within a frequency band coded as intensity of vibration: this type of system is shown as 'time-swept' in Table 6.1. For example, Ifukubea and Yoshimoto (1974) used a 16 × 3 array of piezoelectric reeds to present either identical information on the three rows of tactile stimulators or a time-swept sequence where each row was updated every 15 ms. The time-swept display resulted in modest improvements over the standard spectral display. Clements, Braida and Durlach (1982) investigated two two-dimensional tactile vocoder systems: one a time-swept display, the other a 'frequency + amplitude to place' display, both using an Optacon piezoelectric array. Both displays produce very similar results in discrimination tests of synthetic and natural vowels.

Feature-extracting devices

In contrast to the direct tactile vocoders, where the emphasis has been on providing as much of the information in the 'raw' acoustic signal to the skin as possible, other devices have attempted to process the acoustic information and to extract certain features that the designers consider critical for the recognition of speech phonemes etc. This partially digested information is then presented to the skin. Table 6.2 provides information on several vocoders of this type (called 'feature-extracting systems' here to distinguish them from the more direct acoustic-to-tactile vocoders presented in Table 6.1).

Kirman (1973) developed a system similar in some ways to the time-swept system described above, but instead of presenting a simple frequency × time display he extracted the first and second formants and presented them to the skin in one column of vibrators in the 15 × 15 tactile array. Each 10 ms the formant information was updated and displaced over one column so that eventually a 150 ms time window of the formant information was displayed. This vocoder is described in Table 6.2.

Table 6.2 Feature-extracting devices

Name	Features	Display Type	Location	Presentation
Kirman (1974)	F0, F1	15 × 15 Array, vibrotactile	Fingers	Time swept
Blamey and Clark (1985)	F0, F2 amplitude	8 Electrodes, electrocutaneous	Fingers	(see text)
Upton (1968)	Voiced, fricatives, stops	Visual	Eyeglasses	On/off
Ifukube (1982)	Voiced, nasals semivowels, fricatives, stops, unvoiced	2 × 3 Array, vibrotactile	Fingertip	On/off
Boothroyd (1988)	F0	Linear, 8/16 transducers, vibrotactile	Forearm	Log F0 frequency to place

A rather novel device called the Tickle-Talker has been described by Blamey and Clark (1985, 1987) and evaluated by Cowan et al. (1988) (Table 6.2). It uses electrical stimulation of the digital nerve bundles of one hand (on either side of each finger) to produce eight channels of information. The speech processor, essentially similar to that employed in their multiple-channel cochlear implant system (Blamey et al., 1987), extracts estimates of the frequency of the second formant, the fundamental frequency and the amplitude of the speech envelope, which are coded respectively as electrode position, pulse rate and pulse width.

Although never implemented in a tactile form, the Upton wearable eyeglass speechreading aid (Upton, 1968) illustrates a feature-extraction system that could quite readily have presented output to the skin rather than to the visual system (Table 6.2). The processing unit automatically recognised five classes of speech sound, which were displayed by reflection as individual lights appearing on the lens of a pair of spectacles. This was intended as a device to aid lipreading and consequently the display was positioned so that it would normally be superimposed on the image of the speaker's face. This system is mentioned here only to convey the idea that feature extraction of this sort could as readily be presented to the somatosensory system as to the visual system.

Finally, a device developed to aid intonation reception and production is included in Table 6.2 as an example of single-feature extraction – in this case extraction of voice fundamental frequency F0. Vocoders of this type are designed for a very specific and limited purpose and contrast with those that attempt to provide most of the information necessary for more complete recognition of speech and environmental sounds. This device was one of the first examples of a wearable multichannel tactile system.

Signal Processing Schemes

Direct devices

'Frequency-to-place' devices

This type of tactile vocoder has been the most studied and evaluated class of multichannel device. The signal processing for all vocoders of this type can be described by the 'generic' block diagram shown in Figure 6.1. There are many possible combinations of elements which can be chosen for each of the blocks. In this chapter, discussion will focus on the signal-processing strategies in each of the blocks on some of the more recent and successful examples. A summary of the most important parameters for representative devices is given in Table 6.1.

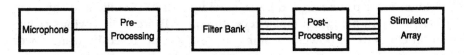

Figure 6.1 'Generic' frequency-to-place vocoder.

Preprocessing

In general, the preprocessing block contains a variable-gain amplifier and a bandpass filter to limit the signal to the frequencies of interest, typically in the range 100 Hz–10 kHz. Several vocoders include a pre-emphasis filter which increases the average gain of the system at higher frequencies. The use of pre-emphasis is based upon the results of Flanagan (1965) who found that the long-term power density for continuous English decreased with increasing frequency above 500 Hz at a rate of 8.67 dB per octave. It was argued that this might make the perception of the higher-frequency components of speech difficult because of their reduced amplitude. Snyder et al. (1982) used pre-emphasis at 6 dB per octave applied from 500 Hz to 5 kHz. Gibson studied the performance of a well-trained subject in a tactile-alone word recognition task using several different pre-emphasis parameters and found that pre-emphasis of 6 dB per octave starting at 1 kHz improved performance over no pre-emphasis, but that pre-emphasis starting at 3 kHz provided the best performance of all conditions tested (Gibson, D.M., 1983, unpublished thesis). He attributed this result to an interaction between the pre-emphasis filter in the preprocessing block and logarithmic compression filters on each channel which were included in the post-processing block. With pre-emphasis starting at 1 kHz, sufficient gain was added to the upper channels that they were close to saturation, making discrimination of the various fricatives difficult

The dynamic range of sounds encountered in life (110 dB) is much greater than the typical dynamic range of the tactile vocoder (20 dB). Several authors have therefore suggested that an automatic gain control be incorporated into the preprocessing block in order to make best use of the limited vocoder dynamic range, but no results of its effects of performance have yet been reported.

Filter bank

The filter bank is what many consider the 'heart' of the vocoder. It separates the speech signal into frequency bands and, in effect, allows a signal to be generated which is proportional to the amount of speech energy in each band at any time. Many parameters of the filter bank can be varied in any vocoder implementation, and include: the number of filters, filter bandwidth, filter spacing, filter sharpness. Several different combinations have been assessed.

The number of filters used has ranged up to 160 (Guelke and Huyssen, 1959), with 16 being a popular recent choice. There is an obvious reduction in complexity, power consumption and size achieved by using fewer filters, but this is achieved at the expense of frequency resolution.

The most common choice for filter bandwidth is one-third of an octave because it closely matches the measured critical bands of the normal auditory system over most of the frequency spectrum of interest. Some authors have increased the bandwidth of the lower-frequency channels to two-thirds of an octave to model the wider critical bands in the ear at frequencies below 400 Hz. Sixth-order filters have been used to achieve the desired sharpness. Other filter arrangements that have been tried include: constant-bandwidth filters (Guelke and Huyssen, 1959), filters with different high- and low-frequency slopes (Sparks et al., 1978, 1979), and filters whose bandwidths and centre frequencies have been chosen to optimize machine speech recognition (Swab, L.W., 1989, unpublished thesis).

To test this latter filter arrangement and compare it with the usual one-third octave filter bank, a monolithic audio spectrum analyser integrated circuit containing 16 second-order Butterworth filters with centre frequencies of 390–8895 Hz was incorporated into a version of the Queen's University Tactile Vocoder. The filter outputs were processed through a half-wave rectifier and second-order low-pass filter. The filter centre frequencies were more concentrated in the region 750–3500 Hz, these filters having Q of 6–7. Higher-frequency filters were wider, with a Q of around 3.

Subjects were able to achieve comparable word learning rates with either filter arrangement, implying that filter spacing and filter sharpness may not be as significant in determining the performance of this type of vocoder as has previously been assumed.

Post-processing

After the filter bank stage, typically the signal in each channel is detected using either half-wave or full-wave rectification and averaged using a low-pass filter. The time constant chosen for the filter affects the temporal characteristics of the vocoder; the choice determines how quickly a channel can respond to a change in the magnitude of a particular spectral component, for example, too low a value of cut-off frequency would result in a slow response and remove some information about rapidly changing speech features such as plosives. The effect on performance of using different time constants does not appear to have been studied in detail.

The Queen's Tactile Vocoder also includes a logarithmic compression filter on each channel in the post-processing stage. This filter was intended to compensate for the fact that the spectral components of the speech waveform have a dynamic range of 40–50 dB whereas that of the tactile display is limited to about 20 dB. Gibson (D.M., 1983, unpublished thesis) compared the performance of a well-trained subject using a vocoder with and without compression and found that compression significantly improved word recognition performance. This improvement was attributed to the fact that, with compression, spectral components with a dynamic range of 54 dB could be displayed on the stimulator array, but with simple linear amplification only 16.3 dB was available between the detection threshold and saturation of the electronics.

Others who also have compressed the filter output include Snyder et al. (1982) and Clements et al. (1982), although neither compared performance with and without compression.

Stimulator array
The design of vibrotactile transducers has been discussed in detail in Chapter 3 and will not be addressed further here.

A variety of different types of stimulator array (electrocutaneous, miniature solenoid, piezoelectric reed) have been used in multichannel devices, as have a number of body locations (see Table 6.1). There do not appear to have been any detailed studies of the effects of changing stimulator type or location on subject's performance. For multichannel devices the issues of transducer size, weight, efficiency, convenience and appearance become more important than they are for single-channel devices, and these considerations are likely to dictate the choice of stimulator array for a device intended to be used outside the laboratory.

'Frequency + amplitude to place' devices

The most extensively studied example of this class of device was reported on by Sparks et al. (1978, 1979) and was called MESA (Multipoint Electrotactile Speech Aid). The speech signal was first filtered into 36 channels by a so-called cochlear filter, designed to be an electronic realization of a theoretical model representing the hydromechanical filtering function of the cochlea. The frequency for maximum power transfer of the filters was 86 Hz–10.9 kHz. The filters had a high-frequency slope of 66 dB per octave and a low-frequency slope of 12 dB per octave. Each filter output was full-wave rectified and averaged in a fashion designed to preserve the delay-line characteristics of the cochlear filter. Each channel output was quantized into one of eight amplitude steps with each step representing an amplitude change of 5 dB (in other words, the output of the filters was logarithmically processed). The information was displayed on an electrotactile belt worn on the abdomen. The rectangular display had a total of 288 electrodes – 36 columns representing frequency and eight rows representing the amplitude of the signal in each frequency band.

The device was tested in vowel recognition, consonant recognition and speech-tracking tasks: vowels were recognized easily with little training; consonant recognition was more problematic and speech-tracking rates after 20 h training were unchanged by the additional tactile information provided by MESA. (Initially, aided speech-tracking was better than lipreading alone.)

Similar attempts to assess this type of device have been reported by Snyder et al. (1978) and Yeni-Komshian and Goldstein (1977): the latter used 18 channels and 6 discrete levels of amplitude and displayed the information on a rectangular array of vibrotactile stimulators in contact with the subject's fingertip (Optacon display).

No significant advantage to using the second spatial dimension to encode amplitude has yet been found.

Time-swept devices

These devices differ from 'frequency-to-place' devices primarily in the way in which spectral information is displayed on the skin: they can be identical until the final processing stage and the stimulator array.

A time-swept device displays not only the present spectral distribution of energy on a column of stimulators but also a fixed number of prior samples of the distribution on parallel columns in a rectangular array. Each time a speech signal is sampled, it is entered into the leading column of the array and all previous samples are shifted to the next column.

Clements, Braida and Durlach (1982) evaluated one such device. The signal was filtered into 18 channels between 100 Hz and 5 kHz. The channel envelopes were detected, logarithmically compressed and sampled every 16 ms. A 24 × 6 array of piezoelectric vibrators was used as the output device (Optacon display) – some channels were represented on multiple rows of the display.

In their experiments Clements, Braida and Durlach compared the time-swept display with the same device used in a 'frequency + amplitude to place' mode using vowels as stimuli. They found that the time-swept display was slightly better than the other display, but considered the overall results to be rather unimpressive.

Ifukube (1982) also tested a time-swept device for the transmission of Japanese vowels and consonants: it had 16 channels, covering 200 Hz to 4.4 kHz, displayed on a 16 × 3 vibrotactile array. It also had a unique post-processing scheme which included lateral inhibition between neighbouring channels in the filter bank in order to sharpen the display of formants at high signal levels. Unfortunately, the effect of this inhibition on performance was not independently assessed.

Duplex frequency-to-place devices

An early attempt at constructing a multichannel tactile vocoder was that of Guelke and Huyssen (1959). This was essentially a 'frequency-to-place' device in which speech frequency was coded as place and also sub-coded as frequency of stimulation. There were a number of interesting aspects to this device:

- The incoming signal was band-limited to the range 410–2880 Hz and then separated into 160 channels, each 15 Hz wide, by means of a combination of electrical and mechanical filters. No mention was made of pre-emphasis.
- Electrical bandpass filters divided the initial signal into eight 300-Hz-wide frequency bands. Each of these bands was mixed with a local oscillator whose frequency was chosen so that the output would be in the range of 100–400 Hz.
- The output from each channel was fed to a mechanical device which had 20 resonant reeds with resonant frequencies at 15 Hz intervals between 100 and 400 Hz. The reeds not only provided high resolution filtering but were also used as the tactile stimulators.
- The eight stimulators (each with 20 resonators) were applied to the five digits of one hand: one to the thumb and little finger and two to each of the other fingers. Therefore, if a slowly increasing tone were presented to the device, the subject would feel the stimulation gradually move up the thumb, increasing in frequency as it did, jump to the bottom of the left side of the index finger and to a low stimulation frequency, gradually move up the finger increasing in frequency, and so on. The frequency of the signal is thus encoded twice, first in the position and finger on which the stimulation occurs and second in the frequency of vibration of the stimulator.

The tests with the device using deaf and temporarily deafened normal subjects showed that it was relatively easy to recognize vowels with very little training; consonants, however, were not well recognized.

Feature-extracting devices

Kirman

Kirman, in 1973, reported on a computer-driven device which displayed previously calculated estimates of fundamental frequency F0 and first-formant frequency F1 on a 'Times Square' type of vibrotactile display (i.e. a time-swept two-dimensional array). He used a 15 × 15 array of stimulators spaced 0.2 in apart.

Recorded samples of a variety of speakers saying 15 common English words (containing no plosives, fricatives or nasals) were processed by computer to estimate the F0 and F1 frequencies at 10 ms intervals. These estimates were then replayed through the stimulator array. Frequency (100–4500 Hz) was represented vertically on the array in 200-Hz-wide bands up to 2500 Hz and wider bands for the last three channels. Every 10 ms all rows were shifted to the right and a new sample was entered on the left column of the display. Thus, the array displayed 150 ms information at any instant: the present formant position and 140 ms of history.

After about 30 h of training, subjects achieved an accuracy of 90% in identifying the 15 words. However, significant persistent confusions remained and the authors concluded that the level of performance was probably too low for the device to be considered as a comprehensive tactile display of all speech sounds.

Blamey and Clark (Tickle-Talker)

The Tickle-Talker is an interesting device, reported on by Blamey and Clark (1987), which was the result of using a signal processing strategy very similar to that used in a successful cochlear implant, but presenting the output to an electrotactile array on the fingers.

The signal processor extracted fundamental frequency F0 (by counting the zero crossings of a low-pass-filtered signal), second-formant frequency F2 (by counting the zero crossings of an 800 Hz to 4 kHz bandpass-filtered signal) and amplitude (from a peak detector). The display consisted of nine electrodes: one common wrist-mounted electrode and eight active electrodes located in rings worn on the fingers of one hand. The F0 parameter controlled the pulse repetition frequency of a biphasic electrical stimulus at one of the active electrodes and controlled what was perceived by the user as the 'roughness' of the stimulation. The F2 parameter was used to select which of the electrodes would be active: the place of stimulation. The choice was made by using a look-up table that had seven preselected frequency boundaries distributed between 900 and 3300 Hz. The peak-detector output was used to control the pulse width of the stimulation, which was perceived as strength of stimulation.

The Tickle-Talker, intended as an aid to lipreading, was evaluated using a speech-tracking task as well as consonant and vowel identification tasks with normal and hearing-impaired subjects. In all situations, significant improvements in performance were noted when the aid was used. In the speech-tracking experiments, average tracking rates were about 50% higher for both sets of subjects when the aid supplemented lipreading, compared with lipreading alone. No measures of the tracking rates of the normal subjects using hearing were reported.

Upton/Ifukube

A number of researchers have attempted to extract electronically from the speech signal those features which are considered to be particularly significant. For each feature extracted, a discrete present/absent signal is presented to the user either tactually or visually. These devices were intended as an aid to lipreading (Upton, 1968) or as an adjunct to a feature-to-place tactile vocoder (Ifukube, 1982).

The features extracted corresponded to voiced sounds, voiced fricatives, unvoiced fricatives, voiced stops and unvoiced stops (in Upton's device) and voiced sounds, nasals, semivowels, fricatives, stops and unvoiced sounds in Ifukube's device). Unfortunately, few details of how these features were extracted are given in the literature and neither of these devices appears to have been evaluated to any extent.

Boothroyd

Boothroyd's wearable device (Boothroyd, 1985) was designed to extract voice fundamental frequency F0 and display it on an 8-channel linear vibrotactile display. The channel number of the active stimulator was logarithmically related to the value of F0. The array, worn on the forearm, was intended as an intonation monitor and as an aid to lipreading. Promising test results were reported from a pilot investigation.

Hanin et al. (1988) have evaluated a 16-channel version of this device with quite encouraging results, although a recent study (Kishon-Rabin et al., 1990) has indicated that transmission of pitch information may be less than satisfactory.

Future Developments

With the widespread availability of very large scale integration (VLSI) implementation schemes, miniaturization to 'Walkman' size units should be possible. For example, the group at Queen's University, Ontario, have made prototypes of the Queen's Tactile Vocoder using custom-integrated circuits. The reduction in size of vocoders and the widespread use of 'Walkman' stereo systems and 'Watchman' televisions also means that the potential stigma associated with wearing this form of electronic apparel has now virtually disappeared.

Alternatively, and perhaps more appropriately for the development of an evolving and versatile vocoder system, would be an implementation using digital signal processing (DSP) chips. Already Engebretson and O'Connell (1986) and the group at Queen's have implemented the Queen's Tactile Vocoder using a Texas Instruments DSP. The obvious advantage of this approach is that it still results in a miniature vocoder, but changes in characteristics can be effected in software as quickly as the appropriate code can be changed. In addition, as the processing speed and power of DSP chips increase (as they inevitably will), more and more of the signal-processing functions can be incorporated into the software and the size and power consumption of the device reduced. This approach could be used to implement most of the different classes of vocoder discussed in this chapter, including both direct and feature-extracting systems.

In terms of direct-coding vocoders it is suggested that, at the preprocessing stage, automatic gain control should always be a switchable option. It is also suggested that 12–16 channels are probably optimal and that pre-emphasis of 3 dB per octave applied from 3 kHz upwards, when combined with logarithmic compression, seems to be the most efficacious (Gibson, D.M., 1983, unpublished thesis; Brooks et al., 1986a,b).

The precise characteristics of the filters used in the filter bank (type, bandwidth, sharpness, etc.) do not appear to be too critical to the vocoder performance. It is important that they cover a large enough range of frequencies (100 Hz–10 kHz) to represent speech sounds adequately and to allow discrimination between them. The extent of training, with realistic tasks, is more critical than filter parameters in determining performance with direct vocoders. Their ultimate usefulness will become evident once individuals, using convenient wearable devices, have had enough experience in using them in their daily lives to demonstrate what discriminations are ultimately possible.

As far as post-processing for direct vocoders is concerned, there is no clear advantage in moving to a two-dimensional array from a unidimensional array. It does not appear that using place on the second tactile dimension for the coding of either intensity or time is particularly helpful. Consequently, for direct-coding vocoders it is probably best at this stage to leave amplitude coded as amplitude of vibration (or amplitude of electrotactile stimulation), and time as time, since the processing capacity of the skin has been shown to be sufficient for extracting substantial information in real-time tests of tracking connected speech (Brooks et al., 1986b; Weisenberger and Miller, 1987).

It is beyond the scope of this chapter to deal extensively with output transducers, but units similar to those developed by Franklin (Audiological Engineering Corporation, Somerville, MA.) are probably the best available. They operate in a relatively non-resonant mode and therefore can be driven efficiently over a range of frequencies.

There have been over the years a few studies employing vibrational frequencies that have been directly transposed and compressed down from the acoustic signal into a much lower frequency range that the skin can handle. For example, the slowed-speech studies of Newman (as reported in Kirman, 1973) and the investigation of the duplex 'frequency-to-place' system of Guelke and Huyssen (1959) both suggest that some frequency information might be extracted directly through the skin. It might be a worthwhile venture to incorporate a duplex coding system into a 'frequency-to-place' vocoder system so that acoustic frequency is also represented by vibrational frequency; for example, if a linear array of vibrotactile units is employed, the end of the array receiving the low-frequency information could be driven at 50 Hz, with the drive frequency systematically increasing across vibrators representing higher filter channels. Of course, drive frequencies above 550–600 Hz should not be used because of the sharp drop-off in the skin's transfer function (Geldard, 1953; Guelke and Huyssen, 1959).

As far as feature-extracting vocoders are concerned, it seems unwise to make suggestions at this time because great strides are currently being made in computer technology and automatic speech recognition. Small, versatile devices will probably be available before too long, which will provide direct speech-to-text translations, and tactile codes of various types may eventually be derived from these devices. Whether researchers in this field attempt to tap into such systems at an early feature-extraction level, phonemic level, syllabic or word level will depend on the individual views about what the somatosensory system is ultimately capable of learning. However, there will undoubtedly be interesting and exciting developments in the future.

References

BLAMEY, P.J. and CLARK, G.M. (1985). A wearable multiple-electrode electrotactile speech processor for the profoundly deaf. *J. Acoust. Soc. Am.* **77**, 1619–1620.

BLAMEY, P.J. and CLARK, G.M. (1987). Psychophysical studies relevant to the design of a digital electrotactile speech processor. *J. Acoust. Soc. Am.* **82**, 116–125.

BLAMEY, P.J., SELIGMAN, P.M., DOWELL, R.C. and CLARK, G.M. (1987). Acoustic parameters measured by a formant-estimating speech processor for a multiple-channel cochlear implant. *J. Acoust. Soc. Am.* **82**, 38–47.

BOOTHROYD, A. (1985). A wearable tactile intonation display for the deaf. *IEEE Trans. Acoust. Speech Signal Proc.* **33**, 111–117.

BROOKS, P.L. and FROST, B.J. (1983). Evaluation of a tactile vocoder for word recognition. *J. Acoust. Soc. Am.* **74**, 34–39.

BROOKS, P.L. and FROST, B.J. (1986). The development and evaluation of a tactile vocoder for the profoundly deaf. *Can. J. Pub. Health.* **77**, 108–113.

BROOKS, P.L., FROST, B.J., MASON, J.L. and CHUNG, K. (1985). Acquisition of a 250-word vocabulary through a tactile vocoder. *J. Acoust. Soc. Am.* **77**, 1576–1579.

BROOKS, P.L., FROST, B.J., MASON, J.L. and GIBSON, D.M. (1986a). Continuing evaluation of the Queen's University Tactile Vocoder, I: Identification of open set words. *J. Rehab. Res. Dev.* **23**, 119–128.

BROOKS, P.L., FROST, B.J., MASON, J.L. and GIBSON, D.M. (1986b). Continuing evaluation of the Queen's University Tactile Vocoder. II: Identification of open set sentences and tracking narrative. *J. Rehab. Res. Dev.* **23**, 129–138.

BROOKS, P.L., FROST, B.J., MASON, J.L. and GIBSON, D.M. (1987). Word and feature identification by profoundly deaf teenagers using the Queen's University tactile vocoder. *J. Speech Hear. Res.* **30**, 137-141.

CLEMENTS, M.A., BRAIDA, L.D. and DURLACH, N.I. (1982). Tactile communication of speech: II. Comparison of two spectral displays in a vowel discrimination task. *J. Acoust. Soc. Am.* **74**, 1131-1135.

COWAN, R.S.C., ALCANTARA, J.I., WHITFORD, L.A., BLAMEY, P.J. and CLARK, G.M. (1988). Speech perception studies using a multichannel electrotactile speech processor, residual hearing, and lip reading. *J. Acoust. Soc. Am.* **85**, 2593-2607.

DUDLEY, H.W. (1939). The Vocoder. *Bell Lab. Rec.* **18**, 122-126.

ENGEBRETSON, A.M. and O'CONNELL, M.P. (1986). Implementation of a microprocessor-based tactile hearing prosthesis. *IEEE Trans. Biomed. Eng.* **33**, 712-716.

ENGELMANN, S. and ROSOV, R. (1975). Tactual learning experiment with deaf and hearing subjects. *Except. Child.* **41**, 243-253.

FLANAGAN, J.L. (1965). *Speech Analysis, Synthesis and Perception*. New York: Academic Press, pp. 137-139.

GAULT, R.H. (1924). Progress in experiments on tactile interpretation of oral speech. *J. Ab. Soc. Psych.* **19**, 155-159.

GAULT, R.H. and CRANE, G.W. (1928). Tactual patterns from certain vowel qualities instrumentally communicated from a speaker to a speaker's fingers. *J. Gen. Psych.* **1**, 353-359.

GELDARD, F.A. (1953). *The Human Senses*. New York: John Wiley.

GUELKE, R.W. and HUYSSEN, R.M.J. (1959). Development of apparatus for the analysis of sound by the sense of touch. *J. Acoust. Soc. Am.* **31**, 799-809.

HANIN, H., BOOTHROYD, A. and HNATH-CHISHOLM, T. (1988). Tactile presentation of voice fundamental frequency as an aid to the speechreading of sentences. *Ear Hear.* **9**, 335-341.

IFUKUBE, T. and YOSHIMOTO, C. (1974). A sono-tactile deaf-aid made of piezoelectric vibrator array. *J. Acoust. Soc. Jpn* **30**(8), 461-462.

IFUKUBE, T. (1982). A cued tactual vocoder. In: Raviu, J. (ed.), *Uses of Computers in Aiding the Disabled*. Amsterdam: North-Holland, pp. 197-215.

KIRMAN, J.H. (1973). Tactile communication of speech: A review and an analysis. *Psych. Bull.* **80**, 54-74.

KIRMAN, J.H. (1974). Tactile perception of computer-derived formant patterns from voiced speech. *J. Acoust. Soc. Am.* **55**, 163-169.

KISHON-RABIN, L., HANIN, L. and BOOTHROYD, A. (1990). *Lipreading enhancement by a spatial tactile display of fundamental frequency*. Paper presented at the International Conference on Tactile Aids, Hearing Aids and Cochlear Implants, Sydney.

LÖVGREN, A. and NYKVIST, O. (1959). Speech transmission and speech training for the deaf child by visual and tactual means using special devices. (Swedish) *Nord. Tidskr. Dövunderv.*, 122-143.

MASON, J.L., SCILLEY, P.L. and FROST, B.J. (1981). A vibrotactile auditory prosthetic device. *IEEE Conf. Digest*, 104-106.

MERZENICH, M.M., KAAS, J.H., WALL, J., NELSON, R.J., SUR, M. and FELLEMAN, D. (1983a). Topographic reorganization of somatosensory cortical areas 3B and 1 in adult monkeys following restricted deafferentation. *Neuroscience* **8**, 33-35.

MERZENICH, M.M., KAAS, J.H., WALL, J.T., SUR, M., NELSON, R.J. and FELLEMAN, D.J. (1983b). Progression of change following median nerve section in the cortical representation of the hand in areas 3B and 1 in adult owl and squirrel monkeys. *Neuroscience* **10**, 639-665.

MERZENICH, M.M., NELSON, R.J., STRYKER, M.P., CYANDER, M.S., SCHOPPMAN, A. and ZOOK, J.M. (1984). Somatosensory cortical map changes following digit amputation in adult monkeys. *J. Comp. Neurol.* **224**, 591-605.

MOORE, B.C.J. (1982). *An Introduction to the Psychology of Hearing*, 2nd edn. London: Academic Press.

PICKETT, J.M. and MCFARLAND, (1985). Auditory implants and tactile aids for the profoundly deaf. *J. Speech Hear. Res.* **28**, 134-150.

PICKETT, J.M. and PICKETT, P.H. (1963). Communication of speech sounds by a tactual vocoder. *J. Speech Hear. Res.* **6**, 207-222.

REED, C.M., DURLACH, N.I. and BRAIDA, L.D. (1982). Research on tactile communication of speech: A review. *Am. Speech Hear. Mon.* **20**.

RICHARDSON, B.L. and FROST, B.J. (1977). Sensory substitution and the design of an artificial ear. *J. Psychol.* **96**, 259-285.

ROE, A.W., PALLAS, S.L., HAHM, J.-O. and SUR, M. (1990). A map of visual space induced in primary auditory cortex. *Science* **250**, 818-820.

RÖSLER, G. (1957). Über die vibrationsemfindung Literaturdurchsicht und Untersuchungen in Tronfrenquenzbereich. *Zeitschr. Exp. Ang. Psych.* **4**, 549-602.

SAUNDERS, F.A., HILL, W.A. and SIMPSON, C.A. (1980). Speech perception via the tactile mode: Progress report. In: Levitt, H., Pickett, J.M. and Houde, R. (eds), *Sensory Aids for the Hearing Impaired*. New York: IEEE Press, pp. 278-281.

SHERRICK, C.E. (1984). Basic and applied research on tactile aids for deaf people: Progress and prospects. *J. Acoust. Soc. Am.* **75**, 1325-1341.

SNYDER, J.C., CLEMENTS, M.A., REED, C.M., DURLACH, N.I. and BRAIDA, C.D. (1982). Tactile communication of speech: I. Comparison of Tadoma and a frequency-amplitude spectral display in a consonant discrimination task. *J. Acoust. Soc. Am.* **71**, 1249-1254.

SPARKS, D.W., ARDELL, L.A., BOURGEOIS, M.R., WIEDMER, B. and KUHL, P.K. (1979). Investigating the MESA (Multipoint Electrotactile Speech Aid): the transmission of connected discourse. *J. Acoust. Soc. Am.* **65**, 810-815.

SPARKS, D.W., KUHL, P.K., EDMONDS, A.E. and GRAY, G.P. (1978). Investigating the MESA (Multipoint Electrotactile Speech Aid): The transmission of segmented features of speech. *J. Acoust. Soc. Am.* **63**, 246-257.

UPTON, H.W. (1968). Wearable eyeglass speechreading aid. *Am. Ann. Deaf.* **113**, 222-229.

WEISENBERGER, J.M. and MILLER, J.D. (1987). The role of tactile aids in providing information about acoustic stimuli. *J. Acoust. Soc. Am.* **82**, 906-916.

WIENER, N. and WEISNER, J. (1949-1951). Felix (Sensory replacement project). *Quarterly Progress Report, RLE*. Cambridge, MA: Massachusetts Institute of Technology.

YENI-KOMSHIAN, G.H. and GOLDSTEIN, M.H. (1977). Identification of speech sounds displayed on a vibrotactile vocoder. *J. Acoust. Soc. Am.* **62**, 194-198.

Chapter 7
The Selection and Training of Tactile Aid Users

GEOFF PLANT

Interest in the use of tactile aids with profoundly deaf children and adults dates from the pioneering work of Robert Gault in the 1920s (Gault, 1926, 1930). The first tactile aids used in the education of hearing-impaired children were desk-top units which were restricted to classroom activities. Goodfellow (1934) described the use of Gault's 'Teletactor' in improving the speech perception and production skills of hearing-impaired children. He concluded that the aid

> helps the child to build a concept of sound, and of certain phonetic elements in speech, such as the length of a vowel; it enables him to grasp the pattern and flow of spoken language and consequently to put more rhythm into his own speech; and it makes it possible for him to compare his speech with that of his teacher and thus to recognise his own particular difficulties.

Despite such success, the development of wearable hearing aids following World War II saw a rapid decline in the use of tactile aids. The major contributing factor to this decline was the widely held belief that there were very few cases of total deafness (Dale, 1962). Proponents of this view cited the fact that almost all profoundly hearing-impaired persons had audiometric thresholds at 250 and 500 Hz, albeit at very high intensities. By the beginning of the 1970s, however, many researchers (Boothroyd and Cawkwell, 1970; Nober, 1970; Ericson and Risberg, 1977) were beginning to question this belief. As a result of their investigations they concluded that many profoundly deaf persons do not have true hearing, but perceive amplified sound via tactile receptors in their ears. The information available via hearing aids for such persons is very limited and, as Risberg (1978) argues, they would be better served by a specifically designed tactile aid.

At about the same time Kirman (1974) published a critical review of tactile research, which concluded that 'neither the results of past work on tactile displays, nor contemporary theories of speech perception, nor psychophysical studies of tactile perception have provided reasonable grounds for believing that the skin lacks the capacity to comprehend a suitable display of speech'. Kirman believed that the major factor contributing to the relatively poor performance obtained with tactile aids up to that time was the use of coding strategies which were not appropriate to the tactual sense.

This view has been supported by studies of experienced deaf-blind users of Tadoma conducted by researchers at the Massachusetts Institute of Technology (Norton et al., 1977; Reed et al., 1982, 1985). Tadoma may be regarded as a manual form of lipreading 'in which the listener receives speech information by placing his hand on the talker's face and monitoring the articulation process' (Durlach et al., 1982). Results reported for nine experienced deaf-blind users of Tadoma by Reed et al. (1985) showed a mean consonant recognition score of 60.3% and scores for W-22 word lists of 26–56%. When testing was carried out using Kalikow, Stevens and Elliott's (1977) SPIN Test the scores for the low predictability sentences were very similar to those obtained with the W-22 words. The scores obtained with the high predictability items were 26–85%. Connected Discourse Tracking (De Filippo and Scott, 1978) rates of 30–40 words per minute were also found during in-depth testing of three of the experimental subjects. Reed believed that the results of their testing provided an 'existence proof for communication of speech through the tactile sense' (Reed et al., 1985).

The awareness that there were people with total or near-total hearing losses, Kirman's (1974) review and the seminal research by the Massachusetts Institute of Technology Tadoma group have all been key factors in the renaissance of tactile aid research. This has led to the widespread availability of tactile aids for profoundly hearing-impaired children and adults. Before the 1980s the only tactile aids available were either desk-top units such as the Siemen's Fonator (Schulte, 1972) or high-powered hearing aids driving bone conductors which were usually held in the hand (Boothroyd, 1972; Plant, 1979, 1982).

This situation changed greatly in the 1980s when a range of wearable, commercial tactile aids became available for the first time. These ranged from simple vibrotactile aids such as the Minivib (Spens and Plant, 1983) and the TAM (Summers, Peake and Martin, 1981), which present time and intensity variations via a single vibrator, to complex multi-channel electrotactile displays such as the Tacticon (Saunders and Franklin, 1982). Comparative studies of available commercial aids (Weisenberger and Miller, 1987; Plant, 1989a; Weisenberger, 1989; Weisenberger and Russell, 1989) have shown that all can provide useful speech information to the profoundly hearing impaired.

Selection of an aid to be fitted to individual hearing-impaired persons may be determined by a number of factors. Different therapists may desire different signal characteristics which will determine, in part, the aid selected. For example, one therapist may wish to use an aid which presents an accurate representation of the syllabic structure of speech, whilst another may wish to give detailed information about segmental structure. Cost is another factor which may preclude the selection of some aids. The size of the aid, the site of stimulation and the aid's overall cosmetic appeal may also be important selection criteria. The type of stimulation may also determine the selection or rejection of a particular aid: for example, some teachers and therapists feel uncomfortable about the use of electrotactile aids with young children and as a result may prefer the use of a vibrotactile aid even when the performance of an electro-tactile aid is demonstrably superior. Finally, the choice of tactile aid may be influenced to a large extent by the communication needs of the person to be fitted. The aid selected for use with a congenitally deaf child may not be suitable for use with an adventitiously deaf adult.

Following the fitting of a tactile aid it is critical that a training programme immediately commence. Training should ensure that the tactile aid user derives optimal benefit from the aid. The tactile training programmes for congenitally hearing-impaired children will necessarily differ from those provided for adults with an acquired hearing loss. Programmes for congenitally hearing-impaired children should concentrate on improving oral communication skills and emphasise both speech perception and production exercises. The major component with adven-titiously hearing-impaired adults should be the development of speech perception skills. Some parts of the program should concentrate on the use of the aid to maintain or improve monitoring of established speech patterns, but the emphasis and type of training will be very different from that provided to profoundly hearing-impaired children.

Selection of Potential Tactile Aid Users

There appear to be two distinct opinions concerning the selection of tactile aid users. One viewpoint is that tactile aids should be fitted only to those profoundly hearing-impaired persons who derive little or no benefit from conventional hearing aids. This has been the policy of the National Acoustic Laboratories (NAL) in Australia, which has restricted the fitting of tactile aids to those clients who appear to gain very limited benefit from hearing aid usage.

Other workers in the field feel that the use of tactile aids should not be so restricted. This is especially true of programmes dealing with profoundly hearing-impaired children. The University of Miami's Mailman Center, for example, fits tactile aids to all children enrolled in their programme (Oller et al., 1986). Proponents of this view argue that the information provided by tactile aids supplements that available via hearing aids, resulting in improved speech perception skills (Alcantara et al., 1990a).

Both points of view have obvious merit, and the use of tactile aids in conjunction with hearing aids and cochlear implants warrants further extensive study. Pending the findings of such studies, however, it is critical that the fitting of a tactile aid be considered for those who derive little or no benefit from hearing aid usage.

The number of profoundly hearing-impaired people who fall into this category is unknown. Lind (1973, cited in Risberg, 1973), for example, in a study of profoundly hearing-impaired Swedish adolescents found that 40% reported receiving little or no benefit from hearing aid usage. This figure rose to 60% for those students who had pure tone averages (at 0.5, 1 and 2 kHz) greater than 105 dB ISO. A smaller, but still substantial number, has been found among profoundly hearing-impaired children in Australia. NAL's policy requires that a tactile aid request be sent in and approved before the fitting of a tactile aid to any NAL client. An examination of these requests revealed that in the period 1986–1990 a total of 223 children under the age of 16 years in New South Wales, Victoria and Queensland were recommended for tactile aid fitting. This represents 18.8% of all profoundly hearing-impaired children (pure tone average greater than 90 dB ISO) in these three states.

In order to select those who would be best served by the fitting of a tactile aid, a series of 'at risk' criteria needs to be established. These should include audiometric data, aided thresholds with hearing aids, speech test results, aided and unaided lipreading comparisons and subjective reports of benefit from the patient and significant others (such as a child's parents and teachers, an adult's spouse, family members or friends). The selection criteria outlined below are those used by NAL in Australia to determine those who would be best fitted with a tactile aid. It should be noted that when tactile aids are fitted by NAL the continued use of hearing aids is actively encouraged. The tactile aid is seen as a supplement to hearing aid usage, not as a substitute. This is especially true with children. It is felt that the use of the tactile aid may alert the child to the acoustic environment and thus improve his or her use of the information provided by hearing aids. Some adults reject the dual use of hearing aids and tactile aids, feeling that the hearing aid provides no benefit.

Audiometric data

A number of researchers (Boothroyd and Cawkwell, 1970; Nober, 1970; Ericson and Risberg, 1977) have attempted to specify those audiometric thresholds which may result from vibratory rather than auditory stimulation. Nober (1970) attempted to obtain air conduction thresholds after he had eliminated 'the participation of the cutaneous-tactile receptors with a local subcutaneous anesthetic block'. He found that five children who had thresholds greater than 65 dB at 125 Hz, 80 dB at 250 Hz and 100 dB at

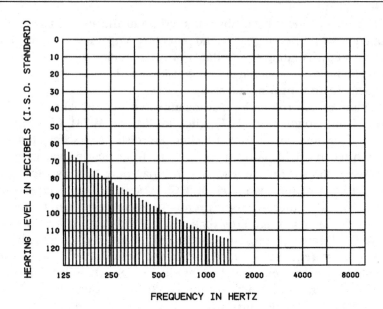

Figure 7.1 Range of hearing level (as a function of frequency) for which tactile detection of acoustic stimuli presented via TDH 39 headphones was reported by Ericson and Risberg, 1977).

500 Hz gave no response to audiometric testing following the anaesthetic block. He concluded that the responses given before the anaesthetic block were attributable to tactile rather than auditory stimulation.

Boothroyd and Cawkwell (1970) tested subjects with profound unilateral hearing losses and asked each to indicate whether they could hear or feel the sound in their impaired ear. As these subjects had normal hearing in one ear, it was felt that they would be able to differentiate between auditory and tactile sensations. The tactile thresholds obtained in this study were 95 dB at 250 Hz, 115 dB at 500 Hz and 120 dB at 750 Hz. On the basis of these findings Boothroyd and Cawkwell concluded that thresholds of 100 dB at 1 and 2 kHz probably indicated the presence of true residual hearing. A later study by Ericson and Risberg (1977), however, indicates that Boothroyd and Cawkwell's (1970) conclusion may have been overly optimistic. Ericson and Risberg's subjects were a group of profoundly hearing-impaired adolescents who were able to give reliable thresholds for hearing, vibration and discomfort. Audiometric testing was carried out with these subjects using TDH 39 headphones with MX41/AR cushions. The subjects were asked to respond when they first felt the sound, first heard the sound and experienced discomfort. The vibratory thresholds obtained are presented in Table 7.1. These tactile thresholds agree closely with those reported by Nober (1970), but are 10-15 dB better than those found by Boothroyd and Cawkwell (1970). Ericson and Risberg's data also differ from

Table 7.1 Vibrotactile thresholds*

	Test frequency (kHz)					
	0.125	0.25	0.5	1	1.5	2
Number of ears	53	51	40	17	3	—
Mean (dB ISO)	65.3	84.5	99.4	111.2	113	—
Standard deviation (dB ISO)	10.4	9.2	7.3	7.7	—	—

*From Ericson and Risberg (1977).

Table 7.2 Audiometric test results for 149 children recommended for tactile aids by NAL audiologists*

	Test frequency (kHz)				
	0.25	0.5	1	2	4
Number of responses	104	86	40	12	3
Mean (dB ISO)	95.1	108.4	113.2	111.2	95.0
Range (dB ISO)	75–110	90–120	95–120	80-120	70–110

*The thresholds given are for the individual child's better ear.

those of Boothroyd and Cawkwell in that a number of subjects reported tactile thresholds at 1 kHz. There were, however, only three tactile responses at 1.5 kHz. They concluded that 'if a detection threshold during pure tone audiometry can be obtained for any frequency above 1,500 Hz, it is very likely that this is a sign of the existence of residual hearing' (Ericson and Risberg, 1977). Potential candidates for tactile aids should have pure-tone thresholds which are equal to or worse than the tactile thresholds determined by Ericson and Risberg (1977). These thresholds are presented in Figure 7.1. It is extremely unlikely that a candidate for a tactile aid would have audiometric thresholds at or above 2 kHz. As Ericson and Risberg note, 'the vibratory sensitivity of the skin falls off very rapidly over 500 Hz. It is, therefore, very difficult to stimulate vibratory receptors in the skin above 1,000 Hz' (Ericson and Risberg, 1977). They also noted that several of their subjects reported tactile sensations before auditory thresholds were obtained. Audiologists should take this into account when testing potential candidates for tactile aids. Attempts should be made wherever possible with such subjects to determine whether they are able to detect any qualitative difference in the stimulus tone which may indicate the presence of true hearing.

A preliminary analysis of requests for tactile aids made by NAL audiologists for 149 children under the age of 16 years supports the use of these audiological criteria. The results of their analysis (Table 7.2) show that for most of the children audiometric thresholds are confined to 0.25, 0.5 and 1 kHz. Only 12 of the children had audiometric thresholds at 2 kHz. Three children had audiometric thresholds at 4 kHz; these children were multiply handicapped and gave no response to amplified sound. Fitting of tactile aids was recommended for these children in the hope that the signal from the tactile aids would alert them to their acoustic environment and thus lead to improved hearing aid usage.

Aided thresholds

Some caution needs to be exercised in using only audiometric test results as the criterion for fitting of a tactile aid. For example, Plant, Galt and Symonds (1986) reported on a subject with an average hearing loss (at 0.5, 1 and 2 kHz) greater than 120 dB ISO who gained great benefit from the use of a high-powered (HAICMPO–147 dB SPL) hearing aid. Aided threshold testing of this subject revealed thresholds of 60 dB SPL at 0.25 kHz, 55 dB SPL at 0.5 and 1 kHz and 50 dB SPL at 2 kHz. The information available to this subject from his hearing aid enabled limited perception of open-set words and sentences via audition alone. When the hearing aid supplemented lipreading the subject's performance was significantly better than that obtained via lipreading alone – for example lipreading alone, using sentence lists from the SPIN Test (Kalikow, Stevens and Elliott, 1977), yielded a score of only 11% correct. When the subject's hearing aid supplemented the lipreading his score rose to 67%. This subject's performance highlights the need to consider aided threshold tests in determining the suitability of tactile aids for individual hearing-impaired people.

There are many profoundly deaf people who appear to derive little or no benefit from conventional hearing aids. Both Erber (1979) and Risberg (1978) have conjectured that some profoundly hearing-impaired persons receive the amplified sound from hearing aids via tactile receptors in their ears. Unfortunately, there have been no studies reported which have specified those aided thresholds which may be attributable to tactile stimulation.

The requests for tactile aids made by NAL audiologists also contained aided threshold test results for the 149 children. These data have been analysed and the results are presented in Table 7.3. The results indicate that for an overall speech level of 70 dB L_{eq} (the typical level experienced by children in classrooms) the mean aided thresholds equalled or

Table 7.3 Aided thresholds for 149 children recommended for tactile aids by NAL audiologists

	Test frequency (kHz)				
	0.25	0.5	1	2	4
Number of responses	91	69	44	14	3
Mean (dB SPL)	72.75	70.4	63.5	65.0	55.0
Range (dB SPL)	50–105	45–110	45–85	50–80	50–60

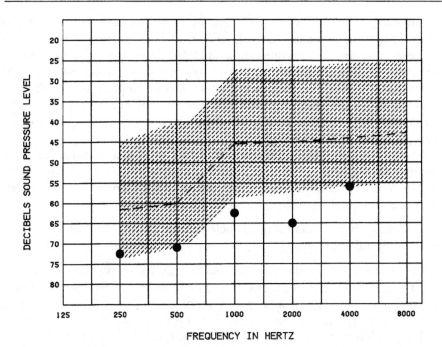

Figure 7.2 The mean aided thresholds in dB SPL (●) for 149 children recommended for vibrotactile aids by NAL audiologists. The shading shows the area covered by the short-term average one-third octave spectrum for Australian English at an overall speech level of 70 dB L_{eq}. The dashed line shows the long-term average one-third octave spectrum.

exceeded the maximum one-third octave speech levels (Figure 7.2). These are the short-term r.m.s. levels exceeded only 1% of the time in each one-third octave band and are 12 dB above the L_{eq} level of each band. That is, for speech input levels typically received in classrooms, hearing aids would provide little or no speech cues for these children.

Based on these data it is recommended that profoundly hearing-impaired persons with aided thresholds greater than 70 dB SPL at 0.25 kHz, 65 dB SPL at 0.5 kHz, 60 dB SPL at 1 kHz and 55 dB SPL at 2 kHz should be considered as potential candidates for tactile aids.

Speech test results

In determining suitability for a tactile aid, speech testing using the patient's hearing aid should be carried out whenever possible. NAL audiologists working with children and adults use the PLOTT Test (Plant, 1984) to evaluate the auditory speech perception skills of potential tactile aid users. This test gives an overview of the client's ability to detect speech sounds using a hearing aid and to discriminate between selected suprasegmental and segmental speech features.

Subtest 1 of the PLOTT Test evaluates the ability to detect the long and short vowels of Australian English, the nasal consonants and voiced and voiceless fricatives. Clients recommended for tactile aids typically are able to detect the vowels and voiced consonants but not the voiceless fricatives.

Subtest 2 is based on Erber's (1980) Auditory Numbers Test (ANT) and requires the client to discriminate between the number strings 1, 12, 123, 1234 and 12345. Most profoundly hearing-impaired clients are able to complete this task successfully.

Subtest 3 of the PLOTT Test is a closed-set word-identification test contrasting monosyllabic, spondaic, trochaic and polysyllabic words. Three words from each of the syllabic categories are presented in the subtest, which is designed to evaluate the client's ability to

1. categorise words according to their syllable number and type
2. identify individual words within the syllable categories.

Clients recommended for tactile aid fittings are usually unable to perform the identification task, but can sometimes categorise the test words by their syllabic type. Those who cannot categorise words by syllable number and type are obvious candidates for tactile aid fitting.

The task presented in Subtest 4 of the PLOTT Test contrasts 12 monosyllabic words. Although it may be possible to correctly identify some of the test words based on the duration and/or intensity of their vowel nucleii, this subtest is byond the capabilities of most potential tactile aid users.

The remaining five subtests of the PLOTT Test evaluate the person's ability to perceive vowel and consonant contrasts of increasing difficulty. The contrasts presented are vowel duration, vowel identification, consonant voicing, consonant manner of articulation and consonant place of articulation. Some clients are able to discriminate between long and short vowels but usually perform at or near chance level for the higher level tasks.

Other closed-speech-test materials which could be used to evaluate the ability of profoundly hearing-impaired adults to understand speech using their hearing aids include the SILL Test from Commtram (Plant, 1984) and selected subtests of the Minimum Auditory Capabilities (MAC) Battery (Owens et al., 1981). Open-set materials such as monosyllabic or spondaic word lists or simple sentence tests such as the HELEN Test (Plant, Phillips and Tsembis, 1982) are usually excessively difficult for most potential users and consequently should be used with caution. The use of open-set materials may, however, be justified in some cases where closed-set testing has yielded equivocal results.

Aided and unaided lipreading

Aided and unaided lipreading testing should also be attempted whenever possible, to determine whether lipreading performance is enhanced when audition supplements vision. This cannot be predicted by auditory alone speech testing. Consider for example the auditory (14%), visual (11%) and auditory-visual (67%) scores for the SPIN Test sentences (Kalikow, Stevens and Elliott, 1977) obtained by the subject in Plant, Galt and Symonds' (1986) study. The improvement in the auditory-visual condition could not be predicted by the subject's auditory test result. Many people who cannot be tested using open-set speech tests presented via audition alone derive considerable benefit when audition supplements lipreading. The degree of benefit offered should be determined before deciding to fit a tactile aid.

The test materials used by NAL audiologists with adult candidates are the HELEN Test (Plant, Phillips and Tsembis, 1982) and Tonisson's (1976) adaptation of the CID Everyday Sentence Test (Davis and Silverman, 1970). Lists are presented via unaided and aided lipreading to determine whether the client derives significant benefit (at the 0.05 level) in the aided condition. Clients whose aided scores are significantly better than their unaided scores may not be suitable candidates. Other testing materials which may be used with adults to compare aided and unaided performance include the SPIN Sentence Lists (Kalikow, Stevens and Elliott, 1977) and Bench and Bamford's (1979) BKB Sentences which were used for assessing lip reading performance by Rosen and Corcoran (1982).

It is more difficult to assess the aided and unaided lipreading performances of children. The materials recommended for adults may be suitable for older children and adolescents, but at present there are few, if any, suitable materials for assessing younger children: the English language level of most tests make them unsuitable for use with young children. NAL is currently working on the development of tests to evaluate aided and unaided lipreading tests for use with children of 5–10 years old. These include a simple token test (Ballge-Kimber and Plant, 1988) and a sentence test requiring a picture-pointing response.

Subjective reports

In assessing whether a tactile aid is to be fitted it is important to consider the opinion of the potential user and any significant others. With children the significant others can include parents, teachers, speech pathologists etc; an adult's significant other persons include their spouse, family members and/or friends.

Wherever possible the opinion of the potential user on the benefit of any hearing aid(s) they have currently should be elicited. Questions should refer to the information available to the user for communication via listening alone – can speech be understood without lipreading? Do hearing aids present information which enhance lipreading performance? Do the aids enable the user to monitor their own voice? Do the hearing aids enable the user to pick up common environmental sounds and warning signals?

Perceptions about the benefit offered by their hearing aid(s) should be compared with the results obtained in the testing of aided performance both with and without lipreading cues. Any conflict should be discussed in detail.

The client's attitude towards tactile aids should also be gauged: this will necessarily involve allowing the person the opportunity to experience the signal provided by a tactile aid. This demonstration may stimulate many questions regarding the aid's long-term benefits and perceived disadvantages. They may also seek information about alternative strategies such as cochlear implantation or the use of another hearing aid. He or she may ask 'How does the performance of the tactile aid compare with that of a cochlear implant? What are the relative costs of the alternative aids? What is involved in the rehabilitation/habilitation process following the fitting of a tactile aid?' All of these issues should be covered before a decision is finally made.

Before deciding to fit a tactile aid to a child, the opinion of the parents, teacher(s) and others involved in their education should be sought. Do the parents feel that the child derives any significant benefit from the hearing aid? Is there a difference in communication skills aided and unaided? The teacher should have had the opportunity to view the child's aided performance in structured listening situations over an extended period and should be aware of any potential benefit offered by the hearing aid(s).

Summary

The criteria listed above set out a systematic basis for determining which profoundly hearing-impaired people should be fitted with tactile aids. Audiometric results should alert the clinician to 'at risk' cases, but cannot be the sole reason for recommending the fitting of a tactile aid. Aided threshold testing, the results of speech tests presented via audition alone, lipreading performance with and without hearing aids and subjective reports all need to be considered.

Finally, the decision to fit should not be seen as meaning that hearing aid use should be discontinued. Rather, continued wearing of hearing aid(s) in conjunction with the tactile aid should be actively encouraged. This is particularly important with children. The parents and teachers may see the decision to fit a tactile aid as proof of total deafness. This view should be discouraged; as previously mentioned the tactile aid may alert the child to the acoustic environment and lead to improvements in hearing aid performance. There will be cases where it is obviously unrealistic to expect the hearing-impaired person to continue to wear a hearing aid. Examples include adults whose hearing losses result from the removal of bilateral acoustic neuromas, or children born without cochleas. In most cases, however, hearing aid usage should continue and should be encouraged at all times.

Training Programmes for Children

Goodfellow (1934) outlined the tactile training programme adopted at the Illinois State School for the Deaf, which emphasised the use of the Gault Teletactor as an aid to lipreading and as a means of enhancing the teaching of speech. Goodfellow also noted that with training the children grew to appreciate music and poetry via the tactile aid. In many ways this resembles programmes currently provided to children fitted with tactile aids. The areas which appear critical in a training programme for children are:

1. discrimination of tactile patterns including both speech and non-speech signals;
2. the development of visual/tactual speech perception skills;
3. use of the tactile aid to improve speech production skills.

The exact form these exercises take will depend on the capabilities of the tactile aid being used. Alcantara et al. (1990), for example, provide a brief overview of a programme used with children fitted with the 'Tickle-Talker' (Cowan et al., 1988). The areas covered in training – vowel duration, vowel place, initial and final /s/, /m/ versus /b/ and /s/ versus /t/ – are those which are transmitted well by the Tickle-Talker. Similarly, the training programme for the Tactaid II developed by Plant (1988a) was based on testing of adult subjects (Plant, 1988b, 1989a) to determine the sensory information provided by the aid. The capabilities of the children being trained will also determine in part the type of training provided. Franklin (1989), for example, has developed a programme for the use of the Tactaid II with deaf-blind children which is very different from the Tactaid II programme developed for sighted children.

The Tactaid II training program

The following summary of Plant's (1988a) Tactaid II Training Program gives an overview of the necessary components of a tactile training programme. It should be stressed that it is aimed specifically at children using the Tactaid II. The Tactaid II is a two-channel vibrotactile aid which presents intensity-time patterns from two bandpass filters (0.1–1.5 kHz, 1.5–6 kHz) as an amplitude-modulated fixed frequency of 375 Hz. Spatial separation of the output transducers enables discrimination between the 'high' and 'low' channels.

The Tactaid II Training Program provides practice in tactile pattern perception. Exercises are divided into four basic areas. These are:

1. sound detection
2. tactile pattern perception
3. word syllable-number and type
4. high-frequency detection.

Sound detection

Exercises at this level are aimed at giving practice in detecting the presence or absence of sound via the tactile aid alone. Initially, simple exercises are used which require the child to indicate whether she or he can detect the presence of sounds ranging from the human voice to a variety of noise makers such as a drum. These exercises gradually increase in difficulty. More complex exercises at this level include having to determine whether the aid is turned on or off, requiring the child to indicate when a sound ceases, and exploring a range of environmental sound inside and outside the classroom.

Tactile pattern perception

This section provides the child with the opportunity to learn to discriminate between a variety of tactile patterns. Areas covered include discriminating between long and short syllables (/baaaaa/ versus /ba/); continuous and repeated syllables (/baaaaa/ versus /ba,ba,ba/); fast and slow rates of speech; differing syllable numbers (/ba/ versus /ba,ba/ versus /ba,ba,ba/) and various intensity levels (soft/normal/loud). The child is provided with visual cues which enable her or him to respond by pointing at an appropriate picture. It is recommended, however, that the child be encouraged to respond verbally wherever possible. The use of the nonsense syllable /ba/ for many of the exercises was deliberate as it can be produced by most hearing-impaired children.

Word syllable-number and type

This section is an extension of the exercises in level 2. The stimuli in this section are real words which differ in their syllabic structure. The contrasts used are monosyllabic, trochaic, spondaic and trisyllabic words. At first the child is required to discriminate between two words, then three and finally four. The exercises provide an opportunity to build up an awareness of syllabic patterning and to generalise this skill. A picture-pointing response is used, although again the child is encouraged wherever possible to give a verbal response.

High-frequency detection

One of the best features of the Tactaid II is its ability to signal the presence of high-frequency consonants. In practice the high-frequency vibrator is triggered by the consonants /s/, /z/, /t/, /tʃ/, /dʒ/, /ʃ/ and /ʒ/. The exercises in this section are designed to alert the child to the presence of high-frequency consonants and require discrimination between words with and without high-frequency consonants. Again, both picture-pointing and verbal responses are encouraged.

Lipreading instruction

There have been numerous studies (Gault, 1930; De Filippo and Scott, 1978; Erber, 1979; Plant, 1979, 1982, 1988b; Weisenberger and Miller, 1987; Cowan et al., 1988) which have shown that tactile aids lead to significant improvements in lipreading abilities. Children fitted with tactile aids should be provided with exercises which provide the opportunity to practise using their tactile aids as supplements to lipreading. There should be some time set aside in each school day to provide practice in aided lipreading. This is especially critical in Total Communication programs where signing and finger spelling are used in conjunction with speech. The long-term aim of this instruction should be to provide the child with the opportunity to communicate with hearing people both socially and vocationally once they have left school.

A lipreading programme is currently being developed to supplement the Tactaid II Training Program. This programme is based around a popular Swedish character 'Bamse, the world's strongest bear', developed by Rune Andersson. The exercises initially contrast single words, with the child responding by pointing to the appropriate picture. Teachers are encouraged, however, to expand complexity and the response expected. For example, the teacher may give the child a limited number of coloured pens and ask her or him to colour in the picture or part of it. Further extensions may require the child to circle an object or draw another object. The complexity gradually increases, with the response set expanding to three words and then to increasingly complex sentence patterns.

A series of short books based on the characters have been written to supplement the programme. These have been designed to enhance the interest level and also to provide the opportunity to use story telling and context-based questions. Sets of cards based on the characters are available and these can be used in lipreading activities based on popular games such as 'Memory', 'Fish' and 'Donkey'. These cards can also be used in referential communication activities such as the 'Barrier Game'. (The Barrier Game is used to develop referential communication skills. A listener and a speaker have a common set of pictures or objects. The speaker places his/her set in a specific order and then attempts to transmit this information to the listener. The listener's task is to place his/her set in the same order as the speaker's. The level of difficulty of the technique can be adapted to meet the communication competence of the listener.)

The teacher need not confine lipreading practice to these activities. Teachers need to be encouraged to provide informal lipreading experiences throughout the school day. Discussions of class topics, news, etc. can be used to provide valuable context-based lipreading practice.

Speech production training

In the mid 18th century the great French teacher Jacobo Rodriguez Periera used 'the sense of touch for noting the vibrations of the voice' (Bender, 1960) with many of his pupils. Teachers of profoundly hearing-impaired children often still use this method in speech teaching. The child is encouraged to place a hand on the teacher's face or throat as a means of perceiving 'invisible' speech features such as voicing and nasality. Much information is available via this method. Plant and Spens (1986), in a study of a subject who had used this method as a supplement to lipreading for over 40 years, found that he was able to perceive with a very high degree of accuracy features such as voicing, the stop/continuant and the oral/nasal contrasts.

In early speech training with tactile aid users it is often useful to use direct contact with the teacher's face and/or throat in conjunction with the tactile aid. The information available from the two sources is complementary and may help reduce the task complexity for the child. Further, some children may find it difficult at first to isolate the source of the signal provided by the tactile aid and may not associate it with speech production. The child should be encouraged to place one hand *lightly* on the teacher's throat with the other placed on their own throat. It is important to ensure that minimal pressure is applied to the throat to avoid the tense voice quality which usually accompanies increased pressure.

Teachers should be encouraged to use tactile aids as a means of enhancing speech acquisition. For many profoundly hearing-impaired children the tactile aid will offer the first opportunity to monitor their own speech. The success of the speech teaching programme described by Oller et al. (1986) highlights the potential of tactile aids in developing intelligible speech. Initially the teacher may need assistance to help determine what information is available via the particular aid being used. It may also be necessary to point out that some information is available by the tactile aid alone while other cues require a combination of tactile and visual inputs.

The Tactaid II can again be used as an example. With this aid the teacher can be confident that the child will be able to detect the presence/absence of voicing: it can thus be a very useful aid in the development of spontaneous voicing. Suprasegmental features such as word and syllable duration, syllable number and type, and syllable rate are all available through the aid; pitch variations, however, are not perceptible. Vowel duration cues are also available and, to a limited degree, so are the intensity variations which accompany vowel height. The acoustic cues to front and back vowels (vowel second formant frequency) are, unfortunately, not provided by the Tactaid II. Limited consonant voicing information is available to the Tactaid II user via the tactile aid alone. This information is greatly enhanced when vision supplements the signal. Many articulation contrasts are provided by the Tactaid II: the stop/continuant, oral/nasal, fricative/stop and sibilant/non-sibilant fricative contrasts are all available via the tactile sense alone. It should be pointed out to the teacher that identification of these contrasts is greatly enhanced in the tactile-visual condition. The acoustic cues to consonant place of articulation are not well signalled by the Tactaid II, or by any other tactile aids so far developed.

This information should help the teacher to plan the order of speech sound acquisition and the mode of presentation to be used. Systematic speech training programmes such as those set out by Calvert and Silverman (1975), Ling (1976) and Siebert (1980) can be greatly enhanced by the use of a tactile aid. Skills learned in other parts of tactile training can also be transferred to assist in speech teaching.

Summary

The essential components of a successful tactile training programme for children must be regarded as interconnected and not as separate entities. The opportunity to have flow-through of learned skills from one area to another is critical. The aim of the teacher should be to use the tactile aid as part of an overall programme to enhance communication skills.

Training Programmes for Adults

Training programmes provided for adults with acquired losses differ considerably from those provided for children. Although the effects of acquired profound hearing loss do include changes in speech production (Leder and Spitzer, 1990; Waldstein, 1990), the major concern for most adventitiously profoundly hearing impaired is their loss of receptive communication skills. As a result the major component of training programmes for adults with acquired losses must be exercises aimed at enhancing receptive communication skills. The exercises should aim to optimise receptive communication skills via taction alone and combined visual-tactile training. Where necessary, the tactile aid user should be alerted to the aid's potential for monitoring of speech production.

Tactile-alone training

Tactile-alone training should highlight the specific suprasegmental and segmental information provided by the tactile aid. Commtram (Plant, 1984) is an example of a programme which provides a wide range of tactile-alone training exercises. These exercises are presented using a closed-set format, that is, the client needs to have a list of the possible responses. This form of training is usually termed *analytic*. Exercises at the suprasegmental level include contrasts of words which differ in their syllable number and stress pattern. For example, the subject may be asked to differentiate between monosyllabic, spondaic and trochaic words such as car, carport and carpet. Other exercises at the suprasegmental level include recognition of sentence patterns in closed sets ranging from two to ten alternatives, contrastive stress patterns, speaker sex and speaker emotion.

The segmental activities in Commtram include both vowel and consonant contrasts. The exercises are graded in order of difficulty and screening tests are provided to pinpoint areas of difficulty. Vowel contrasts covered include vowel duration, vowel height and vowel place. The consonant training exercises concentrate on those contrasts which create difficulty via lipreading alone and include consonant voicing and manner of articulation contrasts. The materials in Commtram all use meaningful words as the training stimuli. The use of nonsense syllables can, however, provide useful practice; for example, a set of consonants may be contrasted in an /aCa/ frame or English vowels presented in a /hVd/ frame.

Another area of tactile-alone training which should be covered is the identification of environmental sounds. Ramsdell (1947) reported on the reactions of American soldiers deafened during war service. He observed that the loss of auditory contact with the environment was a significant factor for many deafened subjects. Commtram provides a series of exercises aimed at providing practice in identifying common environmental sounds. Training is provided via a series of tapes and home exercises involving a family member or friend. Home exercises include the use of a checklist of environmental sounds and assignments detailing noises in the kitchen and the car.

Visual–tactile training

Exercises aimed at improving the tactile aid user's ability to understand face-to-face communication should involve both analytic and synthetic materials. The use of the terms analytic and synthetic dates from lipreading methodologies devised in the early years of this century. *Analytic* exercises concentrate on developing 'bottom-up' skills. The subject is trained using materials which concentrate on developing the ability to discriminate between minimal units such as phonemes or syllables. Exercises contrasting the vowels of English in a /hVd/ frame are an example of the analytic approach. *Synthetic* exercises aim at developing 'top-down' skills through the use of more meaningful materials. Conversational training is an obvious example of the synthetic approach. Analytic materials can include practice using closed sets of consonants and vowels in nonsense syllables, lists of contrasting words, or sentences. These exercises provide invaluable practice in the integration of tactile and visual inputs.

Synthetic exercises which more closely replicate everyday communication are a very important part of visual–tactile training. The hearing-impaired person needs the opportunity to practise the use of visual–tactile integration with connected discourse materials if the tactile aid is to be used successfully in everyday life. Therapists should attempt to provide a variety of synthetic exercises in training sessions. One of the most popular techniques used at this level is De Filippo and Scott's (1978) connected discourse tracking (CDT). In this procedure the therapist reads from a prepared text section-by-section, with the subject repeating exactly what was said. If the response is correct the therapist presents the next section for identification. If an error is made the therapist repeats the section until a correct response is made. This may require the use of repair strategies such as re-wording, or other cues enabling correct word identification. At the completion of a set time period, usually 10 min, the number of words correctly repeated is calculated and divided by the time elapsed to give a words per minute score. This is an extremely useful technique, but it may be excessively difficult for some tactile aid users. A simplified form of CDT has been developed by Plant (1989b): this does not require the client to give a word-perfect response and also provides the written form of the text so that she or he can verify what was presented in each section.

Other techniques which can assist in the development of improved face-to-face communication skills include the use of structured conversations. The subject may be provided with a series of questions around a single theme, their task being to comprehend the therapist's spoken answers. The complexity of response can be modified to suit the communication skills of the individual. Responses can gradually be increased in complexity as proficiency increases. Referential communication tasks such as the 'Barrier Game' can also be used, again providing the therapist with the opportunity to tailor the degree of complexity to meet individual communication competencies.

Summary

Tactile training for adults with acquired hearing losses should concentrate on the development of receptive communication skills. This involves training in both tactile-alone and visual-tactile speech perception. The programme should involve practice with both analytic and synthetic materials. Alcantara et al. (1990b) have shown that subjects unfamiliar with tactile displays derive most benefit when they receive both analytic and synthetic training. The difficulty for the therapist is in finding the right balance between the two approaches. To a large extent, however, this will be determined by the needs, strengths and weaknesses of the individual receiving training.

Training in the recognition of environmental sounds should also be an important component. This can involve the participation of family members and friends through the use of home-based training exercises.

Conclusions

The two aspects covered in this chapter are critical components in ensuring the success of tactile aid fittings. The use of systematic and comprehensive selection criteria pinpoints those individuals who gain limited or no assistance from hearing aids and who would potentially benefit from tactile aid usage. Future research may show that these criteria need to be revised to include a greater number of profoundly hearing-impaired people.

Following the fitting of a tactile aid it is very important that appropriate training be provided. There are general principles which should be followed in almost all cases. The training should involve both synthetic and analytic exercises and provide practice in both tactile-alone and visual-tactile integration. The exact form of the training will differ according to the type of aid used, the age of the tactile-aid user and his or her existing communication skills and needs.

The past decade has seen great advances in the availability of tactile aids. A number of exciting changes have occurred which should have long-term benefits for many profoundly hearing-impaired children and adults. The use of systematic selection procedures and the provision of appropriate training will help consolidate these advances and help ensure that individuals benefit optimally from tactile aid usage.

References

ALCANTARA, J.I., WHITFORD, L.A., BLAMEY, P.J., COWAN, R.S.C. and CLARK, G.M. (1990a). Speech feature recognition by profoundly hearing-impaired children using a multiple-channel electrotactile speech processor and aided residual hearing. *J. Acoust. Soc. Am.* **88**, 1260-1273.

ALCANTARA, J.L., COWAN, R.S.C., BLAMEY, P.J. and CLARK, G.M. (1990b). A comparison of two training strategies for speech recognition with an electrotactile speech processor. *J. Speech Hear. Res.* **33**, 195-204.

BALLGE-KIMBER, P. and PLANT, G. (1988). A lipreading test for profoundly hearing-impaired children. Paper presented at the Speech Science and Technology Conference, Macquarie University, Sydney, November 1988.

BENCH, J. and BAMFORD, J. (1979). *Speech Hearing Tests and the Spoken Language of Hearing-Impaired Children*. London: Academic Press.

BENDER, R. (1960). *The Conquest of Deafness*. Cleveland: Western Reserve University Press.

BOOTHROYD, A. (1972). Sensory Aids Research Project – Clarke School for the Deaf. In: Fant, G. (ed.), *International Symposium on Speech Communication Ability and Profound Deafness*. Washington: A.G. Bell Society, pp. 367-377.

BOOTHROYD, A. and CAWKWELL, S. (1970). Vibrotactile thresholds in pure tone audiometry. *Acta Otolaryngol.* **69**, 381-387.

CALVERT, D.R. and SILVERMAN, S.R. (1975). *Speech and Deafness*. Washington: A.G. Bell Association.

COWAN, R.S.C., ALCANTARA, J.I., BLAMEY, P.J. and CLARK, G.M. (1988). Preliminary evaluation of a multichannel electrotactile speech processor. *J. Acoust. Soc. Am.* **83**, 2328-2338.

DALE, D.M.C. (1962). *Applied Audiology for Children*. Springfield: Charles M. Thomas.

DAVIS, H. and SILVERMAN, R. (1970). *Hearing and Deafness*. New York: Holt, Rinehart and Winston.

DE FILIPPO, C.L. and SCOTT, B.L.R. (1978). A method for training and evaluating the reception of ongoing speech. *J. Acoust. Soc. Am.* **63**, 1186–1192.

DURLACH, N.I., REED, C.M., BRAIDA, L.D., SCHULTZ, M.C. and NORTON, S.J. (1982). Research strategy for the study of tactile speech communication. In: Pickett, J.M. (ed.), *Papers from the Research Conference on Speech-Processing Aids for the Deaf*. Washington: Gallaudet University, pp. 56–63.

ERBER, N.P. (1979). Speech perception by profoundly hearing-impaired children. *J. Speech Hear. Dis.* **44**, 255–270.

ERBER, N.P. (1980). Use of the Auditory Numbers Test to evaluate the speech perception abilities of hearing-impaired children. *J. Speech Hear. Dis.* **45**, 527–532.

ERICSON, L. and RISBERG, A. (1977). Thresholds of hearing, vibration and discomfort in a group of severely hard of hearing and deaf students. *Speech Transmission Laboratory - Quarterly Progress and Status Report*, **1977/4**, 22–28.

FRANKLIN, B. (1989). *A Tactaid II Training Program for Deaf-Blind Children*. San Francisco: San Francisco State University

GAULT, R.H. (1926). Touch as a substitute for hearing in the interpretation and control of speech. *Arch. Otolaryngol.* **3**, 121–135.

GAULT, R.H. (1930). On the effect of simultaneous tactual-visual stimulation in relation to the interpretation of speech. *J. Ab. Soc. Psychol.* **24**, 498–517.

GOODFELLOW, L.D. (1934). Experiments on the senses of touch and vibration. *J. Acoust. Soc. Am.* **6**, 45–50.

KALIKOW, D.N., STEVENS, K.N. and ELLIOTT, L.L. (1977). Development of a test of speech intelligibility using sentence materials with controlled word predictability. *J. Acoust. Soc. Am.* **61**, 1337–1351.

KIRMAN, J. (1974). Tactile communication of speech: A review and an analysis. *Psychol. Bull.* **80**, 54–74.

LEDER, S.B. and SPITZER, J.B. (1990). A perceptual evaluation of the speech of adventitiously deaf adult males. *Ear Hear.* **11**, 169–175.

LING, D. (1976). *Speech and the Hearing Impaired Child: Theory and Practice*. Washington: A.G. Bell Association.

NOBER, E.H. (1970). Cutile air and bone conduction thresholds of the deaf. *Except. Child.* **56**, 571–579.

NORTON, S.J., SCHULTZ, M.C., REED, C.M., BRAIDA, L.D., DURLACH, N.I., RABINOWITZ, W.M. and CHOMSKY, C. (1977). Analytic study of the Tadoma method: Background and preliminary results. *J. Speech Hear. Res.* **20**, 625–637.

OLLER, D.K., EILERS, R., VERGARA, K. and LAVOIE. (1986). Tactual vocoders in a multisensory program training speech production and reception. *Volta Rev.* **88**, 21–36.

OWENS, E., KESSLER, D.K., TELLEEN, C.C. and SCHUBERT, E.D. (1981). *The Minimal Auditory Capabilities Battery*. St Louis: Auditec.

PLANT, G. (1979). The use of tactile supplements in the rehabilitation of the deafened: A case study. *Aust. J. Audiol.* **1**, 76–82.

PLANT, G. (1982). Tactile perception by the profoundly deaf: Speech and environmental sounds. *Br. J. Audiol.* **16**, 233–244.

PLANT, G. (1984). *Commtram. A Communication Training Program for Profoundly Hearing Impaired Adults*. Sydney: National Acoustic Laboratories.

PLANT, G. (1988a). *Tactaid II Training Program*. Sydney: National Acoustic Laboratories.

PLANT, G. (1988b). Speechreading with tactile supplements. *Volta Rev.* **90**, 149–160.

PLANT, G. (1989a). A comparison of five commercially available tactile aids. *Aust. J. Audiol.* **11**, 11–20.

PLANT, G. (1989b). *Commtrac: Modified Connected Discourse Tracking Exercises for Hearing-Impaired Adults.* Sydney: National Acoustic Laboratories.

PLANT, G. and SPENS, K.-E. (1986). An experienced user of tactile information as a supplement to lipreading. An evaluative study. *STL-QASR,* 1/1986, 87–110.

PLANT, G., GALT, J. and SYMONDS, S. (1986). How deaf is totally deaf? A case study. *Aust. J. Audiol.* **8**, 67–75.

PLANT, G., PHILLIPS, D. and TSEMBIS, J. (1982). An auditory-visual speech test for the elderly hearing impaired. *Aust. J. Audiol.* **4**, 62–68.

RAMSDELL, D.A. (1947). The psychology of the hard-of-hearing and deafened adult. In: Davis, H. (ed.), *Hearing and Deafness: A Guide for Laymen.* New York: Murray Hill, pp. 392–420.

REED, C.M., DURLACH, N.I., BRAIDA, L.D. and SCHULTZ, M.C. (1982). Analytic study of the Tadoma method: Identification of consonants and vowels by an experienced Tadoma user. *J. Speech Hear. Res.* **25**, 108–116.

REED, C.M., RABINOWITZ, W.M., DURLACH, N.I., BRAIDA, L.D., CONWAY-FITHIAN, S. and SCHULTZ, M.C. (1985). Research on the Tadoma method of speech communication. *J. Acoust. Soc. Am.* **77**, 247–257.

RISBERG, A. (1978). Requirements on speech processing aids for the profoundly deaf: Some preliminary results. *Scand. Audiol.* (Supplement) **6**, 179–198.

ROSEN, S.M. and CORCORAN, T. (1982). A video-recorded test of lip-reading for British English. *Br. J. Audiol.* **16**, 245–254.

SAUNDERS, F.A. and FRANKLIN, B. (1982). Transmission of information via an electrotactile display. Paper presented at the Tactual Communication Conference, Wichita, Kansas, USA.

SCHULTE, K. (1972). Fonator System: Speech stimulation and speech feed-back by technically amplified one-channel vibrations. In: Fant, G. (ed.), *International Symposium on Speech Communication Ability and Profound Deafness.* Washington: A.G. Bell Association, paper no. 36.

SIEBERT, R. (1980). Speech training for the hearing impaired: Principles, objectives, and strategies for preschool and elementary levels. In: Subtelny, J. (ed.), *Speech Assessment and Speech Improvement for the Hearing Impaired.* Washington: A.G. Bell Association, pp. 102–110.

SPENS, K-E. and PLANT, G. (1983). A tactual 'hearing' aid for the deaf. *Speech Transmission Laboratory Quarterly Progress and Status Report,* 1/1983, 52–56.

SUMMERS, I.R., PEAKE, M.A. and MARTIN, M.C. (1981). Field trials of a tactile acoustic monitor for the profoundly deaf. *Br. J. Audiol.* **15**, 195–199.

TONISSON, W. (1976). Australian standardisation of the CID Everyday Sentence Tests. In: *Second National Conference of the Audiological Society of Australia.* Melbourne: Audiological Society of Australia.

WALDSTEIN, R.S. (1990). Effects of postlingual deafness on speech production: Implications for the role of auditory feedback. *J. Acoust. Soc. Am.* **88**, 2099–2114.

WEISENBERGER, J.M. (1989). Evaluation of the Siemens Minifonator vibrotactile aid. *J. Speech Hear. Res.* **32**, 24–32.

WEISENBERGER, J.M. and MILLER, J.D. (1987). The role of tactile aids in providing information about acoustic stimuli. *J. Acoust. Soc. Am.* **82**, 906–916.

WEISENBERGER, J.M. and RUSSELL, A.F. (1989). Comparison of two single-channel vibrotactile aids for the hearing-impaired. *J. Speech Hear. Res.* **32**, 83–92.

Chapter 8
The Evaluation of Tactile Aids

LYNNE E. BERNSTEIN

This chapter describes work that has been conducted to assess the degree to which tactile aids provide information to benefit speech reception and facilitate children's speech and language development. Since excellent reviews exist for work up to the early 1980s (Kirman, 1973; Reed, Durlach and Braida, 1982; Sherrick, 1984), this chapter focuses on methods and results of assessments of tactile aids over the past decade.

Assessments have primarily been to predict possible benefit of laboratory devices, should they become wearable and generally available. Since most devices have never emerged from the laboratory, little is known about the relationship between laboratory benefit shown with any particular procedure and benefit in 'real life'; also, most 'real life' experience has been logged by profoundly hearing-impaired children and most laboratory experience by hearing adults.

Although more hearing-impaired adults are being tested than in the past, the typical test subject has been a young, normally hearing adult, frequently associated with the research community in which the device is being tested. An advantage with this type of subject is that their speech and language may be presumed normal: when the subject errs in responding, the errors can be attributed to lack of device efficacy, not immaturity or impairment of language or speech. Of course, errors can also be attributed to lack of long-term experience with the device, outside the laboratory (Sherrick, 1984).

One presupposition in the use of hearing subjects is that visual language experience is irrelevant to estimates of device efficacy: this presupposition may be quite inappropriate. Profoundly hearing-impaired adults bring to the evaluation of tactile devices varying levels of reliance on manual or verbal, but always visual, language processing. Visual factors need to be considered, since tactile devices are seen currently as supplements to lipreading (speechreading), and the visible talker is a significant source of speech information.

Procedures Frequently Used with Adult Subjects

Procedures used with adult subjects can be generally categorized by level of the linguistic units used as stimuli. The most frequent types of procedures involve:

1. Closed-set nonsense syllable identification (e.g., all or a subset of the 15 vowels (V) of English in the context /hVd/, or all or a subset of the approximately 23 consonants (C) of English in the context /CV/).
2. Open-set word identification, involving repeated training and testing of words.
3. Closed-set identification of suprasegmental characteristics such as stress or intonation (e.g. tests of the distinction between the intonation of statements and questions).
4. Open-set identification of isolated sentences, usually involving lipreading.
5. Connected discourse tracking (CDT; De Filippo and Scott, 1978), in which the experimenter reads from a prose text and the subject must repeat verbatim what was said.

Some additional procedures have been developed to assess reception of non-verbal sounds in the environment (see Chapter 4, and Eilers, Widen and Oller, 1988).

Nonsense syllable tests

Many experiments have required subjects to identify, within a closed set, a single phoneme* that changes from trial to trial, presented in a fixed syllabic context (e.g. 'ba', 'da', 'ga', etc.). The justification for using nonsense syllables is that if the device in question can convey or aid in conveying a phonemic distinction in isolation, the same information will be available for the perception of running speech. Thus nonsense syllable performance might predict performance with words, phrases or longer linguistic units. There is reason to doubt the soundness of this assumption, not only because longer linguistic units bring into play additional cognitive/linguistic processes, but also because perception of longer units is likely to involve perceptual processes such as masking that may be less important for short isolated stimuli. On the other hand, nonsense syllable tests do provide boundary estimates for information available with the aid; for example, if it is designed to convey information to identify phonemes, and if the target distinction cannot be identified or discriminated in a short isolated stimulus, there can be little hope for better performance when the stimulus becomes more complex.

---

*Phonemes are linguistic units used in the description of the sound system of a language. Phonemes signal the difference between words in a language, e.g. 'mat' versus 'bat'.

The literature provides examples of nonsense syllable testing with live voice, recordings, or synthetic speech; vowels are tested separately from consonants; the size of the closed set and the number of tokens and trials varies from study to study. Devices also vary across studies. In order to discover which devices are most effective, data must be re-analysed in terms of a common measure. For this chapter transmitted information (TI) (Miller and Nicely, 1955) has been chosen for the comparison. One reason for adopting TI is that it accounts for the systematicity in the off-diagonal cells (incorrect responses) of the stimulus–response matrix, in addition to the number of correct responses. TI calculations were made using published data matrices and the SINFA software (Wang and Bilger, 1973; Wang, 1976), unless TI was supplied in the publication (Blamey et al., 1989; Reed et al., 1982). Table 8.1 lists information about the studies that were compared, including phonemes tested and their contexts, and transmitted information in the various conditions for which TI results were available or could be calculated.

The range of tactile aids in Table 8.1 is relatively wide, single- to multichannel. Results for Tadoma were also included. Tadoma (Reed et al., 1982) is a method by which some deaf-blind people communicate. The Tadoma user places a hand on the face and throat of the talker in order to receive speech. This 'natural' method of tactile communication was included here, because it has often been cited as the standard against which tactile aids should be judged. Tan, Rabinowitz and Durlach (1989) state 'The Tadoma method is superior to any artificial tactile display of speech that has been studied to date'. Sufficient information about Tadoma users is available to assert that (at least for some individuals who have had long-term individual training) this method has resulted in normal or near-normal speech and language abilities, including communication at near-normal rates (Chomsky, 1986).

TI results from Table 8.1 are plotted in Figure 8.1. The line labeled TI = $\log_2(x)$ corresponds to the minimal amount of information required to accurately transmit the number of stimulus categories. For example, three binary distinctions are required to transmit eight categories. Data points are categorized as tactile-only, visual-only, tactile–visual, and Tadoma. Figure 8.1 illustrates that, in general, tactile devices alone provide less information than lipreading alone, which in turn provides less information than lipreading with tactile aids. However, the amount of information that tactile aids add to lipreading is extremely small compared with the information transmitted by tactile aids in the absence of visual information (see Table 8.1).

Surprisingly, TI for two normal Tadoma subjects was greater than for deaf-blind subjects (see Table 8.1). But the hearing subjects were highly trained and tested with a single talker (Reed et al., 1982); thus it is possible that the hearing subjects were able to learn idiosyncracies of the talker, which

Table 8.1 Studies providing confusion matrices for consonant and/or vowel identification, stimuli tested, and transmitted information in bits

Authors	Figure/table[a]	Subjects[b]	Speech stimuli	Transmitted information			Tactile stimulation
				T[c]	V[d]	TV[e]	
Reed et al. (1985)	III	9 DB	24 consonants in C-/a/ context: /p,t,k,b, d,g,f,T,s,S,C,v,D,z,Z,J,m,n,r,w,l,j,h,hw/	2.27			Tadoma: receiver's hand is placed on the face and throat of talker
	IV	9 DB	15 vowels in /h/ -V-/d/ context: /i,I,E, ^,@,a,c,U,u,R,e,A,W,o,O/	1.57			Tadoma
Reed et al. (1982)	3	2 NH	24 consonants in C-/a/ context: /p,t,k,b,d, g,f,T,s,S,C,v,D,z,Z,J,m,n,r,w,l,j,h,hw/	3.67			Tadoma
	5	2 NH	15 vowels in /g/-V/-d/ context: /i,I,E, ^,@,a,c,U,u,R,e,A,W,o,O/	3.14			Tadoma
Carney (1988)	7a-c	6 NH	20 consonants in C-/a,i,u/ context: /p,b,m,t,d,s,z,l,n,S,Z,T,D,f,v,w,r,j,k,g/	1.20	2.99	3.29	1-Channel, Fonator (Siemens, Inc.), amplitude 63-8000 Hz
	5a-c	6 NH	9 vowels in /b,d,g/-V context: /i,I,E, @,a,c,U,u,^/	1.01	2.53	2.54	
	8a-c	6 NH	20 consonants in C-/a/ context: /p,b, m,t,d,s,z,l,n,S,Z,T,D,f,v,w,r,j,k,g/	1.18	3.06	3.32	24-channel vibrotactile vocoder, 80-10 000 Hz
	6a-c		9 vowels in /b/-V context: /i,I,E,@,a,c,U,u,^/	1.15	2.73	2.59	
Blamey et al. (1988)	4	7 NH	12 consonants in context /a/-C-/a/: /p,b,m,v,f,t,d,n,s,z,k,g/	1.76			8-channel electrotactile, Tickle Talker, F0, F1 and amplitude.
	5	4 HI	11 vowels in the context /h/-V-/d/: /i,I,E, a,c,U,u,^/				
	4	7 NH		1.76			
	5	4 HI					
Blamey et al. (1989)	6f	4 NH	12 consonants in context /a/-C-/a/: /p,b, m,v,f,t,d,n,s,z,k,g/	1.04	1.90	2.19	Tickle Talker
	4	4 NH	11 vowels in the context /h/-V-/d/: /i,I,E, @,a,c,U,u,^/	1.49	2.59	2.84	
Bernstein (this chapter)		2 HI	23 consonants in context C-/a/: /p,t,k,b,d, g,f,T,s,S,C,v,D,z,Z,J,m,n,r,w,l,j,h/	3.14		3.47	16-channel vibrotactile vocoder
		2 NH		3.10		3.16	

[a]Figure/Table, the figure or table from which data were extracted; [b]subjects, number and hearing status of subjects (NH, normal hearing; HI, hearing impaired; DB, deaf and blind; [c]T, tactile only; [d]V, visual only; [e]TV, visual-tactile; [f]the reference provides transmitted information values but none of the confusion matrices that were used for calculating those values.

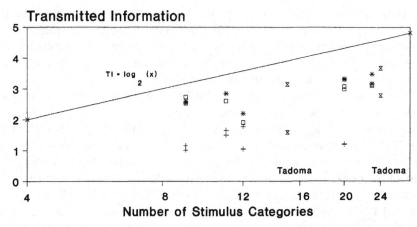

Figure 8.1 Transmitted information as a function of number of stimulus categories in nonsense syllable identification tasks. +, Tactile-only condition; □, visual-only condition; *, tactile–visual condition; X̲, Tadoma.

the deaf–blind subjects could not in the relatively short period of their laboratory experience (Reed et al., 1985). The performance of hearing subjects dropped when additional talkers were introduced. Approximately the same proportion of information about vowels was conveyed by the Tickle-Talker (11 categories; 47.5% for hearing impaired) as by Tadoma used by deaf–blind subjects (12 categories; 47.0% TI). It is generally the case that Tadoma was more effective than any tactile aid used without lipreading. In the only direct comparison between single- and multichannel stimulation (Carney, 1988; see Table 8.1), there were no differences in TI.

What is perplexing about the studies that provide results on all the conditions – tactile, visual and tactile–visual – is the failure to obtain greater increments between the visual and tactile–visual conditions in the presence of reasonably high levels of transmitted information in the tactile condition. Statistical analyses in the Carney (1988) paper showed no difference between tactile–visual and visual conditions, and Blamey et al. (1989) showed that the tactile–visual results were less than predicted on the basis of visual and tactile results. Several explanations can be offered: information available via the tactile sense is reduced in the presence of visual stimulation; information via the visual sense is reduced in the presence of tactile stimulation; information to the visual and tactile senses is mostly redundant, and therefore little advantage is obtained with cross-modal stimulation.

It is possible that at least two processes are affecting cross-modal perception. First, vision may be prepotent to taction in the allocation of attention. Support for this point is found in the study of intonation and stress by Bernstein, Eberhardt and Demorest (1988). Second, when the subjects have normal hearing, they are being required to process speech via two modalities that are not primarily used for that function. In the authors' experiments, subjects sometimes ignore the tactile stimulus and focus on the visual stimulus. Profoundly hearing-impaired subjects already have extensive experience of obtaining information from vision and may be better able to make use of the second modality.

There is some support for the role of hearing status in magnitude of aid benefit of nonsense syllable identification. Plant et al. (1984) tested a hearing-impaired subject who had experience using a single-channel tactile aid. With the experimental device providing voicing duration and overall intensity, the subject achieved 18 percentage points higher in identification of 20 consonants in nonsense syllables in the tactile–visual than the visual conditions, a generally larger gain than reported in Table 8.1. In Table 8.1, the largest increment between the visual and tactile–visual conditions was for Bernstein's hearing-impaired subjects. These few results notwithstanding, the relationship between magnitude of aid benefit and hearing status or individual differences is virtually unknown.

Isolated word recognition

Relatively few studies have required subjects to learn to recognize isolated words in tactile-only conditions. One reason is that the task of learning any sizeable vocabulary is reasonable only with a tactile signal that provides adequate information to specify the phonemes. Vibrotactile vocoders are arguably most capable of providing such information. A reason to study tactile vocabulary acquisition is to determine the shape of the learning curve, that is, how quickly words are acquired at various phases of the experiment.

The most impressive effort to learn words has been the work of Brooks and her colleagues (Brooks and Frost, 1983; P.L. Brooks, 1984, unpublished doctoral dissertation, Queen's University, Kingston, Ontario; Brooks et al., 1986a,b) at Queen's University, Ontario, Canada. Brooks herself has been the main subject of their experiments, and she has perhaps logged more hours with vibrotactile vocoders than any other subject.

Brooks and Frost (1983) reported on an initial word-learning experiment using a 16-channel vocoder with one-third octave spacing across the range 200–8000 Hz, followed by logarithmic compression of the energy in each band. Stimulation was by vibrators. The procedure involved iterative training on sets of five words that were incorporated into a pool of previously learned words. Words from the pool were then randomly selected and tested. One subject learned 70 words in 40.5 h and another 150 words in 55 h. The more proficient subject learned words at the rate of 2.7 per h. Learning curves appear to be linear functions, with no evidence that subjects were approaching an asymptote in their ability to learn new vocabulary. The shape of the curves implies that subjects were not 'learning to learn', an effect that would result in a positively accelerated curve.

Brooks (1984, unpublished doctoral dissertation, Queen's University, Kingston, Ontario) next undertook to learn an additional 100 words via a modified vocoder using a procedure similar to the previous study. Word learning averaged 3.92 words h[-1], the total 250-word vocabulary requiring 80.5 h. The learning rate was higher than in the previous experiment, which suggests that the modified vocoder was more effective, since the previous results did not show that the subjects were 'learning to learn'. Results of testing with the entire vocabulary showed that 23% of the words were identified accurately on every presentation, and 57% of words at least 80% of the time.

After acquiring 196 hours of tactile vocoder experience, Brooks (Brooks et al., 1986a) undertook open-set word identification in visual, tactile, and tactile–visual conditions, and 1000 words were presented in each condition. Word identification was accurate at the level of 8.8% in the tactile condition, 39.4% in the visual condition, and 68.7% in the combined condition. Stimulus response pairs were also analysed in terms of number of phonemes correct, and accuracy levels rose, since many words were partially correct: 36.7% of phonemes correct in the tactile, 64.9% in the visual, and 85.5% in the combined condition. These results suggest that a fairly high level of information was contributed by both modalities in the combined condition, in contrast to the results reported above for nonsense syllables, since here the vocoder appears to have greatly contributed to the subject's tactile–visual performance. The factor most probably responsible for these results is the relatively vast tactile experience of the subject, suggesting that effective processing of bimodal stimulation should not be expected unless the subject is very experienced in at least one of the modalities.

Other investigators have studied word learning, but far less extensively. Using a Queen's vocoder, subjects in a study by Weisenberger and Miller (1987) learned a list of 20 words at the rate of 2.5–3.0 h[-1]. Lynch et al. (1988) enlisted two profoundly hearing-impaired subjects to learn a 50-word vocabulary with the Tacticon 1600, an electrocutaneous vocoder (Saunders, 1985). Subjects were less successful than Brooks had been. Overall, subjects in the Lynch et al. (1988) study correctly identified 42% of the words, in contrast with the 76% overall success reported by Brooks. This result may be due to the vocoder, since in a direct comparison between the Queen's vocoder and the Tacticon Weisenberger, Broadstone and Saunders (1989) found that reception of running text was less accurate with the Tacticon.

The acoustic phonetic manifestations of phonemes vary as a function of their context (i.e. phonemes that precede and/or follow), with the result that tactile phonemes also have context-specific patterns. Other factors affect the tactile stimulation, such as the talker's vocal tract length (which determines certain spectral characteristics) and rate of speech. Therefore subjects in word learning experiments are learning not simply to perceive combinations of a small fixed set of approximately 15 vowels and 23 consonants in English, but a highly varied set of patterns.

Identification of suprasegmental speech characteristics

'Suprasegmental' speech characteristics are those characteristics of the speech code that are produced across more than a single phoneme, such as syllabic stress, word emphasis, and intonation. In general, questions concerning suprasegmental speech characteristics have not been explored in great detail. Voice fundamental frequency (F0), intensity, and timing provide information about intonation, stress, and syllabic structure. Several studies have shown that lipreading performance can be improved substantially by providing F0 *auditorily* to normally hearing subjects (Ardell, 1980; Rosen, Fourcin and Moore, 1981; Breeuwer and Plomp, 1986). For example, Breeuwer and Plomp reported 33% syllables correct in sentences with unaided lipreading and 73% correct with auditory F0. This has suggested that F0 might be a particularly beneficial form of speech information presented tactually.

Not only is F0 potentially valuable to lipreaders, its frequency characteristics appear particularly well suited to the skin, since the range of voice F0 across men, women, and children is approximately 70–500 Hz and because individual talkers produce F0 across approximately 1 octave only (Hess, 1983). Rothenberg et al. (1977) reported several tactile psychophysical experiments that supported the notion that a single vibrotactile channel can convey voice F0. Rothenberg and Molitor (1979) subsequently reported on several transformations of F0 involving frequency scaling and shifting into what they predicted would be the skin's best frequency range. Subjects identified stress (on one of three words) and intonation patterns (question *versus* statement) of a short sentence – 'Ron will win'. The most favorable results were obtained when the center frequency was 50 Hz and the scale factor was 1:1 or 1:0.75 for a male talker whose 80-Hz F0 range centered at 125 Hz. Figure 5 in Rothenberg and Molitor (1979) suggests that intonation judgments were more accurate (approximately 90% correct, chance was 50%) than stress judgments (approximately 51%, chance was 33%).

Bernstein, Eberhardt and Demorest (1989) took this work a step further. They found that stress was fairly visible to the lipreader and reasoned that the combination of high tactile accuracy for intonation and high visual accuracy for stress should result in high tactile–visual performance. Although several of the single-channel transformations that they tested were effective in conveying stress and intonation in the tactile experiment, disappointingly little benefit from tactile stimulation was achieved in the combined condition: a 3% advantage over the visual condition for intonation judgments, and no advantage for stress judgments, once number of trials in which the visual stimulus was presented (i.e. visual practice) was held statistically constant. Subjects were primarily deriving stress information from vision and not learning to use the tactile information. For three of the transformations, tactile identification of intonation was greater than tactile–visual.

Hnath-Chisholm and Kishon-Rabin (1988) measured perception of intonation and word stress with either a single-channel or a 16-channel aid providing voice F0 in normally hearing subjects. The multichannel aid was more effective than the single-channel aid in conveying intonation, in both the tactile-visual and tactile conditions. This is one of the few examples in which any advantage of the multichannel over the single-channel config-uration has been found by investigators from this group working with these aids (Hnath-Chisolm and Kishon-Rabin, 1990, personal communica-tion). But the number of channels was not a factor in identifying stress, for which the difference between visual and tactile–visual identification was small. Also, the addition of the tactile information to lipreading resulted in a significantly lower score than predicted by assuming indepen-dent contributions of taction and vision.

These and the results of Bernstein, Demorest and Eberhardt (1989) support the theory that vision has a significant effect on the level of prosodic information that subjects are able to obtain from tactile aids. The extent to which long-term training or experience affects the integration of the visual and tactile information in a task requiring identification of suprasegmental characteristics is not yet known.

A recent, fairly extensive attempt to determine what suprasegmental characteristics are conveyed by devices not specifically designed to provide voice F0 has been carried out by Carney and Beachler (1986), who compared a 24-channel vocoder with the single-channel Fonator (Siemens Hearing Instruments, Union, NJ, USA) to determine respective efficacy of each device for transmitting the number of syllables per word, the stress pattern within a word, and identification of rising and falling intonation patterns on disyllabic nonsense words. These tasks were performed in the tactile condition. Subjects appeared more successful at identifying the number of syllables in a word using the single-channel device; similar results were obtained when the task was to identify the syllabic stress on words. Intonation patterns were identified at chance levels with both devices. These results can be explained in terms of the signal processing of the two devices: neither was engineered to optimize the transmission of F0 for the skin. The differential advantage of the Fonator for the other two tasks is probably due to the single channel being perceived as an energy envelope (a good indication of syllabic stress and number), whereas the vocoder was providing a much more complex signal that would require integration across all 24 channels to obtain a percept of the energy envelope.

Isolated sentence recognition

Virtually all isolated sentence recognition data have been collected in
tactile-visual conditions (but see Erber and Cramer, 1974; Englemann and
Rosov, 1975) and relatively few data of this kind have been collected,
probably because of the problem of scoring sentence responses.
Identification or discrimination with nonsense syllables or words are
straightforward tasks to devise and score in comparison with tasks involving sentences. The problem can be simplified if subjects are required to
identify sentences from a small closed set when the task becomes formally
similar to closed-set word or nonsense syllable identification. If the task is
open-set sentence identification, in which little if any context is provided
to the subject, numerous errors can arise, some of which render the
scoring extremely difficult.

The following example is typical of stimulus–response pairs in tasks that
involve visual or tactile–visual conditions (Bernstein, Demorest and
Eberhardt, 1989):

Stimulus: Why should I get up so early in the morning?
Response: Watch what I'm doing in the morning.

The response both inserts new words and omits some stimulus words.
One method for scoring is to mark those words that are completely
correct. This method is straightforward as long as words are in the correct
order and/or no words are repeated in the sentence, and as long as various
grammatical characteristics such as verb tense are correct. Another
method is to transcribe the sentences from normal orthography to
phonetic notation, so that the correct phonemes can be counted. But
alignment of the stimulus with response phonemes is not a trivial problem,
since word boundaries are frequently misaligned between stimulus and
response, in addition to the problem of omissions and deletions. For
example,

Stimulus: Do you want to wa-sh up?
Response: Do you want to go sh-opping?

in which 'sh' and 'p' are in two different words in the stimulus and one
in the response. Sequence comparison algorithms exist to obtain such
alignments (Sankoff and Kruskal, 1983), and work has begun with them
(Bernstein, Demorest and Eberhardt, 1989), but it is still typical to report
results in terms of number of words correct.

Another problem that sentences present is response collection. Subjects
must either write down what they think the talker said, or speak the
sentence aloud, in which case an experimenter must transcribe the
subject's response. The latter approach is extremely tedious, and does not
encourage the use of large numbers of subjects in an experiment. It also

introduces the possibility of transcription errors on the part of the experimenter. Bernstein, Eberhardt and Demorest (1989) have automated response collection by presenting stimulus sentences recorded on laser videodiscs and having subjects type their responses at a computer video terminal. Computer software is used to correct spelling and score words correct on a per sentence basis.

Eberhardt et al. (1989) and Hanin, Boothroyd and Hnath-Chisolm (1988) used recorded isolated sentences to evaluate tactile aids that provided subjects with voice fundamental frequency (F0). Both groups tested single-channel transformations, and Hanin et al. also tested a multichannel aid. Transformations were designed to bring the talkers' voice pitch into an optimal range for the skin. Subjects had normal hearing. Each group obtained approximately 4% more words correct with than without an aid, regardless of number of channels or transformation.

Hanin, Boothroyd and Hnath-Chisolm (1988) also reported on a second study in which three hearing-impaired subjects received video-recorded sentences in a story – the difference between supplemented and visual-alone performance ranged between 11% and 20% words correct. The larger benefit could be attributed to the story context, and/or the hearing status of the subjects.

Brooks et al. (1986b) reported on a single normally hearing subject (herself) with 196 hours of practice on the Queen's vocoder, including extensive tactile-alone training with isolated words, being tested in an open-set sentence procedure. The number of words correctly identified in isolated sentences in visual-alone and visual-tactile conditions was reported for the *second* presentation of the sentences. The score was 58% words correct in the visual condition, but rose to 80% words correct in the combined condition.

Recently, Bernstein et al (1991) compared three 16-channel vocoders: a version of the Queen's University vocoder (Engebretson and O'Connell, 1986); the Queen's vocoder with linear output scaling rather than logarithmic scaling; and a new filter bank designed at Gallaudet University. The video-recorded sentences from the experiment by Eberhardt et al. (1990) were used. Significant benefits were not obtained with the Queen's University filter bank, but the Gallaudet aid was effective for both normal and profoundly hearing-impaired subjects. Over the *entire* experiment the mean difference between aided and unaided lipreading scores with the Gallaudent vocoder was 6%. Benefit to the normally hearing subjects was approximately equal to that obtained in the earlier study with the single-channel fundamental frequency aids.

Use of recorded isolated sentences permitted both reception of natural speech and controlled comparisons across experiments and hearing status. There has been relatively little work on tactile aids for which such direct comparisons are possible, due to variations in procedures and stimuli from study to study. It is hoped that with the availability of video-recording technologies, more investigators will conduct research that affords direct comparison across devices, subjects and laboratories.

Connected discourse tracking

In acknowledgment of the complexity of language and in an attempt to import more complex language processing into the laboratory while obviating the need to develop complex scoring methods, the method of connected discourse tracking (CDT) has become popular (De Filippo and Scott, 1978). In this method, the experimenter reads from a text, such as a novel, and the subject is required to repeat verbatim what was said. Correction procedures are used when an error is made, typically including repetition of the target phrase, and if that fails, provision of a phoneme or word clue. The measure obtained is words correctly repeated per minute, or percentage of the normal tracking rate (i.e. tracking by a subject who can hear the experimenter).

Although CDT may be useful in providing the tactile aid user with experience in lipreading with and without the aid, many flaws have been noted for it as an assessment procedure (Pickett, 1983; Robbins et al., 1985; Matthies and Carney, 1988; Tye-Murray and Tyler, 1988; Rosen and Bell, 1989): stimulus materials, talkers and correction procedures vary from study to study; investigators generally choose their own stimulus materials (Matthies and Carney (1988) 'the comparison of tracking results between investigations is virtually impossible because of the differential effects of stimulus materials'); rapport between subject and experimenter may affect tracking rates – since the two participants know which condition is being tested, expectations regarding outcomes may nevertheless affect even the most careful investigators; a flaw less frequently noted is the difficulty of using CDT with profoundly hearing-impaired subjects whose speech is often unintelligible. Nevertheless, since a relatively large assessment effort has relied on CDT, an attempt is made here to summarize and compare the results.

Table 8.2 lists studies from which measures of CDT in visual and tactile–visual conditions were obtained. Results are frequently presented as learning curves, not a convenient form in which to compare across studies. The results in Table 8.2 labeled V and TV were obtained by estimating tracking rates for approximately the final hour of tracking in each condition for each entry in the table. In order to facilitate comparison between results, Figure 8.2 shows relative improvement as a function of visual-only tracking on log–log coordinates, as suggested by Levitt (1986). The line is the relative improvement over unaided tracking rates required to attain 70 words per minute. Tracking with auditory speech is estimated at 100–110 words min[-1]. Levitt has suggested that a

Table 8.2 Studies that measured aided and unaided connected discourse tracking rates

Authors	Figure[a]	Hours[b]	Subject[c]	V[d]	TV[e]	TV/V[f]	Tactile stimulation
De Filippo and Scott (1978)	1	21	NH(1)	43	53	1.23	1-channel 1000 Hz low-pass vibrotactile and 1 high-pass electrotactile
			NH(2)	52	74	1.42	
Sparks et al. (1979)	1	3	NH(LA)	39	43	1.10	8 × 36-channel (amplitude frequency) electrotactile array
			NH(BW)	62	65	1.05	
			NH(MB)	48	50	1.04	
Plant et al. (1984)	3	5.33	HI	46	62	1.35	1-channel fundamental frequency (F0) and 1-channel low-frequency amplitude, vibrotactile
Brooks et al. (1986b)	4	7.5	NH	13	50	3.85	16-channel Queen's University multichannel vibrotactile vocoder
Cholewiak and Sherrick (1986)	2	16 yrs[g]	HI	45	59	1.31	1-channel broad-band low frequency and 1 channel high frequency vibrotactile
Grant et al. (1986)	4	21	NH(S1)	55	60	1.09	10-channel electrotactile, F0
Weisenberger and Miller (1987)	6	5.67	HI(SR)	30	46	1.53	16-channel Queen's University vocoder
			NH(CB)	30	43	1.43	
Cowan et al. (1988)	3	UK[h]	NH(1)	42	60	1.43	8-channel electrotactile, conveying F0, amplitude and F2
		UK	NH(2)	21	44	2.10	
		UK	NH(3)	43	70	1.63	
		UK	NH(4)	24	34	1.42	
		UK	NH(5)	41	56	1.37	
		UK	NH(6)	40	60	1.50	
		UK	NH(7)	41	58	1.41	
		UK	HI(A)	26	39	1.50	
		UK	HI(B)	9	20	2.22	
		UK	HI(C)	30	39	1.30	
		UK	HI(D)	34	49	1.44	
Lynch et al. (1989b)	3	21	HI[i]	52	52	1.00	Tactaid II, 1-channel low-pass 2000 Hz and 1-channel high-pass 2-8 kHz
	4	21		50	55	1.10	Tacticon 1600, 16-channel electrotactile
Weisenberger, Broadstone and Saunders (1989)	9	8.33	NH(LD)	16	38	2.38	16-channel Queen's University vocoder
			NH(KM)	25	52	2.08	
			NH(CD)	24	57	2.38	
			NH(LD)	16	20	1.25	Tacticon 1600
			NH(KM)	25	32	1.28	
			NH(CD)	24	30	1.25	

[a]Figure, the figure in the paper from which data were extracted; [b]hours, the time subjects had practised tracking; [c]subject, whether the subject was normally hearing (NH) or hearing impaired (HI). Parentheses give the subject designation as it appears in the citation; [d]V, lipreading unaided; [e]TV, lipreading aided; [f]TV/V, relative improvement with aid; [g]subject developed his device while a student at Moscow University and used the device for approximately 16 years. 160 min of Russian tracking and 240 min of English tracking were shown in Figures 2 and 3, respectively; [h]the number of hours of tracking is not given in the paper. Hearing-impaired subjects received approximately 35 total hours of training and normal hearing subjects 70, which comprised several different tasks; [i]the same hearing-impaired subject was tested with both the Tactaid II and the Tacticon 1600; the same subjects were tested with both the Queen's University vocoder and the Tacticon 1600.

70 words min[-1] tracking rate corresponds to slow but reasonably effective conversation.

Figure 8.2 suggests that relative improvement is not a function of hearing status, since at almost every level of unaided lipreading both normally hearing and hearing-impaired subjects made equivalent relative gains. Inspection of the figure in conjunction with Table 8.2 suggests that relative improvement may be a function of the device tested, since invariably the highest scores were obtained with multichannel devices. Extreme caution should be taken in reaching such a conclusion, however, since no factors were held constant across the various studies.

Figure 8.2 also reveals that few subjects achieved the 70 words min[-1] level, and those who did were extremely proficient in the visual condition. On the other hand, some very poor lipreaders achieved impressive relative improvements with their aid, the largest of which was made by the subject in Brooks et al. (1986b), who has logged probably the greatest number of tactile hours of training of any normally hearing subject (see Table 8.2). The subject in Cholewiak and Sherrick's (1986) report has greater tactile aid experience but uses a device that in theory provides less speech information, and his relative improvement was lower (Table 8.2).

The CDT measure appears to provide reliable within-subject results. With few exceptions (Figure 8.2), subjects improved tracking with their tactile aid. As investigators move from showing that tactile aids do provide benefit to comparing them for provision of most benefit, it is to be hoped that the CDT procedure is either standardized or abandoned to better controlled procedures.

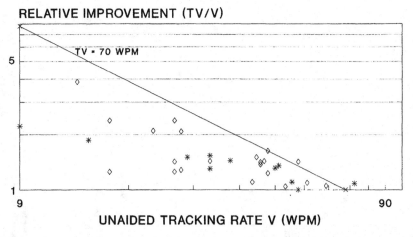

Figure 8.2 Relative tracking improvement (TV/V) as a function of unaided rate (V) on log-log coordinates. ◇, Normal hearing subject; ★, hearing-impaired subject.

Evaluations of Tactile Aids for Children

Frequently the child who is a candidate for a tactile aid has extremely limited oral speech and language abilities, as a direct result of hearing impairment. Testing this child is difficult, not only because of immature or impaired language abilities, but also due to other factors undergoing development such as attention, cognition and perceptual organization. Test interpretation is rendered difficult for the same reasons. The goals of testing may be different from those in studies of adults; the investigator may be concerned with the rate at which the child is developing as a function of device use and secondarily (or not at all) with the difference in performance with the aid on or off (see Friel-Patti and Roeser, 1983; Geers, 1986; Geers and Moog, 1991).

Friel-Patti and Roeser (1983) monitored the duration and type of communicative acts of four profoundly hearing-impaired children (ages 3;10 years to 4;6 years) during an aided Fall school semester and an unaided Spring semester. Their most notable finding was that children's use of vocalization to accompany their signing was increased by the use of the tactile aid. The aid was a three-channel device that transduced the energy passed by filters for low, medium, and high speech frequencies.

The magnitude of the benefit obtained by young children is likely to be a function of the developmental level of their language system, which in turn may be a function of additional unknown factors regulating the development of abilities such as lipreading. One great strength of the work with children is that it typically takes into account the need for long-term experience with the tactile stimuli. Unfortunately, the device given to the child is frequently simpler in design than the laboratory device tested with the adult, a consequence of which devices are available commercially. The Tactaid II has been used most frequently. This device provides indication only of energy in either of a low- or high-pass frequency band, and it cannot provide adequate spectral information for tactile-only phoneme identification, or indication of prosodic characteristics associated with modulation of voice fundamental frequency.

The number of studies of children is quite small. A recent acceleration in their appearance is related to the emergence of cochlear implants as sensory supplements or substitutes for hearing-impaired children.

Two major research efforts in the USA are directed towards comparing tactile aids with cochlear implants: one at Central Institute for the Deaf, in St Louis, Missouri (Geers and Moog, 1991) and the other at the Indiana University School of Medicine (Osberger et al., 1991). Tactile aids do not require the invasive surgery required for implants, yet hold promise of being equally effective for certain children.

Geers and Moog (1991) report on profoundly hearing-impaired children using the Nucleus 22-channel cochlear implant, the Tactaid II (two

channels), or a conventional hearing aid. The experimental design is longitudinal. Subjects are assigned to groups in which there is one implant
patient, one tactile aid user, and one hearing aid user, all matched for
demographic and performance characteristics. The children are all
enrolled in the educational program at Central Institute for the Deaf. They
were tested with a large battery of procedures involving speech perception, lipreading, speech production, and oral language. Results were
obtained before the tactile aids or implants were obtained and 12 months
after. In general, implanted children made the greatest gains on speech
perception measures; speech production gains were about equal between
the implant and the Tactaid groups; language acquisition was greatest
among the tactile aid and hearing aid children. As the authors point out,
it is premature to make conclusions about these results, the first from a
study to be conducted over five years.

The Osberger et al. (1991) study compares three groups of 11
profoundly hearing-impaired children fitted with the 3M/House single-
channel cochlear implant, the Nucleus 22-channel cochlear implant, or the
Tactaid II. A control group of profoundly deaf hearing aid users is also
studied and a longitudinal experimental design is followed. Subjects are
tested on an extensive battery of perception measures: word discrimination, stress identification, word identification, open-set phrase identification, and connected-discourse tracking. Results to date generally favor the
multichannel implant. The single-channel implant is less effective, and
performance with the Tactaid II generally comparable. Tracking data were
obtained on only a subset of the subjects. Both implants appear effective
in increasing tracking rates, in contrast to the tactile aid which was ineffective.

A third effort involving children has been taking place at the Mailman
Center for Child Development in Miami, Florida. Investigators have studied
the question of relative or combined benefit of hearing aids and tactile
aids (Eilers, Widen and Oller, 1988; Lynch et al., 1989a; Geers and Moog,
1991; see also Cowan et al., 1989, with regard to these combinations for
adults). In general, perception of profoundly hearing-impaired children
appears to improve when tactile aids are combined with hearing aids
(Eilers, Widen and Oller, 1988; Lynch et al., 1989a). In one experiment
(Lynch et al., 1989b), children learned to recognize 15 words tactually.
They were then tested on a list that included the original 15 words and
15 tactually new words. Four subjects between 5 and 7 years of age were
assigned to either the 16-channel Tacticon 1600 vocoder or the Tactaid II.
Testing took place in the conditions tactile-only, hearing-aid-only or tactile
and hearing aid combined. Results showed that the tactile aids were effective in raising scores when combined with hearing aids, for both the originally trained list and new words. A similar study was conducted with
slightly older subjects, 9-11 years of age, with similar results. These results

raise the possibility that tactile aids might be not only an alternative to hearing aids or cochlear implants, but also possibly effective used in addition to them.

Conclusions

Work with children sharply illustrates the need for greater availability of sophisticated, wearable tactile aids. Results show that children benefit from the currently available devices, but comparisons with cochlear implants are not as favorable as might be expected considering some of the results obtained with adults. In particular, devices such as the Queen's vocoder (Brooks et al., 1986a,b), the Tickle-Talker (Cowan et al., 1988), and the Gallaudet vocoder (Bernstein et al., 1991) have been shown to provide relatively high levels of tactile information. It is not known what advantage these aids would provide to children over a long period of development, but since they have been shown more beneficial than the devices that have been used, it can be predicted that children would also receive greater benefit with them.

After 70 years of sporadic efforts, tactile aids are clearly entering a more mature period of study. Investigators have shown that these devices can benefit profoundly hearing-impaired children and adults. The challenge now is to move in the direction of more effective and efficient testing as old devices are improved and new ones developed. The most important step in this direction would be to adopt testing methods and analysis procedures that provide for comparison and replication across devices, subjects, and laboratories.

Acknowledgment

This research was supported by NIDCD, DC00695 and DC00023.

References

ARDELL, L.H. (1980). The contribution of fundamental frequency and time-intensity cues to connected-discourse perception by speech-readers. MSc thesis, University of Washington, Seattle, WA.

BERNSTEIN, L.E., DEMOREST, M.E. and EBERHARDT, S.P. (1989). Speechreading sentences I: Development of a sequence comparator. *J. Acoust. Soc. Am.* **85**, Suppl. 1, S59 (abstract).

BERNSTEIN, L.E., EBERHARDT, S.P. and DEMOREST, M.E. (1989). Single-channel vibrotactile supplements to visual perception of intonation and stress. *J. Acoust. Soc. Am.* **85**, 397–405.

BERNSTEIN, L.E., DEMOREST, M.E., COULTER, D.C. and O'CONNELL. (1991). Speechreading sentences with vibrotactile vocoders: Performance of normal-hearing and hearing-impaired subjects. *J. Acoust. Soc. Am.* **90**(in press).

BLAMEY, P.J., COWAN, R.S.C., ALCANTARA, J.I. and CLARK, G.M. (1988). Phonemic information transmitted by a multichannel electrotactile speech processor. *J. Speech Hear. Res.* **31**, 620-629.

BLAMEY, P.J., COWAN, R.S.C., ALCANTARA, J.I., WHITFORD, L.A. and CLARK, G.M. (1989). Speech perception using combinations of auditory, visual, and tactile information. *J. Rehab. Res. Dev.* **26**, 15-24.

BREEUWER, A. and PLOMP, R. (1986). Speechreading supplemented with auditorily presented speech parameters. *J. Acoust. Soc. Am.* **79**, 481-499.

BROOKS, P.L. and FROST, B.J. (1983). Evaluation of a tactile vocoder for word recognition. *J. Acoust. Soc. Am.* **74**, 34-39.

BROOKS, P.L., FROST, B.J., MASON, J.L. and GIBSON, D.M. (1986a). Continuing evaluation of the Queen's University tactile vocoder. I: Identification of open set words. *J. Rehab. Res. Dev.* **23**, 119-128.

BROOKS, P.L., FROST, B.J., MASON, J.L. and GIBSON, D.M. (1986b). Continuing evaluation of the Queen's University tactile vocoder. II: Identification of open set sentences and tracking narrative. *J. Rehab. Res. Dev.* **23**, 129-138.

CARNEY, A.E. (1988). Vibrotactile perception of segmental features of speech: A comparison of single-channel and multichannel instruments. *J. Speech Hear. Res.* **31**, 438-448.

CARNEY, A.E. and BEACHLER, C.R. (1986). Vibrotactile perception of suprasegmental features of speech: A comparison of single-channel and multichannel instruments. *J. Acoust. Soc. Am.* **79**, 131-140.

CHOLEWIAK, R.W. and SHERRICK, C.E. (1986). Tracking skill of a deaf person with long-term tactile aid experience: A case study. *J. Rehab. Res. Dev.* **23**, 20-26.

CHOMSKY, C. (1986). Analytic study of the Tadoma method: Language abilities of three deaf-blind subjects. *J. Speech Hear. Res.* **29**, 332-347.

COWAN, R.S.C., ALCANTARA, J.I., BLAMEY, P.J. and CLARK, G.M. (1988). Preliminary evaluation of a multichannel electrotactile speech processor. *J. Acoust. Soc. Am.* **83**, 2328-2338.

COWAN, R.S.C., ALCANTARA, J.I., WHITFORD, P.J., BLAMEY, P.J. and CLARK, G.M. (1989). Speech perception studies using a multichannel electrotactile speech processor, residual hearing, and lipreading. *J. Acoust. Soc. Am.* **85**, 2593-2607.

DE FILIPPO, C.L. and SCOTT, B.L. (1978). A method for training and evaluating the reception of ongoing speech. *J. Acoust. Soc. Am.* **63**, 1186-1192.

EBERHARDT, S.P., BERNSTEIN, L.E., DEMOREST, M.E. and GOLDSTEIN, M.H. (1990). Speechreading sentences with single-channel vibrotactile presentation of fundamental frequency. *J. Acoust. Soc. Am.* **88**, 1274-1285.

ENGEBRETSON, A.M. and O'CONNELL, M.P. (1986). Implementation of a microprocessor-based tactile hearing prosthesis. *IEEE Trans. Biomed. Eng.* **33**, 712-716.

EILERS, R.E., WIDEN, J.E. and OLLER, D.K. (1988). Assessment techniques to evaluate tactual aids for hearing-impaired subjects. *J. Rehab. Res. Dev.* **25**, 33-46.

ENGLEMANN, S. and ROSOV, R. (1975). Tactual learning experiment with deaf and hearing subjects. *Except. Child.* **41**, 243-253.

ERBER, N.P. and CRAMER, K.D. (1974). Vibrotactile recognition of sentences. *Am. Ann. Deaf.* **119**, 716-720.

FRIEL-PATTI, S. and ROESER, R.J. (1983). Evaluating changes in the communication skills of deaf children using vibrotactile stimulation. *Ear Hear.* **4**, 31-40.

GAULT, R.H. (1926). Touch as a substitute for hearing in the interpretation and control of speech. In: Levitt, H., Pickett, J.M. and Houde, R.A. (eds), *Sensory Aids for the Hearing Impaired*. New York: IEEE (reprinted from *Arch. Otolaryngol.* **3**, 121-135).

GEERS, A.E. (1986). Vibrotactile stimulation: Case study with a profoundly deaf child. *J. Rehab. Res. Dev.* **23**, 111-117.

GEERS, A.E. and MOOG, J.S. (1991). Evaluating the benefits of cochlear implants in an educational setting. *Am. J. Otol.* **12**, 116-125.

GRANT, K.W., ARDELL, L.A.H., KUHL, P.K. and SPARKS, D.W. (1986). The transmission of prosodic information via an electrotactile speechreading aid. *Ear Hear.* **7**, 328-335.

HANIN, L., BOOTHROYD, A. and HNATH-CHISOLM, T. (1988). Tactile presentation of voice fundamental frequency as an aid to the speechreading of sentences. *Ear Hear.* **9**, 335-341.

HESS, W. (1983). *Pitch Determination of Speech Signals, Algorithms and Devices.* Berlin: Springer.

HNATH-CHISOLM, T. and KISHON-RABIN, L. (1988). Tactile presentation of voice fundamental frequency as an aid to the perception of speech pattern contrasts. *Ear Hear.* **9**, 329-334.

HOCHBERG, I., ROSEN, S. and BELL, V. (1989). Effect of text complexity on connected discourse tracking rate. *Ear Hear.* **10**, 192-199.

KIRMAN, J.H. (1973). Tactile communication of speech. A review and analysis. *Psych. Bull.* **80**, 54-74.

LEVITT, H. (1986). Evaluation of a cochlear prosthesis using connected discourse tracking. *J. Rehab. Res. Dev.* **23**, 147-154.

LYNCH, M.P., EILERS, R.E., OLLER, D.K. and COBO-LEWIS, A. (1989a). Multisensory speech perception by profoundly hearing-impaired children. *J. Speech Hear. Dis.* **54**, 57-67.

LYNCH, M.P., EILERS, R.E., OLLER, D.K. and LAVOIE, L. (1988). Speech perception by congenitally deaf subjects using an electrocutaneous vocoder. *J. Rehab. Res. Dev.* **25**, 41-50.

LYNCH, M.P., EILERS, R.E., OLLER, D.K., URBANO, R.C. and PERO, P.J. (1989b). Multisensory narrative tracking by a profoundly deaf subject using an electrocutaneous vocoder and a vibrotactile aid. *J. Speech Hear. Res.* **32**, 331-338.

MATTHIES, M.L. and CARNEY, A.E. (1988). A modified speech tracking procedure as a communicative performance measure. *J. Speech Hear. Res.* **31**, 394-404.

MILLER, G.A. and NICELY, P.E. (1955). An analysis of perceptual confusions among English consonants. *J. Acoust. Soc. Am.* **27**, 338-352.

OSBERGER, M.J., ROBBINS, A.M., MIYAMOTO, R.T., BERRY, S.W., MYRES, W.A., KESSLER, K.S. and POPE, M.L. (1991). Speech perception abilities of children with cochlear implants, tactile aids, or hearing aids. *Am. J. Otol.* **12**, 105-115.

PICKETT, J.M. (1983). Theoretical considerations in testing speech perception through electroauditory stimulation. In: Parkins, C.W. and Anderson, S.W. (eds), *Cochlear Prostheses: An International Symposium. Ann. NY Acad. Sci.* 424-434.

PLANT, G., MACRAE, J., DILLON, H. and PENTECOST, F. (1984). A single-channel vibrotactile aid to lipreading: Preliminary results with an experienced subject. *Aust. J. Audiol.* **6**, 55-64.

REED, C.M., DOHERTY, M.J., BRAIDA, L.D. and DURLACH, N.I. (1982). Analytic study of the Tadoma method: Further experiments with inexperienced observers. *J. Speech Hear. Res.* **25**, 216-223.

REED, C.M., DURLACH, N.I. and BRAIDA, L.D. (1982). Research on tactile communication of speech: A review. *Am. Speech Lang. Hear. Ass. Monograph no. 20*, 1-23.

REED, C.M., RABINOWITZ, W.M., DURLACH, N.I. and BRAIDA, L.D. (1985). Research on the Tadoma method of speech communication. *J. Acoust. Soc. Am.* **77**, 247-257.

ROBBINS, A.M., OSBERGER, M.J., MIYAMOTO, R.T., KIENLE, M.L. and MYRES, W.A. (1985). Speech-tracking performance in single-channel cochlear implant subjects. *J. Speech Hear. Res.* **28**, 565-578.

ROSEN, S.M., FOURCIN, A.J. and MOORE, B.C.J. (1981). Voice pitch as an aid to lipreading. *Nature* **291**, 150-152.

ROTHENBERG, M. and MOLITOR, R.D. (1979). Encoding voice fundamental frequency into vibrotactile frequency. *J. Acoust. Soc. Am.* **66**, 1029-1038.

ROTHENBERG, M., VERRILLO, R.T., ZAHORIAN, S.A., BRACHMAN, M.L. and BOLANOWSKI, JR S.J. (1977). Vibrotactile frequency for encoding a speech parameter. *J. Acoust. Soc. Am.* **62**, 1003-1012.

SANKOFF, D. and KRUSKAL, J.B. (eds) (1983). *Time Warps, String Edits, and Macromolecules: The Theory and Practice of Sequence Comparison.* Reading, MA: Addison-Wesley.

SAUNDERS, F.A. (1974). Electrocutaneous displays. In: Geldard, F.A. (ed.), *Cutaneous Communication Systems and Devices.* Austin, TX: The Psychonomic Society, pp. 20-26.

SAUNDERS F. (1985). *Tacticon 1600 electrocutaneous vocoder.* Concord, CA: Tacticon Corporation.

SHERRICK, C.E. (1984). Basic and applied research on tactile aids for deaf people: Progress and prospects. *J. Acoust. Soc. Am.* **75**, 1325-1342.

SPARKS, D.W., ARDELL, L.H., BOURGEOIS, M., WIEDMER, B. and KUHL, P.K. (1979). Investigating the MESA (multipoint electrotactile speech aid): The transmission of connected discourse. *J. Acoust. Soc. Am.* **65**, 810-815.

TAN, H.Z., RABINOWITZ, W.M. and DURLACH, N.I. (1989). Analysis of a synthetic Tadoma system as a multidimensional tactile display. *J. Acoust. Soc. Am.* **86**, 981-988.

TYE-MURRAY, N. and TYLER, R.S. (1988). A critique of continuous discourse tracking as a test procedure. *J. Speech Hear. Dis.* **53**, 226-231.

WANG, M.D. (1976). SINFA: Multivariate uncertainty analysis for confusion matrices. *Behav. Res. Meth. Instr.* **8**, 471-472.

WANG, M.D. and BILGER, R.C. (1973). Consonant confusions in noise: a study of perceptual features. *J. Acoust. Soc. Am.* **54**, 1248-1266.

WEISENBERGER, J. and MILLER, J. (1987). The role of tactile aids in providing information about acoustic stimuli. *J. Acoust. Soc. Am.* **82**, 906-916.

WEISENBERGER, J., BROADSTONE, S.M. and SAUNDERS, F.A. (1989). Evaluation of two multi-channel aids for the hearing impaired. *J. Acoust. Soc. Am.* **86**, 1764-1775.

Chapter 9
The Potential Benefit and Cost-effectiveness of Tactile Devices in Comparison with Cochlear Implants

PETER J. BLAMEY and ROBERT S.C. COWAN

The use of the word 'potential' in the title of this chapter implies that the discussion must be somewhat speculative in attempting to foresee the benefits and costs of cochlear implants in the future. It is now much easier to do this than it would have been five or ten years ago, although there still remain many unanswered questions about their use, especially for hearing-impaired children. As far as possible, the assumptions and opinions expressed in this chapter are based on fact but in some cases reflect the subjective bias of the authors. (These opinions are not necessarily shared by other contributors to this book.) In particular, one author (PJB) has been involved in cochlear implant research for over ten years and began developing a tactile device in 1984 as a control device in studies of cochlear implants in children. Children and adults using this device have produced results comparable to those for some groups of cochlear implant patients. Despite these results, which exceeded initial expectations, there is still some bias in favour of the cochlear implant.

In this chapter, it will be assumed that the reader is more familiar with tactile devices than cochlear implants, or can find relevant information in other chapters. For this reason, more information will be provided about implant devices and results.

The costs and benefits of any device for the deaf are influenced by many factors: age, needs, previous auditory experience, motivation, financial resources, and health of the individual concerned. Tactile devices and cochlear implants both come in a variety of types with different costs and benefits. It is necessary also to consider the (re)habilitation that may be required to obtain benefit from tactile devices and cochlear implants; clearly, the provision of training will affect the costs as well as the benefits. Prices of commercially available tactile devices and cochlear implants are also affected by market size, competition, marketing strategy, research and development costs, production costs, and profit margins. The question 'who pays?' may also be a major factor affecting the cost and availability.

The Users

Postlinguistically deafened adults

One factor that has contributed greatly to the rapid development and success of cochlear implants has been research identifying potential implant patients who have the greatest chance of benefiting (Brown et al., 1985a; Dowell, Mecklenburg and Clark, 1986). Most successful cochlear implant users are postlinguistically deafened adults, people who lost their hearing after the normal development of auditory speech perception skills was complete. These skills can be applied to speech perception with a cochlear implant to produce substantial benefits with only short periods of experience. Profound or total hearing loss as an adult can occur suddenly, as a result of diseases such as meningitis, through accidental trauma, or following administration of ototoxic drugs. It can also occur more gradually by deterioration of the hair cells in the cochlea. Patients with any of these aetiologies may be treated successfully with a cochlear implant unless the auditory nerve itself is severely affected. The best results are usually obtained with patients who have been profoundly deaf for very short times (Dorman et al., 1989; Blamey et al., 1991b). Most postlinguistically deafened adults achieve substantial benefit from a cochlear implant within a few months of the operation. Typically the benefits include open-set recognition of words and sentences without lipreading, and improvements in speech perception when the implant and lipreading are used together. One-third of postlinguistically deafened adult patients in Melbourne can have a limited telephone conversation without using coded questions or responses (Brown et al., 1985b) and can understand connected speech without lipreading (Dowell et al., 1986). Representative results are given in Table 9.1.

The recognition of open-set speech material without lipreading has become a routine finding with multiple-channel cochlear implants, but has never been achieved by tactile device users. Practised deaf–blind users of the Tadoma method can recognise open-set speech material at reduced rates without lipreading by placing one hand on the face and throat of the speaker. This has been described as an 'existence proof' that speech recognition is possible using only tactile information (Reed et al., 1982). In comparison, the best results for deaf adults using tactile devices include substantial improvements for recognition of open-set speech using the device in combination with lipreading. Representative results from research studies are shown in Table 9.2 for cochlear implant studies, and

Table 9.1 Open-set speech testing results obtained without lipreading in representative multi-channel cochlear implant studies

Implant	Number of patients	Experience with implant (months)	Test	Mean score (%)	Range of scores (%)	Reference
Symbion	50	>12	Monosyllabic words	14[c]	0-60	Dorman et al., 1989
Cochlear	10[a]	3-5	Monosyllabic words	11	3-20	Tyler, Moore and Kuk, 1989
Cochlear	13[b]	3	Monosyllabic words	5		Dowell et al., 1987
	9[a]			12		
Symbion	50	12	CID sentences	44[c]	10-100	Dorman et al., 1989
Cochlear	13[b]	3	CID sentences	16		Dowell et al., 1987
	9[a]			35		

[a]Patients using a later F0F1F2 speech coding scheme. This processor has also been superseded by an improved MSP model described in this chapter.
[b]Patients using an earlier F0F2 speech coding scheme.
[c]Dorman et al. (1989) quote median scores rather than mean scores.

Table 9.2 Lipreading enhancement results from representative multichannel cochlear implant studies

Implant	Number of patients	Experience with implant (months)	Test	Lipreading score	Lipreading + hearing score	Reference
Cochlear	40[a]	3	Speech tracking	19 wpm[d]	49 wpm	Dowell, Mecklenburg and Clark, 1986
Cochlear	13[a]	3	Speech tracking	16 wpm	45 wpm	Dowell et al., 1987
	9[b]			20 wpm	58 wpm	
Symbion	50	>12	CID sentences	64%[c]	99%[c]	Dorman et al., 1989
Cochlear	13[a]	3	CID sentences	59%	88%	Dowell et al., 1987
	9[b]			47%	91%	
Cochlear	8[a]	3	CNC words	25%	50%	Dowell et al., 1985

[a]Patients using an earlier F0F2 speech coding scheme.
[b]Patients using an F0F1F2 speech coding scheme.
[c]Dorman et al. (1989) quote median scores rather than mean scores.
[d]wpm, words min⁻¹.

Table 9.3 for tactile device studies. The enhancements in Table 9.3 are smaller than those in Table 9.2 for comparable tests, with the exception of the speech tracking (De Filippo and Scott, 1978) result for one normally hearing subject reported by Brooks et al. (1986). Speech tracking and other assessments with lipreading tend not to be reported in the recent cochlear implant literature, having been replaced with hearing-alone measures, the results for which have improved as speech coding schemes

Table 9.3 Lipreading enhancement results from representative tactile speech processor studies

Number of channels	Number of subjects[b]	Training with device[a]	Test	Lipreading score	Lipreading + device score	Reference
1	1 deaf	50 h	Speech tracking	26 wpm[d]	35 wpm	Plant, 1986
	1 HI	12 min		40 wpm	56 wpm	Osberger, Rines-Weiss and Kalberer, 1986
1	2 deaf	10 h	Speech tracking	27 wpm	27 wpm	
	2 HI	6 h		34 wpm	41 wpm	
2	1 deaf	9 years[c]	Speech tracking	44 wpm	58 wpm	Cholewiak and Sherrick, 1986
8	7 NH	70 h	Speech tracking	36 wpm	55 wpm	Cowan et al., 1988
	4 HI	35 h		24 wpm	37 wpm	
	7 NH	70 h	CID sentences	54%	68%	
	4 HI	35 h		49%	70%	
8	7 NH	70 h	CNC words	24%	33%	Blamey et al., 1988
	4 HI	35 h		35%	41%	
16	1 NH	200 h	Speech tracking	14 wpm	50 wpm	Brooks et al., 1986
16	1 NH	15 h	Speech tracking	28 wpm	45 wpm	Weisenberger and Miller, 1987
	1 HI	15 h		30 wpm	46 wpm	
36	3 NH	20 h	Speech tracking	43 wpm	46 wpm	Sparks et al., 1979

[a]In some cases, hours of training are estimates.
[b]NH, Normally hearing subjects; HI, hearing-impaired subjects.
[c]Total time of use is given in years for the long-term tactile device user.
[d]wpm, words min⁻¹.

have evolved. It is likely that the lipreading enhancement with implants has also improved.

At the time of writing, financial costs of cochlear implantation in Melbourne are $A17 030 for the implant device and speech processor, $A2945 for surgery and hospitalisation, $A1440 for 12 visits to the clinic for initial programming of the implant speech processor and training, and an estimated annual cost of $A500 for batteries and maintenance. The large initial costs are usually covered by health insurance or the government funded public health scheme. The cost to the user may be up to 10% of the total cost. In comparison, a modestly successful tactile device, the Tactaid II, sells for about $A1200 in Australia. This cost would not be covered by most health insurance funds or by the public health scheme for adults. (In Australia, the National Acoustic Laboratories have supplied Tactaid II free of charge to children meeting their criteria for vibrotactile devices.) The costs of training and habilitation would be similar to those for the implant, but may extend over a much longer period because most postlinguistically deafened adult patients already have well-developed auditory speech perception skills that can be applied directly to an implant, but not to a tactile device. The cost of batteries and maintenance for a tactile device would be similar to that for the implant.

The 'costs' of an implant should also include the medical risks, the pain and inconvenience of surgery, the time and effort required to achieve improved speech recognition, and the cosmetic factors affecting the appearance and comfort of the patient while wearing the device. From this point of view, the tactile device has smaller risks, and no surgical costs. The cosmetic factors are probably similar or slightly better than for an implant that requires a microphone and connector or power transmission coil to be worn on the head. The time and effort required to achieve a substantial improvement in speech recognition with lipreading is greater for the tactile device than for the implant for postlinguistically deafened adults.

In summary, the superior benefits of a multichannel cochlear implant are sufficient to justify the costs for most postlinguistically deafened adults in Australia.

There is also a small number of postlinguistically deafened adults who do not meet criteria for cochlear implant selection because the cause of their deafness is more central (such as an acoustic neuroma) making stimulation of the acoustic nerve ineffective, or for general health reasons. Some potential patients may be unable to use an intracochlear multichannel implant because their cochleae have become obliterated by bone during deafness: these people would be limited to 'extracochlear' implants that are known to be less effective than intracochlear multichannel devices. There are also some potential patients who prefer not to have a cochlear implant operation for personal reasons, such as a preference for a 'non-invasive' approach to rehabilitation: the 'costs' of the implant are too great for these people. The 'costs' of a tactile device may also be too great, or the benefit too small, but this group must be considered a (small) potential market for tactile devices (Cowan et al., 1991).

Prelinguistically deafened adults

Prelinguistically deafened adults have no previously learned auditory skills, and the benefits of a cochlear implant are reduced accordingly. The costs remain the same, or are increased by the need for additional training over a longer period of time. Reports of speech recognition by prelinguistically deafened adults using cochlear implants usually indicate very little benefit (e.g. Clark et al., 1987). In addition to the lack of auditory skills, their communication needs and motivations may contribute to the poorer performance. Most adults will have well-developed alternative non-auditory communication methods such as signing, written messages or lipreading and, with the exception of lipreading, these methods are not easily supplemented by a new auditory (or tactile) input. Thus the prelinguistically deafened adult may have little need or motivation to learn a new communication method. However, there may still be a need for closer contact with the world through the detection and recognition of environmental sounds for safety (approaching vehicles or warning sirens) or for convenience in everyday life (whistling kettles or doorbells). There is no evidence that such sounds are more easily detected or recognised by these patients wearing cochlear implants than tactile devices. Tyler, Moore and Kuk (1989) have recently reported excellent results for recognition of a closed set of 18 environmental sounds for several selected groups of postlinguistically deafened adults using a variety of cochlear implant types; the authors are not aware of similar results for prelinguistically deafened adults. Quite inexpensive tactile devices can provide useful environmental sound detection and recognition (e.g. TAM, Summers, Peake and Martin, 1981; SIGNALON, Uvacek, Ye and Moschytz, 1988). Tactile devices may be more appropriate for the prelinguistically deafened adult because they are less expensive and provide similar benefits. It is also possible for stimulation of the undamaged tactile sense to provide more potentially useful information than stimulation of an impaired auditory system that may have suffered further atrophy through sensory deprivation since birth. This possibility is relevant to the coding of speech and environmental sounds for prelinguistically deafened adults and children.

The alternative communication methods listed above all rely on vision, so that prelinguistically deafened people with Usher's syndrome (a disease that commonly combines total deafness with a progressive loss of sight) have a strong reason to seek communication inputs through cochlear implants or tactile devices. For this reason, several Usher's syndrome patients in Melbourne have received cochlear implants. They have shown closed-set speech recognition abilities and improved speech recognition with lipreading, but no significant open-set speech recognition without lipreading (Blamey et al., 1991a). It is possible that similar results could have been obtained with a modern multichannel tactile device.

Profoundly-to-totally deaf children

There are at least two studies (Geers and Moog, 1989; Miyamoto et al., 1989) comparing tactile devices (Tactaid II, Audiological Engineering Limited, Somerville, MA, USA) with cochlear implants (House/3M; Cochlear 22-electrode implant, House Ear Institute, Los Angeles, CA, USA) for children in the USA. There is also a parallel development of multichannel cochlear implant and electrotactile speech processors for children and adults in progress at the University of Melbourne (Cowan et al., 1990; Blamey et al., 1991a; Dowell et al., 1991). A number of other studies have considered cochlear implants in isolation (e.g. Berliner et al., 1989; Tyler, 1990) or tactile devices in isolation (e.g. Goldstein and Proctor, 1985; Geers, 1986; Lynch et al., 1989). In general, the studies showed improved speech perception with either implants or tactile devices. The largest improvements occurred with implants although the results varied greatly between studies, and between children within studies. The largest published dataset (Berliner et al., 1989) showed that some children using the House/3M single-channel implant achieved limited open-set speech recognition without lipreading. The children with shorter duration of deafness who were enrolled in auditory/oral educational programmes were more likely to achieve this goal than children with longer duration of deafness or in total communication programmes. Tyler (1990) has reported

Table 9.4 Results of open-set tests for children in Melbourne using the cochlear implant without lipreading

Child	AB word score[a] (% phonemes correct)	BKB sentence score[b] (% key words correct)
I1	40	n.a.
I2	47	26
I3	43	34
I4	47	n.a.
I5	72	74
I6	15	0
I7	15	2
I8	n.a.	n.a.

[a]Boothroyd, 1968.
[b]Bench and Bamford, 1979.
n.a. Test not administered.

open-set speech recognition for five children implanted and trained in Sydney with the Cochlear 22-electrode implant, and similar results have been obtained in Melbourne (see Table 9.4). The studies using tactile devices have not reported open-set speech recognition, and preliminary reports from the comparative study (Miyamoto et al., 1989; Osberger, Robbins and Renshaw, 1990) indicated better results for the implant users on closed-set speech discrimination than for the Tactaid II users.

These results are consistent with the interpretation that children form a heterogeneous group including some who are similar to postlinguistically deafened adults, some who are similar to prelinguistically deafened adults, and some who are intermediate. The first group clearly benefit more from the cochlear implant than from a tactile device; the latter groups may obtain similar benefits from cochlear implants and tactile devices provided that both devices encode similar speech information. This is one weakness of the comparative studies using the Tactaid II as the tactile aid of choice: although the Tactaid II has been shown in some studies to provide improved lipreading scores, other tactile devices may convey more speech information (Plant, 1989). Other devices have not been used in comparative studies because they are not available in a commercial form.

In considering deaf children, the total monetary costs of cochlear implants and tactile devices are much greater than for adults because of the amount of time and effort that must be devoted to training them to use the devices effectively. The question of who pays for this training is an interesting one that may have different answers in different circumstances – the parents, educational authorities and clinical bodies may all contribute; the child must also pay a price, in terms of time involved in learning to use the devices. In many cases, parents prefer manual communication alternatives because they are likely to be easier and faster for the child to learn, and the time saved can be spent on normal educational requirements.

There are also emotional and ethical considerations associated with the use of cochlear implants and, to a lesser degree, tactile devices by children. Sometimes they may be at odds with established social patterns in the deaf community or in the child's peer group. The experimental nature of the devices and their unknown potential raise ethical issues that can be stressful for parents, children, teachers and other professionals involved. These indirect costs are likely to be greater for implants than for tactile devices, but should not be overlooked in considering either type of device.

Severely-to-profoundly hearing-impaired adults and children

Historically, cochlear implants and tactile devices have been designed to assist people with profound-to-total hearing losses; however, there is a large population of severely-to-profoundly hearing-impaired people using hearing aids who still have difficulty in understanding speech, particularly in noisy situations. One way to help these people is to supplement auditory and visual (lipreading) information with a tactile input (Cowan et al., 1989a; Lynch et al., 1989; Blamey et al., 1990a). In this case, the tactile processor will need to provide access to the higher frequency, lower amplitude sounds such as consonants that are most difficult for hearing-impaired listeners to detect and recognise. There are obvious ethical and practical reasons why cochlear implants may be less suitable than tactile devices: the implantation of electrodes into the cochlea may destroy residual hearing and prevent future use of a hearing aid, and it is more difficult to guarantee an improvement with the implant if the patient still has some useful hearing. A study of implant use by severely hearing-impaired patients has begun in the USA to address these issues (Food and Drug Administration Investigational Device Exemption no. G880038). In Melbourne, three patients with profound hearing impairment in both ears have been implanted in the poorer ear and are using a hearing aid in the unimplanted ear together with the cochlear implant. Thus, cochlear implants and tactile devices seem destined to compete in this population as well as in the profoundly-to-totally deaf population. No results have yet been published for the implant studies: the tactile results indicate substantial improvements in speech recognition when the tactile device is used to supplement residual hearing, or lipreading, or both.

On the basis of published results and ethical objections to implantation, a tactile device is at present the more appropriate option for this group. It is difficult to predict what is likely to happen in the future: the tactile device has the advantage that it is an additional input and does not require surgery; implants have the disadvantage that they must replace a partially functioning auditory input, but they can make use of already developed auditory speech recognition skills. It is likely that new tactile and implant speech processors will be designed specifically to supplement residual hearing, just as there are tactile and implant speech processors designed to supplement lipreading by coding fundamental frequency (Fourcin et al., 1983; Boothroyd and Hnath, 1986). If this can be done with a small and inexpensive tactile device, the cost saving might make this a more attractive option than a cochlear implant.

This group of potential tactile device and/or cochlear implant users is especially important from a commercial point of view because it represents a larger potential market than the profoundly deaf population (Thornton, 1986). This is more important for tactile devices than for cochlear implants if they are to compete on the basis of cost comparison. To make a fixed amount of profit with a less expensive device, the profit margin must be a larger percentage of sale price, or the sales volume must be greater than for a more expensive device. It would therefore be advantageous for a commercial tactile device to broach this market as quickly as possible.

The Devices

A variety of tactile devices and cochlear implants have been developed: single- and multichannel devices; intracochlear and extracochlear implants; electrotactile and vibrotactile devices; vocoders and feature-extracting processors. For a review of cochlear-implant speech-processor types, see Millar, Tong and Clark (1984) and Millar et al. (1986). The differences in design and construction lead to differences in effectiveness and cost. All of the devices allow detection of sound, and as they increase in complexity, the range of sounds that can be discriminated increases. The ranges of performance for tactile devices and cochlear implants overlap; it is quite possible for a multiple-channel tactile vocoder to provide better results than a single-channel cochlear implant in closed-set speech recognition tests. If compared on the initial financial outlay, the cost ranges do not overlap; the cost of any cochlear implant, implant speech processor, surgery, and hospitalisation is much greater than that of the most expensive tactile device.

It may be concluded from this that the benefit for a given cost is greater for tactile devices than for cochlear implants. However, this argument ignores several significant factors:

1. Multichannel cochlear implants have been shown to be more effective than tactile devices for postlinguistically deafened adults and children who achieve open-set word and sentence recognition without lipreading. For these patients, an equal result cannot be obtained with any device less expensive than a cochlear implant.
2. The cost of training and (re)habilitation: if the implant user has any prior auditory experience, this is likely to reduce the total cost of the implant relative to the total cost of an equivalent tactile device. If the user has no auditory experience, the training time for either device is likely to be quite long so that the initial outlay becomes relatively less important as a proportion of the total cost. Training also introduces variability into the benefit side of the cost-effectiveness relationship by increasing the effectiveness of the device. Oller, Payne and Gavin (1980) have shown that tactile devices can provide useful speech information at a phonetic level to minimally trained subjects, but many other studies have shown substantial gains over longer periods of training (e.g. Brooks et al., 1985; Alcantara et al., 1990). The cost of training in a one-to-one situation with a skilled clinician is very high. To minimise this cost, research into the relative effectiveness of different training methods is required. The development of automated training methods

is also likely to reduce the cost of this component. As training costs are reduced and effectiveness increased, the tactile and implant options will both be enhanced, although the tactile options will probably be affected more.

3. The third factor ignored by the simple analysis above is 'who pays?' Most of the initial cost of cochlear prostheses is likely to be covered by health insurance or government funding, but such funding is more difficult to obtain for tactile devices (in Australia and the USA at least) and so the cost to the user may be greater for the tactile device than the cochlear implant. Without new provision for funding, the market may be reduced to a level that is not commercially viable for any of the more complex multiple-channel tactile devices currently under development. In this context, it is interesting to note that the largest customers of the most successful tactile device manufacturer, Audiological Engineering Limited, are the government-funded National Acoustic Laboratories, who supply the Tactaid II free of charge to profoundly hearing-impaired children in Australia.

4. The human cost in terms of comfort, appearance, safety, and preference: this factor is likely to have a large effect, especially if the monetary cost to the user is similar for different devices. The risk and discomfort of the implant operation is balanced to some extent by the preference for a 'more natural' auditory input. Implant devices also have an advantage over tactile devices in that the present sales are larger, allowing greater expenditure on cosmetic aspects and miniaturisation. To match this level of appearance and comfort with any new tactile processor would require considerable expense.

5. The fifth and final factor is availability. Cochlear implants exist as effective and well-established products. Some tactile devices are on the market, but tend to be the simpler ones that have not produced speech perception results as good as those reported in research studies of multiple-channel devices that are not yet commercially available. Until potential users have easy access to such a device, choices are limited to the relatively expensive and more effective implants, or the less expensive but less beneficial tactile devices.

Comparison of a Cochlear Implant and a Tactile Device

The 22-electrode cochlear implant manufactured by Cochlear Pty Ltd in Australia and marketed by Cochlear Pty Ltd in Australia and Asia, Cochlear Corporation in USA, and Cochlear AG in Europe, was first developed in the Department of Otolaryngology at the University of Melbourne in the 1970s (Tong et al., 1979; Clark et al., 1984). Since its commercialisation, biological, psychophysical, speech processing and clinical studies have continued. The implant has now been approved by the Food and Drug Administration in the USA for use with profoundly deaf adults and children down to the age of 2 years. Over 2500 implants of this type have been sold throughout the world. In 1984, a cochlear implant speech processor was modified to stimulate using electrodes on the fingers instead of in the cochlea (Blamey and Clark, 1985). This electrotactile speech processor was named the 'Tickle-Talker' and has been evaluated in biological, psychophysical, speech processing and clinical studies similar in many ways to the implant studies.

The 22-electrode cochlear implant

The implant receiver/stimulator is a sealed container connected to a circular coil and an electrode array. The array of 22 platinum band electrodes spaced at intervals of 0.75 mm along a Silastic tube is surgically inserted into the scala tympani of the cochlea through the round window. The electrical stimulus is generated by a silicon chip inside the sealed container that is placed in a bed drilled into the mastoid bone behind the ear. Power and control signals are transmitted through the skin by radio waves that are picked up by the coil of the receiver/stimulator.

Speech is encoded as a series of biphasic electrical pulses inside the cochlea that produce hearing sensation by stimulating residual auditory nerve fibres. The electric current flows between selected pairs of electrodes within the scala tympani. The electrodes are usually selected in a bipolar-plus-one configuration such that an inactive electrode lies between the two active electrodes in each pair, yielding a total of 20 (overlapping) pairs along the 22-electrode array. The electrode pairs are numbered from 1 to 20 in order from the basal (high frequency) to the apical (low frequency) end of the electrode array. Psychophysical research has shown that the different electrode pairs produce sensations of different 'place pitch' or 'sharpness' according to a tonotopic ordering of nerves depending on their position in the cochlea, and that different electrical pulse rates produce a sensation of 'rate pitch' (Tong and Clark, 1985). The loudness of the sensation depends mainly on the charge per pulse, which can be varied by changing the electric current level or the duration of the pulse. These stimulus parameters are used to encode speech parameters according to the scheme outlined in Table 9.5. Typically, electrode pairs 20 to 14 are used to code first formant (F1) frequencies and pairs 14 to 7 are used to code second formant frequency (F2). Charge per pulse on electrode pairs 7, 4, and 1 are used to code A3, A4 and A5 respectively. In each period corresponding to the voice fundamental frequency (F0) four electrode pairs are stimulated, corresponding to F1, F2, A3 and A4. For voiceless sounds, the pulse rate is pseudo-random, and four electrode pairs are stimulated to code F2, A3,

Table 9.5 MPEAK speech coding scheme used in the latest processor for the Cochlear 22-electrode cochlear implant

Speech parameter	Electrical parameter	Sensation
Fundamental frequency, F0	Pulse rate	Rate pitch
First formant frequency, F1[a]	Apical electrode position	Lower place pitch
First formant amplitude, A1[a]	Charge per pulse	Loudness
Second formant frequency, F2	Basal electrode position	Higher place pitch
Second formant amplitude, A2	Charge per pulse	Loudness
Amplitude 2–3 kHz, A3	Charge/pulse on electrode 7[c]	Loudness
Amplitude 3–4 kHz, A4	Charge/pulse on electrode 4[c]	Loudness
Amplitude 4–6 kHz, A5[b]	Charge/pulse on electrode 1[c]	Loudness

[a]F1 and A1 are presented only for voiced sounds.
[b]A5 is presented only for voiceless sounds.
[c]Electrodes 1, 4 and 7 are at the more basal or higher pitched end of the electrode array.

A4 and A5. Thus stimulation of a low-pitched electrode pair for F1 indicates a voiced sound, and stimulation of electrode pair 1 indicates a voiceless sound.

The speech parameters are obtained from the acoustic speech signal picked up by a behind-the-ear directional microphone. The signal is analysed by a digital signal processor that measures the amplitudes and frequencies of peaks in the speech waveform, and the fundamental frequency or voice pitch. The speech processor in use at the time of writing is known as the MSP processor (for miniature speech processor, and/or multiple-peak speech processor). This processor was released by Cochlear Pty Ltd in November 1989 to replace the previous WSP3 (wearable speech processor) that was larger and did not measure as many speech parameters. Both processors use the same implanted receiver/stimulator.

The Tickle-Talker

The Tickle-Talker is an eight-electrode electrotactile speech processor, also developed at the University of Melbourne, invented in 1984 for use as a control device in a study of the cochlear implant with deaf children. The experimental design of the study required an initial preoperative period in which the children would be trained with the control device. This scheme turned out to be impractical because of difficulties in fitting and maintaining the electrotactile device on children, and the short time constraints in carrying out the implant study. However, initial speech perception results for normally hearing adults were sufficiently encouraging for a separate trial to be funded by the Australian Commonwealth Department of Industry, Technology and Commerce, who had previously funded initial trials of the cochlear implant. Results from this trial, and from subsequent studies are described below. At present no commercial version of the Tickle-Talker is available.

Novel aspects of the Tickle-Talker compared with previous tactile devices are the speech coding scheme and the electrical stimulation of nerve bundles in the fingers. Electrical stimulation was chosen in preference to vibration in order to minimise power requirements and size of the wearable device. The site of stimulation was chosen to take advantage of the superior tactile capabilities of the hands and the logically ordered array of nerve bundles in the fingers; initial studies had shown that stimulation of nerve bundles produced a more comfortable sensation than stimulation of nerve endings in the skin (Blamey and Clark, 1987). The design criteria used were based on recommendations by Spens (1980) and Sherrick (1984) that tactile devices should use multiple transducers, preferably on the hand, with processing to match the sensory properties of the tactile sense, and should be wearable to create an opportunity for extended use by hearing-impaired people.

The tactile processor is very similar in concept to the cochlear implant and uses the same processing to measure speech parameters that are then encoded in terms of biphasic electrical pulses to the finger electrodes. Table 9.6 shows the tactile speech coding scheme. The scheme used by the Tickle-Talker is much simpler than the present MSP cochlear-implant coding scheme, but is almost identical to an earlier 'F0F2' coding scheme used with the implant. The reasons for this are partly historical, because it was considered more important to investigate the clinical usefulness of a scheme that had been demonstrated to work with the implant, and partly practical because of the smaller number of electrodes in the tactile device. Newer coding schemes providing F1, voiced/voiceless information, and high frequency amplitude are now being investigated, but no speech perception results are yet available. The Tickle-Talker is usually used with an omnidirectional lapel microphone because many of the users have some residual hearing and use the device in combination with behind-the-ear hearing aids.

Table 9.6 F0F2 speech coding scheme used in the Tickle-Talker speech processor

Speech parameter	Electrical parameter	Sensation
Fundamental frequency, F0	Pulse rate[a]	Roughness
Second formant frequency, F2	Electrode position	Place of stimulation
Speech amplitude, A0	Charge per pulse	Strength of sensation

[a]The pulse rate used is approximately half of the fundamental frequency of the voice because changes of rate above about 150 pulses s^{-1} produce no noticeable changes in electrotactile sensation.

Psychophysical comparison of devices

In comparing potential benefits of the cochlear implant and Tickle-Talker, the difficulty lies in choosing a fair basis on which to make the comparison, because there are no tactile equivalents to the postlinguistically deafened adults who do so well with the cochlear implant. Similarly, many of the better results with tactile devices have been obtained with normally hearing subjects, and there are no equivalent results for implants. On the other hand, it hardly seems fair to compare the two devices on the basis of results for children and adults who have used them for a limited time and may improve considerably in the future. Comparisons of psychophysical results and speech feature recognition, rather than word and sentence recognition, involve less linguistic processing and are therefore less affected by learning effects. However, the main objective is to improve speech communication skills, and these are best measured using word and sentence testing. Comparisons will therefore be made from a variety of points of view and the implications of the results defined as precisely as possible.

The first point of view is the psychophysical one. Previous reviews (Geldard, 1960; Kirman, 1973; Sherrick, 1984) have compared the discrimination and recognition of tactile and auditory stimuli with the aim of assessing the possibility of transmitting speech information by the sense of touch. Although some differences between the senses have been found, none of the reviewers found reason to doubt that speech information could be conveyed by touch. Comparisons of psychophysical results for the implant and Tickle-Talker yield even closer results because of the similar electrical stimuli and the impairment of the auditory sense relative to normal hearing. Detailed comparisons have been published elsewhere (Blamey and Clark, 1987; Blamey et al., 1990) and are summarised here.

The dynamic range of electrical stimulation of the auditory and tactile nerves is approximately equal, with values of 6–12 dB being most common and larger ranges occurring for some subjects. Discrimination of different intensities indicates a difference limen of about one-third of a decibel, so that a dynamic range of 10 dB would correspond to about 30 'just-noticeable' steps for both senses. Absolute identification of stimuli differing in intensity (charge per pulse) across the full dynamic range also indicates similar sensitivity.

Identification of the position of stimulation (electrode identification) is almost perfect for the eight electrodes of the Tickle-Talker. In a similar experiment using the implant, some patients could identify electrodes very well when they were separated reasonably widely in the cochlea, but had difficulty when the electrodes were close together (Tong and Clark, 1985). Thus the smaller number of electrodes in the tactile device is compensated for by the better electrode identification on the fingers.

Pulse rate identification and discrimination have been found to vary widely with the Tickle-Talker. In general, the better tactile subjects had results close to the average cochlear implant patients for pulse rates less than about 150 pulses s^{-1}. Above this rate, further increases in pulse rate produced little perceptible change in the sensation. A similar saturation occurs for implant patients, but at a higher rate, typically about 300 pulses s^{-1}.

Discrimination and identification of duration for streams of pulses were similar for electrotactile and electroauditory stimuli. Gap detection is another measure of temporal processing that has been found to correlate with some speech test results (Tyler et al., 1982; Hochmair-Desoyer, Hochmair and Stiglbrunner, 1985). Gap detection with the implant is easier than with the Tickle-Talker, but both devices allow detection of gaps of about 10 ms or less in streams of pulses.

These psychophysical results indicate that neither device is capable of providing the same degree of accuracy in amplitude, spectral or temporal judgments as normal hearing; nevertheless, the results are close enough to suggest that similar levels of speech recognition are achievable. The poorer perception of pulse rate differences with the Tickle-Talker suggests that perception of fundamental frequency variations is likely to be poorer with the Tickle-Talker than with the implant.

As indicated earlier, the people for whom a tactile device may be most suitable include prelinguistically hearing-impaired adults and profoundly-to-totally deaf children. Psychophysical studies on implant patients from these groups indicate that they have poorer auditory skills than postlinguistically deafened adult patients (Tong, Busby and Clark, 1988). This may arise from the unfamiliarity of the auditory sensations, atrophy or imperfect development of auditory neural processes, or from degeneration of physical structures within the cochlea. None of these considerations apply to the tactile sense, which is fully developed and functional in these groups. It is likely, therefore, that a tactile device may offer real advantages over a cochlear implant in terms of the information carrying potential of the two devices.

Speech feature recognition

The second comparison is from the point of view of transmission of segmental speech information. This has been assessed with identical closed-set vowel and consonant recognition tests in the two devices (Blamey et al., 1987, 1988). The Tickle-Talker subjects were seven normally hearing adults who had received 70 hours of speech perception training, and four hearing-impaired adults who had received 35 hours of training plus some everyday use. The implant results are for patients following 3 months of everyday use with the F0F2 and F0F1F2 coding schemes. In the case of the MPEAK coding scheme, the four patients had

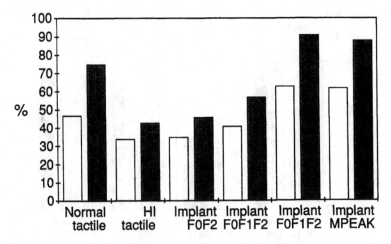

Figure 9.1 Percentage correct scores for closed-set vowel ■ and consonant □ recognition using the Tickle-Talker and the 22-electrode cochlear implant without lip reading. Tactile results are shown for seven normally hearing adults who had 70 h training (Normal), and four hearing-impaired adults who had 35 h training (HI). Results are also given for three speech coding schemes with the implant, and for three groups of patients. The first two groups were tested 3 months after implantation with the F0F2 (n = 13 and n =11 for consonants and vowels, respectively) and F0F1F2 (n = 5 and n = 6, respectively) schemes. The third group (n = 4) were tested with the F0F1F2 and MPEAK coding schemes after 1.5-5 years' implant experience.

1.1-4.5 years' experience with the F0F1F2 coding scheme, and 3-6 months' experience with the MPEAK coding scheme.

The vowel test consisted of 11 vowels spoken in /hVd/ context ('hid, head, had, hud, hod, hood, heed, heard, hard, who'd, hoard'). The consonant test consisted of 12 consonants in /aCa/ context (p, b, m, s, z, f, v, t, d, k, g, n). The items were presented four times each in random order by an audiologist who was familiar to the subjects. No lipreading was used. Feedback was given after each item.

Figure 9.1 shows the results for the different subject groups. Results for three different speech processors are shown for the implant patients. The F0F2 coding scheme is the one closest to the Tickle-Talker coding scheme. The F0F1F2 scheme includes the first formant frequency coded as a second electrode in addition to the electrode representing F2. The MPEAK scheme includes stimulation of three higher pitched (basal) electrodes in the cochlea to represent the amplitude of high frequency regions of the speech spectrum as shown in Table 9.5.

The results show that the Tickle-Talker and implant provide similar amounts of segmental speech information when the same speech parameters are coded. When additional parameters are coded by the implant, the segmental information is increased. The direct comparison of F0F1F2 and MPEAK coding schemes for the same four patients showed no

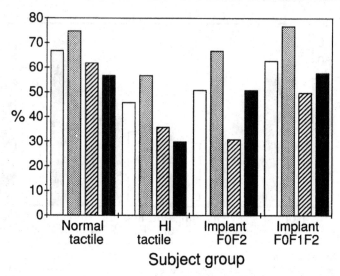

Figure 9.2 Percentages of information transmitted for vowel features using the Tickle-Talker and the 22-electrode cochlear implant without lipreading. Tactile results are shown for seven normally hearing adults who had 70 h training (Normal), and four hearing-impaired adults who had 35 h training (HI). Results are also given for two groups of implant patients who were tested 3 months after implantation with the F0F2 (*n* = 13) and F0F1F2 (*n* = 7) schemes. □, Total; ▨, duration; ▨, F1; ■, F2.

difference in the scores for vowels and consonants. The large difference in the F0F1F2 scores for the two implant groups is due to the selection of patients with more implant experience (18 months to 5 years) with good speech recognition scores for this study. The other groups of implant patients were not selected in this way, and had only 3 months of implant use. The differences between the two tactile groups and between the two implant groups tested with the F0F1F2 coding scheme illustrate the variations that may arise when devices are compared using groups of subjects with different histories and experience.

Information transmission analyses shown in Figures 9.2 and 9.3 show similar patterns for the two devices when similar speech processing strategies are employed. Improvements in the implant speech coding scheme have improved perception at the feature level, but it is not known whether similar improvements will occur for changes in the Tickle-Talker encoding.

Comparative results for tests of suprasegmental speech information from the Minimal Auditory Capabilities (MAC) Battery (Owens et al., 1981) are shown in Figure 9.4. This figure indicates some differences between the devices: in particular, the implant patients performed much better on male/female speaker identification than the Tickle-Talker subjects. This difference may be due to the poorer tactile pulse rate discrimination noted above.

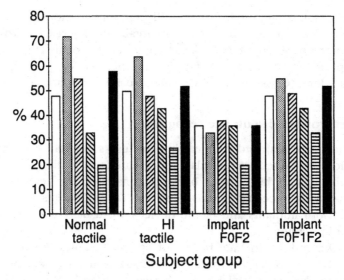

Figure 9.3 Percentages of information transmitted for consonant features using the Tickle-Talker and the 22-electrode cochlear implant without lipreading. Tactile results are shown for seven normally hearing adults who had 70 h training (Normal), and four hearing-impaired adults who had 35 h training (HI). Results are also given for two gropus of implant patients who were tested 3 months after implantation with the F0F2 ($n = 11$) and F0F1F2 ($n = 8$) schemes. □, Total; ▨, voicing; ▧, Nasality; ▨, affrication; ▤, place; ■, amplitude envelope.

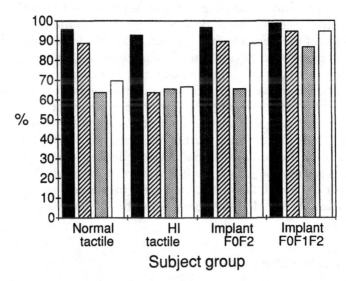

Figure 9.4 Percentage scores on prosodic tests from the Minimal Auditory Capabilities Battery for Tickle-Talker and cochlear implant users without lipreading. Tactile results are shown for seven normally hearing adults who had 70 h training (Normal), and four hearing-impaired adults who had 35 h training (HI). Results are also given for two groups of implant patients who were tested 3 months after implantation with the F0F2 ($n = 13$) and F0F1F2 ($n = 9$) schemes. ■, One/two syllables; ▧, same/different spondee; ▨, question/statement; □, male/female.

The results illustrate the fact that tactile and implant devices can convey speech information in similar ways to obtain similar results. Vowel and consonant recognition of early-deafened users of cochlear implants are usually poorer than those shown in the figures for postlinguistically deafened adults (Clark et al., 1987; Tong, Busby and Clark, 1988).

Open-set word and sentence recognition

Postlinguistically deafened cochlear implant users commonly obtain some recognition of open-set words and sentences without lipreading. Comparable results have never been demonstrated for hearing-impaired users of a tactile speech processor, and the Tickle-Talker is no exception. However, both implants and tactile devices are usually used in combination with lipreading.

Tables 9.2 and 9.3 include results of open-set Central Institute for the Deaf (CID) sentences (Tonnison, 1974) and Consonant-Nucleus-Consonant (CNC) monosyllabic words (Peterson and Lehiste, 1962) with the cochlear implant and Tickle-Talker for adult subjects. Some of the results for speech tracking, CID sentences, and CNC words from Dowell et al. (1985; Dowell, Mecklenburg and Clark, 1986) were obtained using the F0F2 encoding scheme similar to the Tickle-Talker speech encoding scheme. In every case, the lipreading enhancement was greater for the implant than for the Tickle-Talker, regardless of whether the enhancement is expressed as the difference between the scores in the two conditions, or as a ratio of the lipreading plus device score divided by the score with lipreading only. In comparing the open-set scores, the differences in experience between the postlinguistically deafened cochlear implant patients and the incompletely trained tactile subjects must be taken into account. Although the results indicate a clear advantage to the implant users, there are several unanswered questions about the potential benefit from the Tickle-Talker: after further training, would the tactile scores improve? If the Tickle-Talker users had experienced tactile speech inputs as children learning language, would their scores be greater? If the coding scheme for the Tickle-Talker included extra parameters as in the implant MSP processor, would the improvement be as great as it is for the implant?

Results with children

Quite recently, results have become available for groups of children using the cochlear implant (Blamey et al., 1991a) and the Tickle-Talker (Cowan et al., 1990). These studies include results for similar test protocols. In one way, these data are critical for any comparison of tactile and implant devices because the overwhelming effect of prior auditory experience is

Table 9.7 Details for eight implanted children (see text)

Child	Aetiology	Onset of profound loss (years; months)	Duration of profound deafness (years; months)	Educational programme	Age at implantation (years; months)	Duration of implant use (years; months)
I1	Meningitis	3;3	6;9	Auditory/oral	10;2	3;10
I2	Meningitis	3;0	2;5	Cueing supplement	5;5	3;1
I3	Unknown	Congenital	8;0	Cueing supplement	8;0	2;5
I4	Meningitis	2;4	5;10	Auditory/oral	8;2	1;10
I5	Cytomegalovirus	Progressive left ear	6;10	Auditory/oral	14;8	1;5
		Progressive right ear	0;7			
I6	Usher's syndrome	Congenital	14;11	Cueing supplement	14;11	2;2
I7	Mondini malformation	Congenital	14;8	Total communication	14;8	2;9
I8	Meningitis	1;4	12;7	Cueing supplement	13;11	5;7

Table 9.8 Details of the eight children using the Tickle-Talker (see text)

Child	Aetiology	Age at onset of profound loss	Duration of Tickle Talker use (years; months)	Educational programme	Age (years)
T1	Unknown	Birth	2;10	Aural/oral	13
T2	Unknown	Birth	2;10	Integrated with signed English	13
T3	Unknown	Birth	2;10	Aural/oral	10
T4	Genetic	Birth	2;10	Cueing supplement	10
T5	Rubella	Birth	2;10	Cueing supplement	10
T6	Viral	2 years	2;10	Cueing supplement	10
T7	Unknown	Birth	0;10	Cueing supplement	8
T8	Unknown	Birth	0;10	Cueing supplement	13

Table 9.9 Pure-tone hearing thresholds in the better ear in dB HL re: ANSI-1969 for the 16 children whose results are shown in Figure 9.5[a]

Child[b]	Frequency (Hz)				
	250	500	1000	2000	4000
I1	85	NR	NR	NR	NR
I2	85	110	NR	NR	NR
I3	85	100	110	120	NR
I4	70	110	110	115	115
I5	NR	NR	120	115	NR
I6	NR	NR	NR	NR	NR
I7	NR	NR	NR	NR	NR
I8	85	100	NR	NR	NR
T1	100	100	105	105	105
T2	100	100	110	115	115
T3	90	100	110	120	115
T4	110	NR	NR	NR	NR
T5	90	100	110	115	NR
T6	75	95	105	115	105
T7	85	100	105	110	110
T8	100	105	105	115	110

[a]The values for implanted children were measured preoperatively.
[b]Children I4 and T1–T8 continue to use hearing aids in addition to their devices.
NR, No threshold was reached at the output limit of the audiometer.

not present, and the conditions for comparison are more evenly matched. On the other hand, any evaluation of the speech perception of hearing-impaired children is complicated by the developing nature of their speech perception, production and language skills. It is therefore impossible to establish a static level of performance on which to base the comparison. There are other factors, such as educational programme, audiological history and parental support, that may affect the results. The group of implanted children listed in Table 9.7 includes all children implanted for at least 1 year with sufficient spoken language to attempt an open-set sentence test (BKB sentences, Bench and Bamford, 1979). Similarly, the group of young Tickle-Talker users listed in Table 9.8 includes all children who have used the device in Melbourne for at least 1 year and have been tested with the same open-set test. These groups were not matched in other respects.

The preoperative hearing thresholds in the better ear are given for each child in Table 9.9. Child I4 has continued to use a hearing aid in the unimplanted ear, and all children using the Tickle-Talker also wear hearing aids. Figure 9.5 shows the results on the open-set BKB sentence test in the combined lipreading plus device conditions, including the use of hearing aids for the children that wear them. Also included in the figure is the score without the Tickle-Talker or implant, so that the

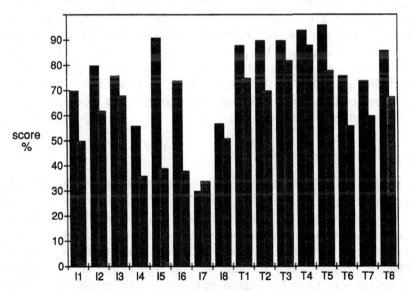

Figure 9.5 Percentage correct scores on the open-set BKB sentence test for eight implanted children and eight children who are Tickle-Talker users. Scores are shown for lipreading plus the device (plus hearing aids if they were usually worn) ■ and for lipreading (plus hearing aids) but without the device ▨.

contribution of the device can be evaluated. Comparison of the overall aided performance suggests that the Tickle-Talker users are performing at a higher level than the implant users (t=2.773, df=14, P=0.015). Three of the implant users (I2, I3, and I5) are able to score on this test without lipreading, scoring 26, 34, and 74% respectively; none of the Tickle-Talker users has attempted this test without lip reading. The 'without device' scores for the Tickle-Talker users in Figure 9.5 are also higher than for the implant users because of the contribution made by the hearing aids (t=4.219, df=14, P=0.001). The lipreading enhancement (expressed as the difference between the two scores for each child) is not significantly different for the two groups (t=0.745, df=14, P=0.469). Child I5 is clearly the one who gains most benefit from the device. This child had a progressive profound hearing loss for 6 years before suffering a sudden total loss of hearing 7 months before implantation at the age of 15 years. In many respects, I5 is closer to the postlinguistically deafened adult patients than to the other children. Further comparisons based on other speech tests have been included in Cowan et al. (1990), but do not alter the conclusion that may be drawn from the BKB sentence results, which is that the Tickle-Talker, used with hearing aids, offers as great an improvement to most children and adolescents as the cochlear implant. This result must be considered a preliminary one because of the highly variable implant results, and the fact that the children in both groups are likely to achieve better speech perception results in the next few years. The unmatched nature of the two groups may also act in favour of one group or the other, depending on the relative importance of the different factors such as age, educational programme, and residual hearing levels. It is clear, however, that both devices offer potential benefits to children and it is important that both should be developed to the stage where they are freely available to suitably selected children. The implant has progressed much further than the Tickle-Talker in achieving this goal.

Summary

The results indicate that postlinguistically deafened adult cochlear implant patients perform better on all open-set tests, with and without lipreading, than normally hearing or hearing-impaired adults using the Tickle-Talker. In the case of children who do not have good speech and language skills, the comparison is not so clear cut. The Tickle-Talker and the implant both provide improved speech recognition with lipreading, at similar levels. The implant also provides limited open-set speech recognition without lipreading for children who have been profoundly deaf for a short time. For children and adults who cannot have, or do not want, an implant the Tickle-Talker is a viable alternative.

Costs of the two devices

The cost of the cochlear implant for a postlinguistically deafened adult has been described earlier. The cost for a child includes the same components, with the addition of a much higher cost for (re)habilitation, extending over several years. The additional time appears necessary to fit the device effectively and to maintain appropriate auditory input to the child while spoken language becomes established.

The Tickle Talker is not commercially available, although it has been used on an everyday basis in Melbourne by five adults and 15 children. The device was provided free to these users. The expected cost of the device is probably $A4000–6000. Although this is relatively expensive compared with simpler tactile devices on the market, its performance is also better (Cowan et al., 1989b). The Tickle-Talker also incorporates similar speech processing hardware to the cochlear implant speech processor which is sold for $A6600 (without the implantable receiver/stimulator). Added to the cost of the device is the cost of (re)habilitation and audiological support similar to the services required for children using the cochlear implant.

Costs for the Tickle-Talker and the implant will be affected greatly by market forces such as sales volume, and support by health insurance companies and government health schemes. At present, implants have gained a significant advantage over tactile devices from a commercial point of view. They are likely to increase this advantage unless industry and/or government funding can be found to develop a truly wearable and effective tactile device to the stage where it can be marketed widely and profitably.

From the point of view of non-monetary costs, such as inconvenience, stress, disruption of normal routine, and medical risk, the Tickle-Talker has obvious advantages over the implant. These differences will always remain, but are likely to be reduced in importance as the potential benefits of cochlear implants in children become better known and the procedures for selection, implantation and (re)habilitation are refined. Cosmetically, both devices incur a definite cost, one being worn on the hand, and the other worn on the head with a cord connected to a body-worn processor. The inconvenience of the devices has been reduced sufficiently, and the appearance improved sufficiently for them both to be accepted for everyday use by children and adults. Further reductions in size and weight will undoubtedly occur in the next few years.

The Future

In the authors' opinions, present knowledge supports the following statements:

1. Cochlear implants are more suitable than tactile devices for most postlinguistically profoundly deafened adults and children.
2. Tactile devices can be an effective supplement to lipreading and residual hearing for postlinguistically profoundly deafened adults and children who cannot or will not have a cochlear implant. Considerable training is required to achieve good speech perception results on open-set tests in combination with lipreading.
3. For profoundly deaf children and adults with little prior auditory experience, multiple-channel tactile devices can be as effective as multichannel cochlear implants when used with lipreading or in closed-set perception tasks, provided that they encode similar speech information. Considerable training is required to achieve good open-set speech perception results in combination with lipreading.
4. Tactile devices can be used effectively to supplement hearing aids and lipreading for severely-to-profoundly hearing-impaired children and adults without affecting their residual hearing.
5. Cochlear implants have greater sales at present, are technically more sophisticated, and are developing faster than tactile devices. This gives cochlear implants a real commercial advantage.
6. Tactile devices are less expensive than cochlear implants. When the cost to the user is considered, and (re)habilitation is included, the costs of the two device types may be much more similar, or even reversed.

These statements are different from the conclusions reached in an earlier comparison of implants and tactile devices by Pickett and McFarland (1985). Both types of device have changed, with implants progressing more rapidly than tactile devices, and with market forces playing a much more significant role. These trends are likely to continue, with tactile devices becoming a 'second best' option unless research and development efforts can be intensified to match the cochlear implant progress. Sherrick (1984) identified a crucial need for wearable tactile processors to provide opportunities for long-term use. The situation has changed a little with the Tactaid I and II and a number of other relatively simple tactile devices on the market, but not enough to match the levels of speech information potentially available from cochlear implants. To do this, small multichannel tactile devices are required.

Apart from direct competition with cochlear implant technology, several other avenues for tactile device development are being pursued.

● The first is development of single-channel devices for purposes other than speech perception. There seems to be a need for this type of device, and a tactile device is less expensive, more easily accessible, and possibly just as effective as a cochlear implant. As multichannel implants and tactile devices become more effective, it seems likely that fewer people will be satisfied with a device that does not help communication as well as awareness of sound.

● The second avenue for development is as a multimodal speech perception aid. Many authors have suggested this possibility and there is no reason why tactile information could not be integrated with auditory information from a hearing aid or cochlear implant as well as lip reading. A logical step in this direction is the introduction of tactile devices specifically designed to complement auditory devices, or even incorporating auditory output signals derived from the same processor.

Acknowledgements

Many people from the Department of Otolaryngology at the University of Melbourne and from Cochlear Pty Ltd in Sydney have contributed to the results for implants and tactile devices reported in this chapter. Their input is gladly acknowledged by the authors. In particular, Joseph Alcantara, Lesley Whitford, Julia Sarant and Karyn Galvin have made important contributions to the Tickle-Talker research. Financial support for the research has come from many sources, including the National Health and Medical Research Council of Australia; the Commonwealth Department of Industry, Technology and Commerce; the Commonwealth Department of Employment, Education and Training; Cochlear Pty Ltd; the Victorian Lions Foundation; the Victorian Deafness Foundation; and the Australian Bionic Ear and Hearing Institute.

References

ALCANTARA, J.I., COWAN, R.S.C., BLAMEY, P.J. and CLARK, G.M. (1990). A comparison of two training strategies for speech recognition with an electrotactile speech processor. *J. Speech Hear. Res.* **33**, 195-204.

BENCH, J. and BAMFORD, J. (1979). *Speech-hearing tests and the spoken language of hearing-impaired children.* London: Academic Press.

BERLINER, K.I., TONOKAWA, L.L., DYE, L.M. and HOUSE, W.F. (1989). Open-set speech recognition in children with a single-channel cochlear implant. *Ear Hear.* **10**, 237-242.

BLAMEY, P.J. and CLARK, G.M. (1985). A wearable multiple-electrode electrotactile speech processor for the profoundly deaf. *J. Acoust. Soc. Am.* **77**, 1619-1620.

BLAMEY, P.J. and CLARK, G.M. (1987). Psychophysical studies relevant to the design of a digital electrotactile speech processor. *J. Acoust. Soc. Am.* **82**, 116-125.

BLAMEY, P.J., COWAN, R.S.C., ALCANTARA, J.I. and CLARK, G.M. (1988). Phonemic information transmitted by a multichannel electrotactile speech processor. *J. Speech Hear. Res.* **31**, 620-629.

BLAMEY, P.J., DOWELL, R.C., BROWN, A.M., CLARK, G.M. and SELIGMAN, P.M. (1987). Vowel and consonant recognition of cochlear implant patients using formant-estimating speech processors. *J. Acoust. Soc. Am.* **82**, 48-57.

BLAMEY, P.J., COWAN, R.S.C., ALCANTARA, J.I., WHITFORD, L.A. and CLARK, G.M. (1990a). Speech perception using combinations of auditory, visual, and tactile information. *J. Rehab. Res. Dev.* **26**, 15-24.

BLAMEY, P.J., ALCANTARA, J.I., COWAN, R.S.C., GALVIN, K.L., SARANT, J.Z. and CLARK, G.M. (1990b). Perception of amplitude envelope variations of pulsatile electrotactile stimuli. *J. Acoust. Soc. Am.* **88**, 1765-1772.

BLAMEY, P.J., DAWSON, P.W., ROWLAND, L.C., DETTMANN, S.J., CLARK, G.M., BUSBY, P.A., BROWN, A.M., DOWELL, R.C. and RICKARDS, F.W.R. (1991a). Speech perception, production, and language results in a group of children using the 22-electrode cochlear implant. In: *Proceedings of the International Conference on Tactile Aids, Hearing Aids, and Cochlear Implants*, Sydney, May 1-3, 1990.

BLAMEY, P.J., PYMAN, B.C., GORDON, M., CLARK, G.M., BROWN, A.M., DOWELL, R.C. and HOLLOW, R.D. (1991b). Factors predicting postoperative sentence scores in postlinguistically deaf adult cochlear implant patients. *Ann. Otol. Rhinol. Laryngol.* (in press).

BOOTHROYD, A. (1968). Developments in speech audiometry. *Sound* 2, 3-10.

BOOTHROYD, A. and HNATH, T. (1986). Lipreading with tactile supplements. *J. Rehab. Res. Dev.* 23, 139-146.

BROOKS, P.L., FROST, B.J., MASON, J.L. and CHUNG, K. (1985). Acquisition of a 250-word vocabulary through a tactile vocoder. *J. Acoust. Soc. Am.* 77, 1576-1579.

BROOKS, P.L., FROST, B.J., MASON, J.L. and GIBSON, D.M. (1986). Continuing evaluation of the Queen's University Tactile Vocoder. II. Identification of open-set sentences and tracking narrative. *J. Rehab. Res. Dev.* 23, 129-138.

BROWN, A.M., DOWELL, R.C., CLARK, G.M., MARTIN, L.F.A. and PYMAN, B.C. (1985a). Selection of patients for multiple channel cochlear implants. In: Schindler, R.A. and Merzenich, M.M. (eds), *Cochlear Implants*. New York: Raven Press, pp. 403-405.

BROWN, A.M., CLARK, G.M., DOWELL, R.C., MARTIN, L.F.A. and SELIGMAN, P.M. (1985b). Telephone use by a multi-channel cochlear implant patient: An evaluation using open-set CID sentences. *J. Laryngol. Otol.* 99, 231-238.

CHOLEWIAK, R.W. and SHERRICK, C.E. (1986). Tracking skill of a deaf person with long-term tactile aid experience: A case study. *J. Rehab. Res. Dev.* 23, 20-26.

CLARK, G.M., TONG, Y.C., PATRICK, J.F., SELIGMAN, P.M., CROSBY, P.A., KUZMA, J.A. and MONEY, D.K. (1984). A multi-channel hearing prosthesis for profound-to-total hearing loss. *J. Med. Eng. Tech.* 8, 3-8.

CLARK, G.M., BUSBY, P.A., ROBERTS, S.A., DOWELL, R.C., BLAMEY, P.J., MECKLENBURG, D.J., WEBB, R.L., PYMAN, B.C. and FRANZ, B.K. (1987). Preliminary results for the Cochlear Corporation multielectrode intracochlear implant in six prelingually deaf patients. *Am. J. Otol.* 8, 234-239.

COWAN, R.S.C., ALCANTARA, J.I., BLAMEY, P.J. and CLARK, G.M. (1988). Preliminary evaluation of a multichannel electrotactile speech processor. *J. Acoust. Soc. Am.* 83, 2328-2338.

COWAN, R.S.C., ALCANTARA, J.I., WHITFORD, L.A., BLAMEY, P.J. and CLARK, G.M. (1989a). Speech perception studies using a multichannel electrotactile speech processor, residual hearing, and lipreading. *J. Acoust. Soc. Am.* 85, 2593-2607.

COWAN, R.S.C., BLAMEY, P.J., ALCANTARA, J.I., WHITFORD, L.A. and CLARK, G.M. (1989b). Speech feature recognition with an electrotactile speech processor. *Aust. J. Audiol.* 11, 57-75.

COWAN, R.S.C., BLAMEY, P.J., GALVIN, K.L., SARANT, J.Z., ALCANTARA, J.I. and CLARK, G.M. (1990). Perception of sentences, words, and speech features by profoundly hearing-impaired children using a multichannel electrotactile speech processor. *J. Acoust. Soc. Am.* 88, 1374-1384.

COWAN, R.S.C., BLAMEY, P.J., SARANT, J.Z., GALVIN, K.L. and CLARK, G.M. (1991). Role of a multi-channel electrotactile speech processor in a cochlear implant program for profoundly-totally deaf adults. *Ear Hear.* 12, 39-46.

DE FILIPPO, C.L. and SCOTT, B.L. (1978). A method for training and evaluating the reception of ongoing speech. *J. Acoust. Soc. Am.* 63, 1186-1192.

DORMAN, M.F., HANNLEY, M.T., DANKOWSKI, K., SMITH, L. and MCCANDLESS, G. (1989). Word recognition by 50 patients fitted with the Symbion multichannel cochlear implant. *Ear Hear.* **10**, 44-49.

DOWELL, R.C., MECKLENBURG, D.J. and CLARK, G.M. (1986). Speech recognition for 40 patients receiving multichannel cochlear implants. *Arch. Otolaryngol.* **112**, 1054-1059.

DOWELL, R.C., MARTIN, L.F.A., CLARK, G.M. and BROWN, A.M. (1985). Results of a preliminary clinical trial on a multiple channel cochlear prosthesis. *Ann. Otol. Rhinol. Laryngol.* **94**, 244-250.

DOWELL, R.C., CLARK, G.M., SELIGMAN, P.M. and BROWN, A.M. (1986). Perception of connected speech without lipreading using a multiple-channel hearing prosthesis. *Acta Otolaryngol.* **102**, 7-11.

DOWELL, R.C., SELIGMAN, P.M., BLAMEY, P.J. and CLARK, G.M. (1987). Speech perception using a two formant 22-electrode cochlear prosthesis in quiet and in noise. *Acta Otolaryngol.* **104**, 439-446.

DOWELL, R.C., DAWSON, P.W., DETTMAN, S.J., SHEPHERD, R.K., WHITFORD, L.A., SELIGMAN, P.M. and CLARK, G.M. (1991). Multichannel cochlear implantation in children: A summary of current work at the University of Melbourne. *Am. J. Otol.* **12**(Suppl.), 137-143.

FOURCIN, A.J., DOUEK, E.E., MOORE, B.C.J., ROSEN, S., WALLIKER, J.R., HOWARD, D.M., ABBERTON, E. and FRAMPTON, S. (1983). Speech perception with promontory stimulation. *Ann. NY Acad. Sci.* **405**, 280-294.

GEERS, A.E. (1986). Vibrotactile stimulation: Case study with a profoundly deaf child. *J. Rehab. Res. Dev.* **23**, 111-117.

GEERS, A.E. and MOOG, J.S. (1989). Evaluating speech perception skills: Tools for measuring benefits in cochlear implants, tactile aids, and hearing aids. In: Owens, E. and Kessler, D.K. (eds), *Cochlear Implants in Young Deaf Children.* Boston: College Hill Press, pp. 227-256.

GELDARD, F.A. (1960). Some neglected possibilities of communication. *Science* **131**, 1583-1588.

GOLDSTEIN, M.H. and PROCTOR, A. (1985). Tactile aids for profoundly deaf children. *J. Acoust. Soc. Am.* **77**, 258-265.

HOCHMAIR-DESOYER, I.J., HOCHMAIR, E.S. and STIGLBRUNNER, H.K. (1985). Psychoacoustic temporal processing and speech understanding in cochlear implant patients. In: Schindler, R.A. and Merzenich, M.M. (eds), *Cochlear Implants.* New York: Raven Press, pp. 291-304.

KIRMAN, J.H. (1973). Tactile communication of speech: A review and an analysis. *Psychol. Bull.* **80**, 54-74.

LYNCH, M.P., EILERS, R.E., OLLER, D.K. and COBO-LEWIS, A. (1989). Multisensory speech perception by profoundly hearing-impaired children. *J. Speech Hear. Dis.* **54**, 57-67.

MILLAR, J.B., TONG, Y.C. and CLARK, G.M. (1984). Speech processing for cochlear implant prostheses. *J. Speech Hear. Res.* **27**, 280-296.

MILLAR, J.B., TONG, Y.C., BLAMEY, P.J., CLARK, G.M., DOWELL, R.C. and SELIGMAN, P.M. (1986). Speech processing for electrical stimulation of the auditory nerve. In: *Proceedings of International Conference on Speech Input/Output: techniques and applications.* London: Institute of Electrical Engineers, pp. 178-183.

MIYAMOTO, R.T., OSBERGER, M.J., ROBBINS, A.J., RENSHAW, J., MYRES, W.A., KESSLER, K. and POPE, M.L. (1989). Comparison of sensory aids in deaf children. *Ann. Otol. Rhinol. Laryngol.* (Suppl. 142) **98**, 2-7.

OLLER, D.K., PAYNE, S.L. and GAVIN, W.J. (1980). Tactual speech perception by minimally trained deaf subjects. *J. Speech Hear. Res.* **23**, 769-778.

OSBERGER, M.J., RINES-WEISS, D. and KALBERER, A. (1986). Speech tracking performance of deaf adults using a vibrotactile aid. Convention of the American Speech-Language Hearing Association, November, Detroit.

OSBERGER, M.J., ROBBINS, A.M. and RENSHAW, J.J. (1990). Speech perception skills of deaf children with cochlear implants and tactile aids. Paper presented at International Conference on Tactile Aids, Hearing Aids and Cochlear Implants, Sydney, May 1–3, 1990.

OWENS, E., KESSLER, D.K., TELLEEN, C.C. and SCHUBERT, E.D. (1981). Minimum Auditory Capabilities (MAC) Battery. *Hear. Aid J.* **34**, 9–34.

PETERSON, G.E. and LEHISTE, I. (1962). Revised CNC lists for auditory tests. *J. Speech Hear. Dis.* **27**, 62–70.

PICKETT, J.M. and MCFARLAND, W. (1985). Auditory implants and tactile aids for the profoundly deaf. *J. Speech Hear. Res.* **28**, 134–150.

PLANT, G. (1986). A single-transducer vibrotactile aid to lipreading. *Speech Transmission Laboratories Quarterly Progress & Status Report 1/1986*, 41–63.

PLANT, G.L. (1989). A comparison of five commercially-available tactile devices. *Aust. J. Audiol.* **11**, 11–19.

REED, C.M., RABINOWITZ, W.M., DURLACH, N.I., BRAIDA, L.D., CONWAY-FITHIAN, S. and SCHULTZ, M.C. (1982). Research on the Tadoma method of speech communication. *J. Acoust. Soc. Am.* **77**, 247–257.

SHERRICK, C.E. (1984). Basic and applied research on tactile aids for deaf people: Progress and prospects. *J. Acoust. Soc. Am.* **75**, 1325–1341.

SPARKS, D.W., ARDELL, L.A., BOURGEOIS, M., WIEDMER, B. and KUHL, P.K. (1979). Investigating the MESA (Multipoint Electrotactile Speech Aid): The transmission of connected discourse. *J. Acoust. Soc. Am.* **65**, 810–815.

SPENS, K-E. (1980). Tactile speech communication aids for the deaf: A comparison. *Speech Transmission Laboratories Quarterly Progress & Status Report 4/1980*, 23–39.

SUMMERS, I.R., PEAKE, M.A. and MARTIN, M.C. (1981). Field trials of a tactile acoustic monitor for the profoundly deaf. *Br. J. Audiol.* **15**, 195–199.

THORNTON, A.R.D. (1986). Estimation of the number of patients who might be suitable for cochlear implants and similar procedures. *Br. J. Audiol.* **20**, 221–229.

TONG, Y.C. and CLARK, G.M. (1985). Absolute identification of electric pulse rates and electrode positions of cochlear implant patients. *J. Acoust. Soc. Am.* **77**, 1881–1888.

TONG, Y.C., BUSBY, P.A. and CLARK, G.M. (1988). Perceptual studies on cochlear implant patients with early onset of profound hearing impairment prior to normal development of auditory, speech, and language skills. *J. Acoust. Soc. Am.* **84**, 951–962.

TONG, Y.C., BLACK, R.C., CLARK, G.M., FORSTER, I.C., MILLAR, J.B. and O'LOUGHLIN, B.J. (1979). A preliminary report on a multiple-channel cochlear implant operation. *J. Laryngol. Otol.* **93**, 679–695.

TONNISON, B. (1974). *National Acoustic Laboratories: Standardisation of CID everyday sentence tests.* Sydney: N.A.L. Publications.

TYLER, R.S. (1990). Speech perception with the Nucleus cochlear implant in children trained with the auditory/verbal approach. *Am. J. Otol.* **11**, 99–107.

TYLER, R.S., MOORE, B.C.J. and KUK, F.K. (1989). Performance of some of the better cochlear-implant patients. *J. Speech Hear. Res.* **32**, 887–911.

TYLER, R.S., SUMMERFIELD, A.Q., WOOD, E.J. and FERNANDES, M. (1982). Psychoacoustic and phonetic temporal processing in normal and hearing-impaired listeners. *J. Acoust. Soc. Am.* **72**, 740–752.

UVACEK, B., YE, H. and MOSCHYTZ, G.S. (1988). A new strategy for tactile hearing aids: Tactile identification of preclassified signals (TIPS). In: *Proceedings of the IEEE Conference*, pp. 2500-2503.

WEISENBERGER, J.M. and MILLER, J.D. (1987). The role of tactile aids in providing information about acoustic stimuli. *J. Acoust. Soc. Am.* **82**, 906-916.

Chapter 10
Natural Methods of Tactual Communication

CHARLOTTE M. REED, NATHANIEL I. DURLACH and LORRAINE A. DELHORNE

The challenges to communication faced by persons with combined auditory and visual deficits are enormous. Not only is the normal communication channel of audition unavailable to such individuals, but alternative methods traditionally employed by the deaf (e.g. speechreading and sign language) are also inaccessible due to their heavy reliance on vision. Apart from sensory information provided by smell and taste, the main source of information about the outside world for those with severe auditory/visual impairments is through touch. The use of the tactual sense for communication has been pioneered by deaf-blind individuals, together with those involved in their education and rehabilitation. As a result, a variety of methods of communication that rely on touch have evolved within the deaf-blind community.

Typically, tactual communication methods are based on direct application to the skin of a communication system originally intended for use by either the auditory or visual system. Examples of the wide variety of communication methods that may be observed in a gathering of deaf-blind individuals include palm spelling, tactual reception of manual alphabets, tactual reception of sign languages, tactual speech reading (Tadoma), and tactual reception of Morse code, as well as use of artificial devices that decode typed text into Braille. The particular method used by an individual depends on several factors, including age at onset of deafness and blindness and educational background. The methods themselves differ widely with regard to the type of information presented and the manner in which it is displayed to the skin, as well as to the amount of specialized training required on the part of both the sender and the receiver.

In addition to the primarily 'natural' methods of tactual communication developed within the deaf-blind community, there is a growing effort in the scientific and technological communities to develop artificial devices for encoding acoustic signals and displaying them on the skin. Such devices have several potential advantages over natural methods of tactual communication: first, no special training would be required on the part of the sender; second, acoustic signals, including both speech and environmental sounds, could be perceived at a distance, thus eliminating the need for direct physical contact between sender and receiver. The availability of such devices could have a tremendous impact on the lives of individuals who become skilled in their use. While substantial progress has been made in this area (see Reed et al., 1989b; also refer to Chapters 4, 5, 6 and 8 of this book), there are still no artificial tactual devices that can replace the communication function of any of the natural methods of tactual communication used by deaf-blind persons.

Despite the various limitations of the 'natural' methods of tactual communication (direct physical contact must be established between the sender and receiver and often very specialized training is required on the part of the sender), these techniques are none the less highly interesting and important. In particular, they clearly demonstrate that the tactual sensory system can be used effectively for purposes of communication. In addition, a deeper understanding of the properties of these methods, as well as the detailed performance characteristics of individuals highly trained in their use, can provide important background information for the development of artificial tactual devices. An interesting account of natural tactual communication used by a sighted individual to supplement lipreading is given by Plant and Spens (1986).

This chapter describes research on three 'natural' methods of tactual communication carried out in cooperation with deaf-blind individuals who are expert users of these systems. These methods are the Tadoma method of speech reading, the tactual reception of finger spelling, and the tactual reception of sign language.

The Tadoma Method of Speech Reading

In the Tadoma method, contact is made between the hand of the deaf-blind person and the face and neck of the talker. By monitoring various actions associated with speech production (e.g. lip and jaw movements, airflow at the mouth, vibrations on the neck) an experienced Tadoma user is able to comprehend connected speech with an accuracy that allows for a relatively easy flow of conversation. The hand position used in Tadoma is shown in Figure 10.1.

The origins of the Tadoma method can be traced to a Norwegian teacher named Hofgaard in the late nineteenth century (see Hansen, 1930). The method was introduced into the USA in the 1920s by Alcorn (1932) and was subsequently employed in the education of deaf-blind children throughout the country. Many of these individuals became deaf and blind in early childhood as a result of meningitis, and attended schools where Tadoma formed the basis of their early education. The use of the method

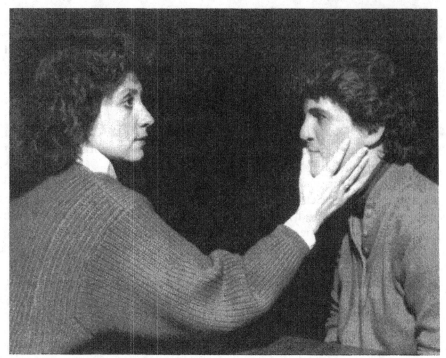

Figure 10.1 Use of the Tadoma method of speechreading.

for teaching both speech reading and speech production has declined in recent years (from the 1960s) due to changing characteristics of the deaf-blind population; the results of a recent survey (Schultz et al., 1984) indicate that there are perhaps 20 deaf-blind adults in the USA who are competent in the use of Tadoma. Although these individuals represent only a very small percentage of the total deaf-blind population, the Tadoma method is of great theoretical interest due to its use of naturally produced speech for communication through the tactual sense alone.

The speech reception, speech production, and linguistic abilities of Tadoma users have been documented in a number of recent studies (Norton et al., 1977; Reed et al., 1982, 1985; Chomsky, 1986; Tamir, T.J., 1989, unpublished SB thesis, Massachusetts Institute of Technology). Speech reception results indicate that performance is highly dependent on the contextual nature of the materials. For example, the reception of key words in conversational sentences (roughly 80% correct at slow speaking rates) exceeds predictions of performance based solely on segmental scores (roughly 55% for consonants or vowels in fixed-context syllables), using an assumption of independence for segmental recognition in words. The ability of Tadoma users to take advantage of contextual information is similar to that documented for normal-hearing subjects in adverse listening conditions (e.g. Miller, Heise and Lichten, 1951; Kalikow, Stevens and

Elliott, 1977) and implies a certain level of linguistic competence on the part of the Tadoma user. In fact, in-depth evaluations of the linguistic abilities of two Tadoma users who became deaf and blind in infancy indicate that their knowledge of a range of semantic and syntactic features of English, while not perfect, generally compares well to that of persons with normal hearing (Chomsky, 1986).

The reception of connected discourse through Tadoma is sensitive to changes in speaking rate. For conversational sentence materials, results from three experienced Tadoma users indicate substantial decrease in performance for rates greater than 3-5 syllables s^{-1}, depending on the individual subject. Speaking rates that are consistent with good intelligibility across listeners are roughly 60-75% of normal speaking rates (estimated at roughly 4-5 syllables s^{-1} by Picheny, Durlach and Braida, 1986, for sentences spoken in isolation). Rates for the tracking of connected discourse (using the procedure described by DeFilippo and Scott, 1978) on a group of three Tadoma users ranged from 30 to 40 words min^{-1}, or roughly one-third of the rates typically reported for auditory reception of textual material for normal-hearing listeners. This measure of the rate at which connected discourse is transmitted through Tadoma, relative to that for normal auditory reception, reflects the reduced speaking rates of both the sender and the receiver as well as the need for repetition due to misperceived components.

In addition to speech reception and linguistic abilities, the acquisition of speech production skills was a major component in the education of deaf-blind children through Tadoma. Results of both acoustic and intelligibility measurements of segmental and sentence productions of Tadoma users are consistent with those reported for sighted deaf speakers.

Additional research on Tadoma has focused on understanding the perceptual basis for the reception of speech through this method. The structure of confusion matrices derived from segmental identification tests indicates that certain articulatory features are better perceived than others through Tadoma. For example, consonants that differ on voicing are rarely confused, whereas many clusters of consonant confusions appear to occur as a result of misclassification of place of articulation within a given manner of production and, to a lesser degree, misclassification of manner of production for sounds with similar places of articulation. For vowels, the most salient cues appear to be lip rounding and vertical lip separation, with many confusions arising as a result of misclassifications of tongue height and position within the oral cavity. The relation of these features to the physical properties of the Tadoma display have been explored through experiments in which the Tadoma user's access to the various articulatory signals was altered by imposing systematic limitations on the contact of the hand with the face (Reed et al., 1989a). The results of these experiments generally support the notion that the reception of specific features is related to particular physical properties (e.g. voicing perception is highly dependent on access to laryngeal vibration on the neck), while at the same time indicating that several physical properties may carry relevant information concerning a given feature.

Research on Tadoma has led to the development of a synthetic Tadoma system that incorporates motorized lip and jaw movements, airflow regulation at the mouth, and vibratory stimulation at the neck into a plastic model of a human skull. Experiments have been conducted with this system both to verify the level of understanding of the cues used in natural Tadoma (Leotta et al., 1988; Rabinowitz et al., 1990) and for use in more general studies concerned with the transfer of information through the tactual sense (Tan, Rabinowitz and Durlach, 1989).

Tactual Reception of Finger Spelling

In this method, the deaf–blind person places a hand in contact with the hand of the sender to feel and interpret the letters of a manual alphabet. The sender transmits a letter-by-letter representation of the words that would occur in the spoken language. The manual alphabet most commonly used in the USA is the American One-Handed Manual Alphabet (AOHMA). Each letter of the English alphabet is associated with a unique handshape; the handshapes for 24 letters are generally static and (except in the formation of the letters J and Z) movement occurs primarily in transitions between letters. The specific type of contact made varies depending on the preference of the receiver. Some deaf–blind individuals prefer to have the sender make primary contact with the palm, while others wrap their fingers and palm around the side and back of the sender's hand. The tactual reception of fingerspelling is shown in Figure 10.2.

Tactual reception of finger spelling as a primary means of communication is generally used by deaf–blind persons whose native language was spoken. Many of these people were either deaf (and attended oral schools) or blind early in life and acquired the second component of their sensory impairment in adulthood. In some cases, deafness and blindness occurred simultaneously in adulthood. Many Tadoma users are also competent in the use of tactual finger spelling. In general, individuals who use tactual finger spelling have excellent speech production skills, and communicate expressively through either finger spelling or speech.

Studies have been conducted to determine the accuracy and rates at which tactual finger spelling can be received by experienced deaf–blind subjects (Reed et al., 1990), and results indicate that conversational sentences can be received at very high levels of accuracy (generally 90–100% correct key-word reception) throughout the range of finger-spelling rates employed. Different rates were achieved by asking the interpreter to vary her finger spelling production from 'slow' to 'very fast' (range

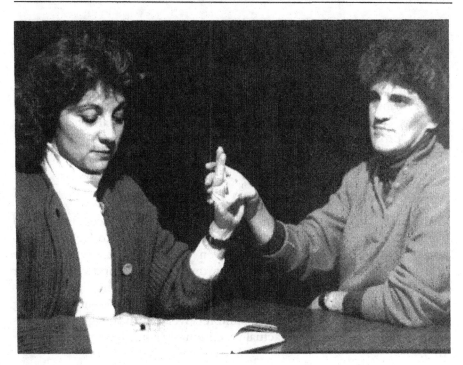

Figure 10.2 Use of the tactual reception of finger spelling.

roughly 2-6 letters s⁻¹). Previous studies have reported comfortable rates of finger spelling between sighted deaf subjects of roughly 5 letters s^{-1} (Bornstein, 1965; Hanson, 1982). Thus, the reception of tactual finger spelling is highly accurate at rates that are comparable to those used for the visual reception of finger spelling.

For purposes of comparison with the results of tactual reception of finger spelling, as well as to permit manipulations of rate beyond those that could be achieved naturally, an analogous study was conducted for the visual reception of finger spelling (Reed et al., 1990). The subjects were sighted deaf adults who were highly experienced in the reception of connected discourse through finger spelling. The test sentences were videotaped and manipulated using variable-speed playback to achieve rates in the range of 3-22 letters s^{-1}. The results for conversational sentences indicated nearly perfect reception of key words up to 8-12 letters s^{-1}, above which performance decreased steadily, reaching 50% correct at 11-16 letters s^{-1}. These results suggest that the visual reception of finger spelling is restricted by the rate at which finger spelling can be produced manually. Although this proposition could not be tested directly for tactual reception, the high performance at natural rates of production suggests that reasonable levels of reception accuracy would be achieved at rates in excess of those that can be produced naturally.

Rates of communication through natural production of finger spelling (for both tactual and visual reception) are slow compared with normal speaking rates. A fast finger spelling rate of 6-7 letters s⁻¹ corresponds to roughly 2 syllables s⁻¹. Such a rate of communication, while slow compared with normal speech, requires the production of a new letter once every 140-170 ms, and taxes the ability of the hand to produce the necessary complex changes in configuration. The development of artificial devices for the production of finger spelling may offer solutions for increasing communication rates (Gilden and Jaffe, 1987; Kramer and Leifer, 1988).

Tactual Reception of Sign Language

In the tactual reception of sign language, the receiver places one or two hands in contact with the hand (or hands) of the sender to feel and interpret the signs associated with a given sign language. Typically, the deaf-blind receiver places one hand on the dominant hand of the signer such that his or her fingertips rest lightly on the back of the signer's hand. The one-handed reception of sign appears to be most common among observations of experienced deaf-blind receivers, even though many signs are two-handed. The use of tactual reception of sign is illustrated in Figure 10.3.

In the USA, the use of sign language among deaf-blind individuals varies along a continuum from American Sign Language (ASL) to Pidgin Sign English (PSE) to Sign English (SE). ASL is a separate language with its own syntax and semantics, whereas SE attempts to represent English manually by employing signs for vocabulary items as they occur in English syntax and finger spelling for syntactical markers which cannot be translated directly into signs (Bornstein, 1978). The type of sign language preferred by a given user is frequently dependent on sociolinguistic considerations (see Woodward, 1980). According to many descriptions, the signs themselves result from the simultaneous variation of four basic parameters: handshape, location, palm orientation, and movement (see discussions in Stokoe, 1960; Battison, 1978; Wilbur, 1979).

The tactual reception of sign is most common among deaf-blind individuals with early onset of deafness and exposure to sign language. For many of these individuals, the onset of visual impairment occurred later in life and necessitated the adaptation of sign reception from the visual to the tactual sense. In addition, many programs for deaf-blind children currently employ sign language (as opposed to Tadoma or finger spelling) in their education.

A study of the tactual reception of sign language (Delhorne et al., 1988) was performed with a group of ten deaf-blind teenagers and adults, roughly half of whom used ASL and half PSE. For isolated signs, correct repetition was 73-96% across the subjects. Typically, incorrect responses

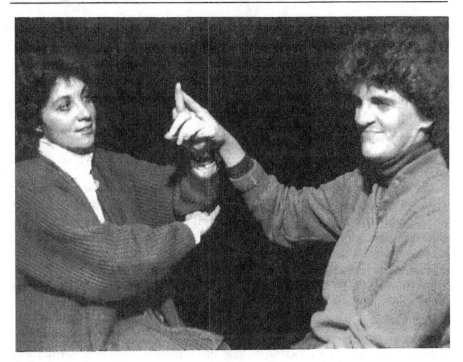

Figure 10.3 Use of the tactual reception of sign language.

arose from misperception of one of the four major cues that define a sign; for example, the two-handed signs 'make' and 'work' (which were confused with each other) are nearly identical in their handshape, movement, and location, but differ in the orientation of the palm. The reception of conversational sentences (translated from English into ASL and PSE) was examined as a function of rate of presentation. The production rates of the interpreters were roughly 0.75–2.6 signs s^{-1}, similar to the rates obtained by Grosjean (1979) when he asked native, sighted ASL signers to vary their rate of signing from slow to fast (normal signing rate averaged roughly 1.5 signs s^{-1}). Correct reception of key signs in conversational sentences was 65–90% across subjects and was relatively independent of rate of production. An analogous study of the visual reception of signed sentences as a function of rate of presentation (controlled through variable-speed playback of videotaped materials) has been conducted on a group of native sighted users of ASL. Preliminary analysis of these data indicate that the visual reception of ASL is insensitive to signing rate for rates up to twice the normal rate of production.

The communication rates that occur in the natural production of sign language have been shown to be roughly equivalent to those that occur in speech. Bellugi and Fischer (1972) have shown that although the basic articulation rate for sign is roughly half of that for speaking (2.4 signs s^{-1}

compared with 5 syllables s^{-1}), fewer signs than syllables are necessary to communicate a given message. In fact, the rate at which simple conceptual units (or propositions) are produced is roughly equivalent for both sign and speech. The normal rates of communication for both sign and speech is approximately 0.8 proposition s^{-1}.

Comparisons Across Natural Methods of Tactual Communication

A key issue that arises when considering the tactual sense for purposes of communication is whether sufficiently high rates of information transfer are possible through the skin. The research described above for three very different natural methods of tactual communication strongly supports the conclusion that the tactual sense is capable of receiving continuous discourse at near-normal communication rates.

A comparison of accuracy-rate functions for Tadoma and for the tactual reception of finger spelling and sign language is shown in Figure 10.4. Using data obtained under each method for the reception of conversational CID sentences (Davis and Silverman, 1970), accuracy of reception can be examined as a function of rate of communication across the three methods. Accuracy of reception is expressed in terms of the percentage correct reception of key words (for Tadoma and finger spelling) or key signs (for sign language), while communication rate is expressed in terms of proposition s^{-1} (Bellugi and Fischer, 1972). By describing the sentences in terms of propositions, a measure of rate may be derived that can be applied to both the original English sentences and to their translations into ASL or PSE. Each sentence is described in terms of the number of main concepts (which is constant whether the sentence is presented in English, ASL, or PSE); the duration of each sentence as actually presented to each subject is measured; and the proposition rate is calculated by dividing the number of propositions by the duration of the presentation. Individual subject data obtained under each method are plotted in Figure 10.4.

Finger spelling yields the highest accuracy of reception, but is accomplished at the slowest rate (0.1–0.3 propositions s^{-1}). Normal-to-fast finger spelling rates (5–6 letters s^{-1}) correspond to proposition rates roughly one-third of normal speaking rates. Communication rates for Tadoma and tactual sign reception are higher than for finger spelling, with some sacrifice in accuracy of reception. For both Tadoma and sign language, reception scores were roughly 60–90% correct for rates in the range 0.2–0.55 propositions s^{-1}, which is nearly three-quarters of normal speaking rate. The highest proposition rates (0.7–1.1 propositions s^{-1}) were obtained through the Tadoma method, but performance through Tadoma dropped at rates above roughly 0.5 propositions s^{-1}. In the small range of rates at

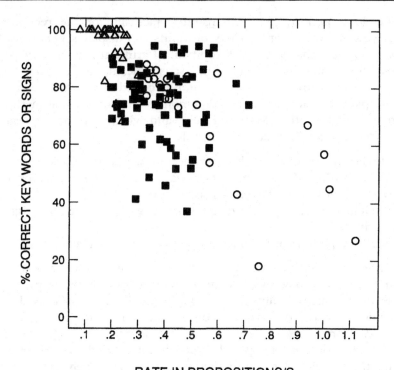

RATE IN PROPOSITIONS/S

Figure 10.4 Comparison of tactual reception rates for three methods of tactual communication. Percentage correct identification of key words or signs in CID sentences is plotted as a function of communication rate in propositions s⁻¹. △, Tactual reception of finger spelling; ○, reception of speech through Tadoma; ■, tactual reception of sign language.

which data are available for all three methods (i.e. 0.2–0.3 propositions s⁻¹), performance appears to be comparable across the three methods.

Discussion

Accurate reception of continuous discourse has been demonstrated for three different natural methods of tactual communication at rates comparable to those associated with slow speaking rates. None of these methods conveys a signal that was initially designed for tactual communication and both the type of information being conveyed and the manner in which it is displayed are quite different across methods. For Tadoma, the dimensions that are monitored in the reception of the oral speech signal include lip and jaw movements, airflow at the lips and laryngeal vibration. In finger spelling, an alphabetic code is transmitted by different handshapes associated with each letter. In sign language, the tactual cues used to monitor signs include the orientation, location, and movements of the hands in addition to handshape.

The good performance demonstrated tactually for the reception of connected discourse for a variety of inputs and display schemes leads to several implications for the development of artificial tactual devices. One general observation is that the tactual sense does not appear to be particular about either the type of information encoded or the manner in which it is displayed. Features that *are* common to all three natural methods of tactual communication described here, and which may be important to the success of artificial devices, include:

- The use of the hand for the reception of tactual stimulation.
- The activation of both the cutaneous and the kinesthetic/proprioceptive branches of the tactual sensory system.
- Simultaneous presentation of information along a number of different dimensions.
- Extensive periods of training in the use of a particular method.

Further research is necessary to determine the relative importance of such factors as body site, cutaneous versus kinesthetic/proprioceptive stimulation, dimensionality and training in the design of successful tactual communication devices; also to address issues related to the cognitive and emotional aspects of experiencing the world solely through the tactual sense. Very little is currently understood about either the cognitive organization that results from input that is almost exclusively tactual or the relation between the emotional needs of deaf–blind individuals and the use of technological devices. Such concerns must be addressed in the design of technological devices with the potential for broadening access to communication and helping relieve the severe isolation faced by most deaf-blind individuals.

Acknowledgments

This work was supported by a grant from the National Institutes of Health (NIH Grant No. 5-R01-DC00126). The authors are grateful to W.M. Rabinowitz and P.M. Zurek for their helpful comments on an earlier version of the manuscript, and to John Cook of the Research Laboratory of Electronics, Massachusetts Institute of Technology for the photographs.

References

ALCORN, S. (1932). The Tadoma method. *Volta Rev.* **34**, 195–198.

BATTISON, R. (1978). *Lexical Borrowing in American Sign Language*. Silver Spring, Maryland: Linstock Press.

BELLUGI, U. and FISCHER, S. (1972). A comparison of sign language and spoken language. *Cognition* **1**, 173–200.

BORNSTEIN, H. (1965). *Reading the Manual Alphabet*. Washington, DC: Gallaudet College Press.

BORNSTEIN, H. (1978). Sign language in the education of the deaf. In: Schlesinger, I.M. and Namir, L. (eds), *Sign Language of the Deaf and Psychological, Linguistic, and Sociological Perspectives.* New York: Academic Press, pp. 333-361.

CHOMSKY, C. (1986). Analytic study of the Tadoma method: Language abilities of three deaf-blind subjects. *J. Speech Hear. Res.* 29, 332-347.

DAVIS, H. and SILVERMAN, S.R. (1970). *Hearing and Deafness.* New York: Holt, Rinehart, and Winston.

DEFILIPPO, C.L. and SCOTT, B.L. (1978). A method for training and evaluating the reception of ongoing speech. *J. Acoust. Soc. Am.* 63, 1186-1192.

DELHORNE, L.A., REED, C.M. and DURLACH, N.I. (1988). The reception of sign language through the tactile sense. *ASHA* 30, 136(A).

GILDEN, D. and JAFFE, D.L. (1987). Speaking in hands. *Soma* 2, 7-13.

GROSJEAN, F. (1979). A study of timing in a manual and a spoken language: American sign language and English. *J. Psycholing. Res.* 8, 379-405.

HANSEN, A. (1930). The first case in the world: Miss Petra Heiberg's report. *Volta Rev.* 32, 223.

HANSON, V.L. (1982). Use of orthographic structure by deaf adults: Recognition of finger-spelled words. *Appl. Psycholing.* 3, 343-356.

KALIKOW, D.N., STEVENS, K.N. and ELLIOTT, L.L. (1977). Development of a test of speech intelligibility in noise using sentence materials with controlled word predictability. *J. Acoust. Soc. Am.* 61, 1337-1351.

KRAMER, J. and LEIFER, L. (1988). The talking glove: A communication aid for deaf, deaf-blind and nonvocal individuals. *Human-Machine Integration: Communication, Report* 55, 123-124.

LEOTTA, D., RABINOWITZ, W.M., DURLACH, N.I. and REED, C.M. (1988). Preliminary speech-reception results obtained with the synthetic Tadoma system. *J. Rehab. Res. Dev.* 25, 45-52.

MILLER, G.A., HEISE, G.A. and LICHTEN, W. (1951). The intelligibility of speech as a function of the context of the test materials. *J. Exp. Psychol.* 41, 329-335.

NORTON, S.J., SCHULTZ, M.C., REED, C.M., BRAIDA, L.D., DURLACH, N.I., RABINOWITZ, W.M. and CHOMSKY, C. (1977). Analytic study of the Tadoma method: Background and preliminary results. *J. Speech Hear. Res.* 20, 574-595.

PICHENY, M.P., DURLACH, N.I. and BRAIDA, L.D. (1986). Speaking clearly for the hard of hearing II. Acoustic characteristics of clear and conversational speech. *J. Speech Hear. Res.* 29, 434-446.

PLANT, G. and SPENS, K.-E. (1986). An experienced user of tactile information as a supplement to lipreading. An evaluative study. *Speech Transmission Laboratories Quarterly Progress & Status Report 1.* Stockholm: Royal Institute of Technology, pp. 87-110.

RABINOWITZ, W.M., HENDERSON, D.R., REED, C.M., DELHORNE, L.A. and DURLACH, N.I. (1990). Continuing evaluation of a synthetic Tadoma system. *J. Acoust. Soc. Am.* 87, S88 (A).

REED, C.M., DELHORNE, L.A., DURLACH, N.I. and FISCHER, S.D. (1990). A study of the tactual and visual reception of fingerspelling. *J. Speech Hear. Res.* 33, 786-797.

REED, C.M., DURLACH, N.I., BRAIDA, L.D. and SCHULTZ, M.C. (1982). Analytic study of the Tadoma method: Identification of consonants and vowels by an experienced Tadoma user. *J. Speech Hear. Res.* 25, 108-116.

REED, C.M., DURLACH, N.I., BRAIDA, L.D. and SCHULTZ, M.C. (1989a). Analytic study of the Tadoma method: Effects of hand position on segmental speech perception. *J. Speech Hear. Res.* 32, 921-929.

REED, C.M., DURLACH, N.I., DELHORNE, L.A., RABINOWITZ, W.M. and GRANT, K.W. (1989b). Research on tactual communication of speech: Ideas, issues, and findings. In: McGarr, N.S. (ed.), *Research on the Use of Sensory Aids for Hearing-impaired People*. Washington, DC: A.G. Bell Association for the Deaf, pp. 65-78.

REED, C.M., RABINOWITZ, W.M., DURLACH, N.I., BRAIDA, L.D., CONWAY-FITHIAN, S. and SCHULTZ, M.C. (1985). Research on the Tadoma method of speech communication. *J. Acoust. Soc. Am.* **77**, 247-257.

SCHULTZ, M.C., NORTON, S.J., CONWAY-FITHIAN, S. and REED, C.M. (1984). A survey of the use of the Tadoma method in the United States and Canada. *Volta Rev.* **86**, 282-292.

STOKOE, W. (1960). Sign language structure: An outline of the visual communication system of the American deaf. *Studies in Linguistics, Occasional Papers No. 8.*

TAN, H.Z., RABINOWITZ, W.M. and DURLACH, N.I. (1989). Analysis of a synthetic Tadoma system as a multidimensional tactile display. *J. Acoust. Soc. Am.* **86**, 981-988.

WILBUR, R. (1979). *American Sign Language and Sign Systems: Research and Applications*. Baltimore: University Park Press.

WOODWARD, J. (1980). Some sociolinguistic aspects of French and American sign languages. In: Lane, H. and Grosjean, F. (eds), *Recent Perspectives on American Sign Language*. Hillsdale, NJ: Lawrence Erlbaum Associates, pp. 103-118.

Chapter 11
A Comparative Trial of
Four Vibrotactile Aids

A. ROGER D. THORNTON and ANDREW J. PHILLIPS

In this chapter, a comparative trial of four vibrotactile aids will be detailed and their performance and design evaluated.

When the study was being planned (1986) there were four types of vibrotactile aid available that differed from each other and that represented the full available range of signal-processing and stimulus-delivery methods. These were the Minivib 3, the Tactaid II, the Minifonator and the TAM. Two of the devices, the TAM and the Minivib 3, make no attempt to convey frequency information to the wearer but pass prosodic components of speech at the resonant frequency of the vibrator. The other two devices, the Tactaid II and the Minifonator, pass frequency information to the wearer, the Minifonator via a single channel and the Tactaid II with two channels.

Description of the Four Aids

TAM

This is a single-channel aid, where the input sound is encoded to 220 Hz causing a piezoelectric crystal to vibrate at its resonant frequency. It has no automatic gain control or noise suppression circuitry. The user may set the appropriate input sensitivity with a continuously variable control. Output vibration intensity is fixed. It has an input telecoil, a facility for external microphone input and can be used with FM trainers. It has a light-emitting diode which indicates when the unit is delivering vibrations. The battery is rechargeable and the unit is supplied with a charger. The processor is connected to the vibrator via a cord which may be ordered to any length. The vibrator is mounted on either a good quality leather strap or a soft plastic one and is in direct contact with the skin. The unit weighs 74 g. The dimensions of the processor box are 65 × 45 × 20 mm and those of the vibrator 38 × 18 × 8 mm. The documentation supplied was

231

adequate to meet the needs of the user. There is good information available to teachers and fitters.

Tactaid II

This is a two-channel vibrotactile aid, the lower channel responding to frequencies within the range 100 Hz to 1.8 kHz, the upper channel covering 1.5-7 to 8.1 kHz (±6 dB). In the processing paradigm employed, the incoming signal is amplified and then separated into high- and low-frequency channels. In each channel the waveform is envelope-detected and the resultant envelope in each channel is multiplied into a sinusoidal signal (at 400 Hz in the version used for this study) to provide the drive for the two vibrators, thus retaining input amplitude information. Front-end automatic gain control and auto-threshold noise suppression circuitry are built in. Sensitivity may be adjusted by the user. The device has an inbuilt telecoil and is compatible with FM systems via an external input; the external input may also be used with an external microphone. The rechargeable battery is an integral part of the unit, which is supplied with a battery charger. The processor is connected via a cord (1.1 m) to the two vibrators which are attached to an expansible nylon strap. The vibrators may be worn next to the skin or the vibrations may be transmitted via the strap. The system weighs 187 g and the processor measures 93 × 57 × 23 mm. The vibrators each measure 28 × 25 × 10 mm. The system is well engineered and was supplied as a grey case with red lettering. There is an impressive amount of documentation including useful instruction manuals for teachers, parents, users and those fitting the aid. The Tactaid II is referred to as Tactaid throughout the rest of this chapter.

Minivib 3

This is a single-channel system that responds to mid-frequency incident sound that causes the output vibrator to be activated at its resonant frequency of around 250 Hz. The system is responsive to different intensities but does not respond to high frequencies. It has no automatic gain control but does have noise-suppression circuitry. The sensitivity may be set by the user. It has no telecoil input and no facilities for an external microphone. The battery is rechargeable. The processor unit is a robust and attractively packaged grey and black plastic unit. The vibrator is supplied attached to a black leather wrist strap and is connected to the processor by a 90 cm long cord. The system, including the battery, weighs 70 g. The dimensions are 65 × 43 × 19 mm for the main unit and for the vibrator 22 × 17 × 10 mm. The vibrator is not in direct contact with the skin, vibrations being transmitted through the leather strap. Documentation is rudimentary. The Minivib 3 is referred to as Minivib throughout the rest of this chapter.

Minifonator

This is a single-channel vibrotactile aid employing a processing paradigm that, up to 1 kHz, causes the vibrator to vibrate at the same frequency as the incident sound. As an optional facility (not used in this study) frequencies above 4 kHz, transposed to the region 0–500 Hz, may be transmitted also. Output vibrations are proportional to input sound intensity. It has neither automatic gain control nor noise-suppression circuitry. It has an input for use with FM receivers and an output that can be used with hearing aids; the microphone may be used remotely. Rechargeable batteries may be used with the aid and a charger is supplied. The vibrator appears very similar to a wristwatch and is mounted on a Velcro strap, directly in contact with the skin. There is a 1.25 m cord connecting the vibrator to the processor. The system weighs 270 g, the processor measures 84 × 82 × 30 mm and the vibrator 45 × 35 × 10 mm. The vibrator has been particularly well engineered but the battery cover on the processor unit was a problem for some patients. It was supplied as a light grey unit. The accompanying documentation is minimal. The user is able to adjust both input sensitivity and output vibration intensity.

Description of the Comparative Trial

Objectives

This study was designed to answer the following questions:

1. Do vibrotactile aids benefit profoundly hearing-impaired patients?
2. If they do, which of the test procedures reflect that benefit?
3. Do vibrotactile aids with more complex coding strategies give greater benefit than those with simpler coding strategies?
4. How does any benefit from vibrotactile aids compare with that obtained from hearing aids?
5. What factors influence the patient's choice of vibrotactile aid?

Design

Patients were selected from the profoundly hearing-impaired group of patients who had taken part in previous research studies at the MRC Institute of Hearing Research at Southampton. Full audiometric data were available for these patients and three groups, each of four patients, were selected:

1. postlinguistically impaired who do not use hearing aids
2. postlinguistically impaired who use hearing aids
3. prelinguistically impaired who do not use hearing aids.

A group of prelinguistically impaired patients who used hearing aids and were willing to participate in the study could not be found.

This study was carried out in conjunction with the speech therapy and hearing therapy departments of the Royal South Hants Hospital. Staff from these departments developed a ten-week training programme for the patients who would participate in the trial (Day, Worsfold and Thornton, 1990). The aims of the programme included: reintroducing users to the auditory environment; training using Visispeech (a device which provides a visual display of voicing, pitch, high-frequency energy and/or overall speech intensity) to show the aspects of speech with which the vibrotactile aid will help; exercises in consonant/vowel discrimination; and familiarisation with other aspects of speech components. In order to familiarise patients with the sensations that they would receive and the judgements that they would be required to make, some form of vibrotactile device was needed during the training programme; however, if one of the four aids that were to be used in the main study were used in the training period then, inevitably, there would be bias introduced into the design. It was decided therefore to use a high-powered body-worn aid designed for acoustic output, giving tactile stimulation via a bone-conduction transducer, as the device for the training period.

The allocation of vibrotactile aids was planned using a balanced Latin-Square design corrected for carry-over effects. Each patient was tested in an unaided condition and was then issued with their first vibrotactile aid. The aid was used for at least 2 weeks before testing with the vibrotactile aid. The next aid was then issued to the patient, and the process repeated a further three times. A final unaided test session completed the experiment.

The initial and final unaided tests enabled any learning effects to be assessed and corrected. Those patients who had hearing aids were also tested for each vibrotactile aid, under the conditions hearing aid alone, vibrotactile aid alone and vibrotactile aid and hearing aid together. The initial and final sessions, for these patients, comprised both an unaided condition and an aided-with-hearing-aid condition.

Patients' audiograms gave thresholds that were nearly all beyond the audiometer limits but with a little low-frequency hearing in some cases. The group that used hearing aids had slightly better low-frequency thresholds that averaged 88 dB HTL at 250 Hz, 107 dB HTL at 500 Hz and 118 dB HTL at 1000 Hz.

With each vibrotactile aid the patient was given a diary containing questions about the aid similar to those contained in a questionnaire given at the end of the test session for a particular aid. One purpose of the diary was to maintain a daily record of the patient's experiences for the particular areas which would be addressed in the questionnaire and so avoid too large a reliance on the patient's recollections of what had happened during the trial period. In addition, the patient could use it for any comments or notes that could be discussed at the clinic.

Once all the vibrotactile aids had been tried and the final unaided test session completed, the patients were shown all of the aids and given a comparative questionnaire on the relative merits of each aid. Patients were asked if they would like to have a vibrotactile aid for full-time use; if the answer was yes he or she was asked to choose one.

The test material comprised:

- The BKB sentence lists (1–17) on video, with 16 sentences per list and scored on three or four keywords per sentence (Rosen and Corcoran, 1982).
- The VCV or twelve-intervocalic-consonant test, which was supplied by the EPI group in London (University College, London) and had two lists each of 48 items. Subjects watched a video screen on which a female speaker presented /aCa/ (e.g. /aTa/,/aGa/). The consonants were b, p, s, z, f, v, n, m, g, k, t and d (Rosen, Moore and Fourcin, 1979; Faulkner et al., 1989).
- An environmental sounds test and an intonation test, which were supplied on audio tape by Dr J.C. Stevens of Sheffield University (Dodgson et al., 1983). The environmental sounds were a toilet flushing, washing up, speech, a vacuum cleaner, an alarm bell and pop music. There were 30 repeats with randomised presentation and the subject was required to make a six-alternative forced choice. The intonation test involved the identification of stress placements on one of the three words in the sentence 'Ron will win'. There were 30 repeats with the subject having to make a three-alternative forced choice.
- Connected discourse tracking (CDT), in which the tester, visible to the patient, read from an appropriate text and the patient was required to repeat the words.
- Various Visispeech measurements, including voice pitch and the percentage of the time that voicing occurred.

Results and Discussion

Patient groups

The data obtained for the unaided and vibrotactile-aided conditions were compared for all three patient groups. Overall there were no statistically significant differences between the groups and so, for many of the analyses, the three groups may be coalesced.

Learning effects

All data were examined for learning effects. Only for the BKB sentences was a statistically significant learning effect found (Wilcoxon matched-ranks signed-pairs test, $P<0.01$). The effect was examined for each test session and approximated to a linear function. Accordingly the number of words correct was reduced by 0.75 per visit (that is by 0.75 for the first visit, by 1.5 for the second visit, by 2.25 for the third visit and by 3.00 for the fourth visit).

Evaluation of the test material

It was felt that if the patients reported at least some benefit from the vibrotactile aids, the test results should reflect those reports. Whilst particular tests may better reflect particular aspects of benefit, the tests whose results most consistently agree with the patients' reports are the tests that should be given most weight in arriving at an overall conclusion.

A further criterion was that the test answers should be consistent if the test is to be of use; that is, a test showing that the hearing-aid condition is better than an unaided condition should consistently show that result on each occasion that it is measured.

Table 11.1 shows the change in score between the unaided condition and the aided condition for each of the four vibrotactile aids. The BKB test could be scored strictly, BKB(S), or loosely, BKB(L), and the VCV test could be scored in full, VCV(F), or as the confusion score, VCV(C).

The various tests differ in evaluating the vibrotactile aids: of all these tests only the BKB(L), the VCV(F and C), the CDT and the environmental sounds gave at least one statistically significant difference between the unaided and the vibrotactile-aided conditions.

Table 11.1 The mean change in score between the unaided condition and the vibrotactile-aided condition for all tests and all vibrotactile aids

| Test | Vibrotactile aid | | | |
	TAM	Tactaid	Minivib	Minifonator
BKB (S)	5.79	3.69	-1.96	-0.54
BKB (L)	8.92	4.51	-1.83	-0.17
VCV (F)	4.50	5.00	3.50	3.00
VCV (C)	2.88	5.13	3.63	2.46
%VC (read)	-0.13	-0.54	0.13	-2.38
%VC (monl)	1.33	-0.25	0.42	2.00
%VC (conv)	0.08	0.08	0.58	-0.92
CDT	33.29	40.04	13.87	35.96
Environ	5.25	5.17	3.55	6.25
Inton	0.33	-0.25	0.36	6.42

BKB, BKB sentences strictly (S) and loosely (L) scored; VCV, the vowel-consonant-vowel test scored fully (F) and as the confusion score (C); %VC, the percentage of voicing for reading (read), saying a monologue (monl) and for conversation (conv); CDT, connected discourse tracking; Environ, the environmental-sounds test; Inton, the speech-intonation test.

Table 11.2 Evaluation of test material tests that gave statistically significant results for change in score between the unaided condition and the vibrotactile-aided condition*

	Vibrotactile aid			
Test	TAM	Tactaid	Minivib	Minifonator
BKB (L)	0.012	0.050		
VCV (F)	0.020			
VCV (C)		0.050		
CDT	0.006	0.012		0.010
Environ	0.013	0.013	0.040	0.003

Abbreviations as in Table 11.1. *Each cell entry is the significance level at which the aided condition is better than the unaided.

Table 11.2 shows those tests which indicated a statistically significant change in score between the unaided condition and the vibrotactile-aided condition. Figure 11.1 shows the data summarised in Table 11.2, together with mean unaided scores and maximum available scores.

The environmental sounds test is the only one to show significant differences for each vibrotactile aid. The percentage-voicing measurements and the intonation tests, whilst giving some significant results for other test conditions (such as the difference between the score obtained using a vibrotactile aid plus hearing aid and the unaided score), gave no significant results for the change between scores obtained from the unaided and vibrotactile aided conditions. These results indicate that the tests shown in Table 11.2 are those that should be given most weight when trying to assess the benefit from a vibrotactile aid.

Table 11.3 The mean change in score between the unaided condition and the hearing aid condition, the vibrotactile-aided condition and the condition in which both the vibrotactile aid and hearing aid are used

	Test condition								
Test	Hearing aid alone	TAM	TAM plus hearing aid	Tactaid	Tactaid plus hearing aid	Minivib	Minivib plus hearing aid	Minifo-nator	Minifo-nator plus hearing aid
BKB (S)	4.88	5.79	9.54	3.69	7.97	-1.96	1.54	-0.54	0.62
BKB (L)	7.69	9.88	9.92	4.72	8.69	-0.88	2.00	0.75	1.67
VCV (F)	12.00	5.19	8.31	7.44	11.56	4.81	8.94	3.19	11.56
VCV (C)	7.31	3.94	4.56	6.69	6.81	4.94	2.69	3.31	8.31
CDT	72.5	36.8	119.1	50.2	103.6	2.4	108.2	40.8	120.6
Environ	10.94	5.25	10.63	5.17	13.38	3.55	11.50	6.25	13.75
Average rank	3=	6=	3=	6=	1	9	5	8	2

Data are given for all tests that showed a statistically significant difference between the unaided and aided conditions. These data were ranked for each test and the average rank is shown in the bottom row.

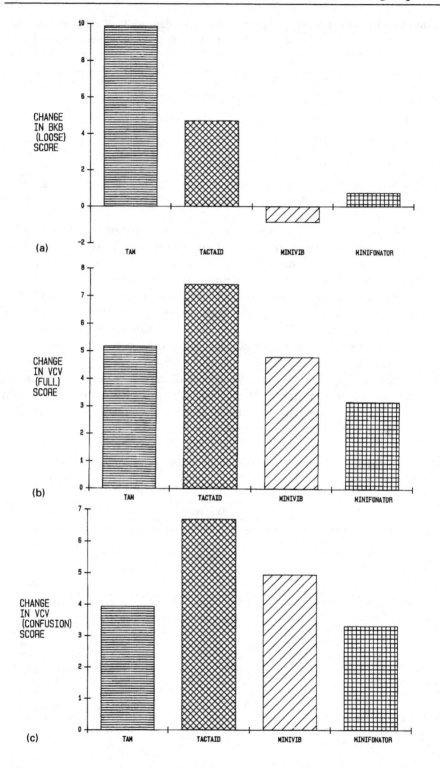

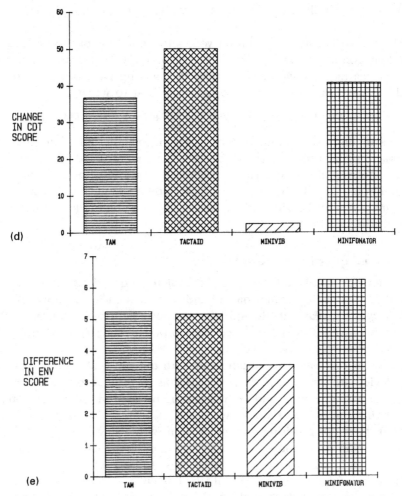

Figure 11.1 Difference between mean test scores in the vibrotactile-aided and unaided conditions (12 subjects) for each of the vibrotactile aids. (a) BKB sentences (scored loosely), mean unaided score 17.17 key words, maximum available score 50; (b) VCV nonsense syllables (scored fully, i.e. on the basis of the number of consonants identified correctly), mean unaided score 15.75 consonants, maximum available score 48; (c) VCV nonsense syllables (confusion score, i.e. incorrect responses weighted according to the degree of confusion expected between the incorrect and correct response), mean unaided score 29.29; (d) connected-discourse tracking over 3 min, mean unaided score 166.54 words; (e) environmental-sounds test, unaided score taken as chance score (5 items), maximum available score 30.

Vibrotactile aids and hearing aids

The group of patients who wore hearing aids were tested in four conditions: unaided, hearing aid alone (HA), vibrotactile aid alone (VTA) and hearing aid and vibrotactile aid together (VTA+HA) (see Table 11.3). Again, not all tests showed a statistically significant difference between the aided and unaided conditions and only those which did were used in the overall assessment.

The hearing-aid-alone condition was better than any of the vibrotactile-aid-alone conditions. However, the Tactaid and the Minifonator, when used with a hearing aid, were better than the hearing aid alone. The overall rankings gave the following sequence from best to worst:

TC+HA > MF+HA > HA = TM+HA > MV+HA > TC = TM > MF > MV

It is of interest to note that the two vibrotactile aids that use more complex signal processing are the two that, when used in conjunction with a hearing aid, give a greater benefit than the hearing aid alone. The two vibrotactile aids that use the simpler coding strategies, when used in conjunction with hearing aids, give the same or slightly less benefit than the hearing aid alone.

Individual questionnaire data

For each vibrotactile aid the patient completed a questionnaire which first asked for the average time that the aid was used each day, how comfortable it was to wear initially and how comfortable it was after an hour or so. It also asked if people noticed the vibrotactile aid; if so, whether they reacted positively or negatively to it.

Six questions followed which dealt with the physical characteristics of the device: its size, the size of the controls, if the controls were easy to use, the vibrator area and output strength, and whether replacing or recharging the batteries was easy.

Four questions covering communication with a single person in a quiet room, talking in a group, talking to a person in the open and talking to someone in a large room or hall were next to be answered.

How helpful the vibrotactile aid had been for awareness of environmental sounds was dealt with in the next four questions: use with the television and telephone, and voice control were covered next.

The final section dealt with whether skin sensitivity decreased after the patient had worn the aid for a while and whether the patient had to move the aid to regain the original sensitivity.

The data were then analysed.

How easy was it to wear the vibrotactile aid?

The questions on comfort, hours of use per day, whether people noticed the aid and how they reacted, together with the skin sensitivity questions and the patient's feeling about wearing the aid were included. Responses are summarised in Table 11.4.

The TAM device was generally considered comfortable and light, with the vibrator closely resembling a wristwatch. It was considered unobtru-

Table 11.4 Summary of patient responses to ease of wear of the vibrotactile aid (ranking)

Question	TAM	Tactaid	Minivib	Minifonator
How many hours use per day	2	2	1	4
How comfortable was the aid initially?	1	2	3	4
How comfortable after an hour or so?	1	3	2	4
Did people notice the aid?	1	3	2	3
If so, did they react positively or not?	2	3	4	1
How did you feel about wearing the aid?	3	2	1	4
Did you have to move aid after a while?	1	3	2	4
If so, what was the time interval?	4	3	1	2
Average rank	1	3	2	4

1, Best; 4, worst.

sive, but some patients complained that the cord easily became entangled and that they would only wear it with long sleeves. Only six patients wore it for more than 4 h a day and three felt uneasy about being seen with it.

The Minivib was considered light, but the wrist strap made it very uncomfortable for some patients; ten found it 'uncomfortable' and two found it 'very uncomfortable'. It scored very well in questions concerning its intrusiveness; ten patients said it was not noticed and two said it was noticed 'only a little'. Only two felt uneasy about being seen with the aid and one thought that others reacted negatively to it.

The Tactaid performed slightly worse than the Minivib but scored well on how patients felt about wearing it; two felt uneasy and one said that others reacted negatively to it, six patients said it was noticed 'only a little'. It was considered reasonably comfortable when first put on by ten of the patients, but after an hour of use three found it 'uncomfortable' and four 'very uncomfortable'; one patient would not wear it for longer than an hour. Six patients used it for more than 4 h each day. Generally, it was thought of as awkward, restricting freedom of movement and in need of a better strap.

The Minifonator was consistently the least comfortable aid, being thought too big, cumbersome and heavy, with the wrist strap attracting much criticism for being uncomfortable. Five patients found the aid 'uncomfortable' and two found it 'very uncomfortable'. Only five used it for more than 4 h a day and seven had to move it after wearing it for some time. It was considered very instrusive; four patients said that others reacted negatively and seemed disturbed by it, whilst two felt uneasy about being seen with the aid and two positively disliked being seen with it.

How well was the vibrotactile aid designed?

Questions on the size of the device, the size and ease of use of the controls, the vibrator area and its output and the ease of replacing or

Table 11.5 Ranks for each vibrotactile aid for the questions on how well the aid was designed

Question	TAM	Tactaid	Minivib	Minifonator
How do you like the size of the device?	2	3	1	4
How do you like the size of the controls?	1	4	1	1
How easy are the controls in use?	1	4	3	1
How do you like the vibrator output?	4	3	1	2
Is the area of the vibrator appropriate?	1	1	1	1
How easy is it to replace batteries?	1	3	4	2
Average rank	1	4	2	2

1, Best; 4, worst.

recharging the batteries were included in this section. Responses are summarised in Table 11.5.

The TAM device was judged the best, with the Minifonator and Minivib close behind. The TAM aid did come in for some criticism about battery charging, with several patients saying that it did not hold its charge for very long although ten felt charging to be easy and two felt that it was 'just manageable'. It was generally thought to be a good size; 11 patients said that the box size was 'about right' and one that it was 'too large'. The wrist vibrator was considered small and light; 11 patients felt that the controls were of a convenient size but one felt that they were too small. Some patients commented that the controls were poorly labelled and easily displaced from their assigned positions; the cord sometimes got caught and the pocket clip was badly designed and often broke off. One patient commented that the controls were not very sensitive and had difficulty in attaining a position between a continual buzz and no vibrator output; however, ten patients found the controls easy to use, with one 'just manageable' and one 'difficult'. Seven patients considered vibrator output 'just right', four that it was too weak and one that it was too strong.

The Minivib was joint second with Minifonator, scoring well on factors related to its physical size. However, the strap came in for some criticism for being too wide and, particularly, for attenuating vibrations, several people commenting that this made vibrator output too weak. Battery life was inadequate, the cord intrusive and rubbed annoyingly on clothes. Eleven patients felt the box to be the right size, one that it was too small. The same numbers applied to the size of the controls: 11 'convenient', one 'too small'. The controls were well designed; nine patients judged that they were 'easy to use', two that they were 'manageable' and one that they were 'difficult'. Six people stated that the vibrator output was 'just right', five that it was 'too weak' and one that it was 'too strong'. For battery replacement and recharging this was the least effective of the devices: eight patients said it was 'easy', three that it was 'just manageable' and one that it was 'difficult'. The vibrating area was considered to be the right size by ten patients and too small by two.

The Minifonator's size and weight posed practical problems, with several patients indicating that it was incompatible with their clothing. Some felt it to be so intrusive that they would not wear it in public. Others commented on the feedback, which made it impossible to wear in public. However, one user, a professional engineer, thought it had engineering potential. All said the Minifonator's box was too large and two felt the controls to be too small (this is consistent with the result that ten found the controls easy to use, one that they were just manageable and one that they were difficult to use). Seven said that vibrator output was too weak and five that it was just right. Ten patients found battery recharging and replacement easy and two that it was difficult. Three felt that the vibrating area was too large, one that it was too small and eight that it was about the right size.

The Tactaid scored well on questions concerning the vibrator but poorly on those about the control box/battery. The design of the strap was criticised and opinion was divided about whether there was any advantage to having low- and high-frequency channels. There were some comments that the vibrator produced a continuous humming (possibly feedback). Ten of the twelve thought that the Tactaid was cumbersome. Eleven felt the controls to be a convenient size, only one that they were too small. Tactaid scored least well on ease of control; eight subjects found the controls easy to use, three that they were manageable and one that they were difficult to use. The Tactaid was considered the best aid with respect to vibrator output: eight people found it 'just right', one 'too weak' and three 'too strong'; ten thought that the vibrating area was the right size and two that it was too large. Replacing/charging the batteries was considered easy by nine, just manageable by two, and one found it too difficult.

How good is the aid for environmental sounds?

Here responses to questions about awareness of traffic noise, pedestrian-crossing sounds, people knocking at the door, environmental sounds such as machine noise and rainfall, and how useful the aid is when watching television or using the telephone were analysed. The data are summarised in Table 11.6.

The TAM aid again performed best, scoring particularly well on questions relating to street noise: five patients found it very helpful in increasing awareness of traffic when crossing the street, three thought it to be of some help and four of no help. In common with the other aids, TAM was not thought helpful in detecting the beeping sound made at pedestrian crossings (eight found it no help, two some help and two said it was very helpful). The TAM aid was considered particularly useful in listening for environmental sounds; six said it was 'very helpful' and six

Table 11.6 Ranks for each vibrotactile aid for the questions on how well the aid helps with environmental sounds

Subject	TAM	Tactaid	Minivib	Minifonator
Street noises	1	3	2	3
Pedestrian crossings	1	3	1	4
People knocking at the door	2	1	4	2
Listening for machine noise etc.	1	2	2	2
Watching the television	3	1	2	3
Using the telephone	3	4	1	2
Average rank	1	3	2	4

1, Best; 4, worst.

said it was 'of some help'. In the home, TAM was of less help than some of the other aids as only two people found it 'very helpful', seven found it of some help in watching television and two found it unhelpful. One did not use it with the television. In common with the other devices, most (eight people) did not use it when using the telephone, although two found it very helpful and one tried it with the telephone but found it of no help. Two people found it very helpful in indicating that people wanted to attract attention, nine found it of some help and one found it to be unhelpful.

The Minivib scored comparatively well on the questions concerned with crossing the street, as five people found it very helpful in awareness of traffic, two found it of some help and five of no help at all. When asked how much help it provided when listening to environmental noises, four said 'very helpful', five 'of some help' and three 'no help at all'. It had the lowest score for the question about people at the door wanting to attract the patient's attention; four found it very helpful, three of some help and four said that it gave no help at all. Patients commented on the ability of the Minivib to pick up noises in the home such as paper rustling, and that the television sounded better when wearing it. One patient commented that she felt more 'connected' in the home when wearing the aid and that it helped in showing her how much noise she made in the kitchen. Another commented that he could pick up vibrations related to the wind and rain.

The Tactaid scored well on the questions about help given in hearing sounds in the home; six found it very helpful in giving awareness of people trying to attract attention whilst three found it of some help and three thought it to be of no help. For watching television, five found it very helpful, four found it to be of some help and two thought it not very helpful. For listening for environmental noises, three patients found it to be very helpful, seven thought it was of some help and two found it was of no help. It scored worst of all the aids in awareness of traffic when crossing the road: four said it was very helpful, two that it was of some help and six that it was of no help at all. Outdoors, Tactaid was felt generally to perform poorly and to pick up too much background noise. One person commented that radio and television sounded more alive when wearing the device, another that wearing the device in conjunction with a hearing aid made her hearing more alert.

The Minifonator was the worst in this category but was quite close to the Tactaid. Three found it helpful in providing awareness of people trying to attract attention, six found it of some help and two found it unhelpful. It scored worst on the question concerning watching the television, for which six stated that it was no help, two that it was of some help and four that it was very helpful. It scored badly on help it gave in detecting the beeping sound made at pedestrian crossings; nine said it was of no help.

How much does the aid help lipreading?

Responses to questions about how much the aid helped lipreading and communication in various circumstances were analysed (Table 11.7).

Table 11.7 How well each aid helps lipreading and communication

Subject	TAM	Tactaid	Minivib	Minifonator
Talking to a person in a quiet room	1	2	4	3
Talking in a group	1	2	2	4
Talking to a person in a quiet open space	1	2	2	4
Talking to a person in a large room	1	2	4	3
Average rank	1	2	3	4

The TAM device was clearly the best here: it was ranked first for all questions. In talking with one person in a quiet room five patients found it helpful and seven said that it was very helpful. The TAM also proved a boon when lipreading in a quiet, open space; six said it was very helpful and six said it was of some help. However, in common with all the aids, it fared less well in group situations, for it was of 'no help' to six patients, 'of some help' to four, and only two said it was 'very helpful'. One patient commented that it helped tremendously in discriminating between words that sound alike, and one said that when she had tinnitus and was unable to use her hearing aid the vibrotactile aid helped her lipreading.

The Tactaid was ranked second for each question. When lipreading in a quiet, open space three patients considered it very helpful, seven said that it was of some help and two that it was of no help. This aid attracted favourable comments: one patient wrote that although he thought it no help when lipreading, if he turned it off, he was a little lost when in conversation; two patients could recognise the differing tones in people's voices and one of these said that he could recognise the difference between deaf and normal speakers. However, one patient indicated that it gave a poor response with ordinary conversation.

The Minivib performed comparatively poorly. When talking to one person in a quiet room three patients found it was very helpful, six said it was of some help and three considered it to be of no help at all. Similarly, when lipreading in a quiet open space four individuals found it very helpful, five of some help and three said it was of no help. The Minivib was the worst aid in the group for lipreading in a large room: nine subjects considered it to be no help. Several patients thought this aid helped their lipreading, with one saying that it made him aware of the more rhythmically precise response of vibration in relation to speech in quiet. Another said it was of some help in talking to one person without a hearing aid and that a friend had remarked that she seemed to be 'hearing better'.

The Minifonator was again the worst of the group. When asked about the help it gave in talking with one person in a quiet room, four patients found it very helpful, five said it was of some help and three said it was no help. It was worst among the devices at giving help when lipreading in a quiet open space; only three people said it was very helpful. Again, one patient could differentiate between deaf and hearing people's voices. One found the vibrations confusing, but they made him more sociable.

How much does the aid help in voice control?

Here the question about voice control was included: in addition a relative or friend, who was present at all test sessions, had been asked to complete a form detailing the patient's speech production, with and without the vibrotactile aid. This comprised questions about the clarity of the speech, whether the voice is monotonous and whether the voice level is appropriate to the circumstances. The data are summarised in Table 11.8.

The TAM device was again ranked first: four patients considered it very helpful in controlling their voice level, six that it was some help and two said that it gave no benefit. When a friend was asked to give an opinion regarding clarity of speech, all eight who were asked said that it was always clear, four out of five said the speech was never monotonous and

Table 11.8 How well the aid helps voice control

Subject	TAM	Tactaid	Minivib	Minifonator
Use in controlling voice level	1	3	1	4
Help make speech clear*	1	3	4	1
Help if voice is monotonous*	2	3	4	1
Help keep voice at correct loudness*	2	1	4	3
Average rank	1	3	4	2

*Relative's or friend's opinion.

one that it was sometimes monotonous; five out of eight considered that the patient's voice was always the correct loudness and three said it was sometimes. One patient commented that people understood her better when she wore the aid.

The Minifonator was second in this group; however it was the worst at helping patients control their voice level (five patients said that it gave no help, two that it gave some help and five that it was very helpful). Out of five friends asked about the patient's speech, all five found speech clearer when wearing the vibrotactile aid, four out of five said the patient's speech was never monotonous when wearing the aid. Three out of five said that the patient's speech was always at the correct loudness when using the aid and two said this was sometimes not the case.

When asked to state how much help the Tactaid gave them in controlling voice level, four patients said it was very helpful, five that it was of some help and three that it was of no help. Out of eight friends, seven said that the patient's speech was always clear when they wore the aid; five out of seven said the patient's speech was never monotonous; four out of six considered the patient's voice always the correct loudness when wearing the aid, and two said this was sometimes true.

The Minivib was worst in this category; in particular, it was rated the lowest by friends of the person wearing the device. However, when asked how useful it was in controlling their own voice level four patients found it very helpful, six of some help and only two said it was not helpful.

Overall results from the individual questionnaire

The data from the previous sections are summarised in Table 11.9.

Overall, the two vibrotactile aids that use the simpler output codings were rated higher than the two that produce more complex outputs. Clearly cosmetic and practical considerations such as weight and the possibility of feedback played a large part in the decision. It is possible to test this tentative conclusion by examining the comparative questionnaire data and the results from the test procedures (below) to see if such a finding is repeated.

Table 11.9 Overall ranking of vibrotactile aids

Question groups	TAM	Tactaid	Minivib	Minifonator
Ease of wear	1	3	2	4
Design	1	4	2	2
Help with environmental sounds	1	3	2	4
Help with lipreading and communication	1	2	3	4
Help with voice control and speech	1	3	4	2
Average rank	1	3	2	4

Table 11.10 Results of the comparative questionnaire

Comparative questions*	TAM	Tactaid	Minivib	Mini-fonator	None
Which is the best vibrotactile aid? (%)	50	20	30	0	
Mean rank (1=very poor, 9=very good)	6.2	6.1	5.1	3.0	
Most useful for controlling voice (%)	36	36	18	0	9
Most useful talking to a person (%)	36	27	18	0	18
Most useful for environmental sound (%)	36	27	18	0	18
Most useful for someone at the door (%)	22	33	22	0	22
Vibrotactile aid chosen for use (%)	55	18	27	0	
Average rank	1	2	3	4	

*Not all subjects replied to all questions; percentage returns correspond to 9, 10 or 11 replies.

Comparative questionnaire data

After the final test session, the patient was asked to complete a questionnaire comparing the four vibrotactile aids. The data are summarised in Table 11.10.

In reply to the question 'Which is the best vibrotactile aid?', 50% chose the TAM device, 30% the Minivib, and the remaining 20% picked the Tactaid. To see if the choices were consistent with other ways of obtaining this information, the patient was also asked to rank each aid on a scale from 1 (very poor) to 9 (very good). The mean ranks for the first three vibrotactile aids were relatively close: 6.2 (TAM), 6.1 (Tactaid) and 5.1 (Minivib), with a larger drop to the Minifonator (3.0). Both methods gave the TAM device the top position with the Tactaid and the Minivib in positions two and three and the Minifonator definitely ranking lowest. The results therefore indicate a good degree of self-consistency in the answers.

The TAM and the Tactaid devices were judged to be the most useful in controlling the patient's voice level. When talking to another person the TAM was judged to be the best followed by the Tactaid, Minivib and Minifonator. The same order was maintained for the use of the device in the street in order to be aware of cars and other environmental sounds.

The Tactaid device was judged best for home use when people wanted to attract the attention of the patient (such as someone knocking at the door). The TAM and Minivib were ranked equally next, followed by the Minifonator.

The mean rank of all the questions asked so far in this questionnaire produced the following order: TAM, Tactaid, Minivib, Minifonator. When patients were asked to choose a vibrotactile aid for their use, the order changed; the Minivib and the Tactaid swapped places. This is probably due to the emphasis that the patients put on size and weight.

The average rank, including the choice of aid for use by the patient, is TAM, Tactaid, Minivib, Minifonator.

Table 11.11 Ranks of the mean change in score between the unaided condition and the vibrotactile-aided condition. Data are given for all tests that showed a statistically significant difference between the unaided and aided conditions

Test	TAM	Tactaid	Minivib	Minifonator
BKB (L)	1	2	4	3
VCV (F)	2	1	3	4
VCV (C)	3	1	2	4
CDT	3	1	4	2
Environ.	2	3	4	1
Average rank	2	1	4	3

BKB(L), BKB sentences loosely scored; VCV, the vowel-consonant-vowel test scored fully (F) and as the confusion score (C); CDT, connected discourse tracking; Environ. the environmental-sounds test.

Comparative test data

The test data may be examined so that the vibrotactile aids can be compared. As before, the tests selected were those that had shown a statistically significant difference between the aided and unaided conditions. Table 11.11 contains the ranked data for these tests.

The test data give a different assessment of the vibrotactile aids than do the questionnaire data. The mean rank of the connected discourse tracking and the environmental-sounds tests show what might have been expected from the signal-processing properties of the aids: the two aids providing more complex output are now ranked higher than those using a simpler strategy. Even when all the test data shown here are considered, it is now the Tactaid, the most complex, two-channel device, that ranks first. The TAM device (which had led the field in all the questionnaire data) now comes second and the Minifonator, assessed very badly by the questionnaire data, now comes up to third place*.

Conclusions

The three main methods for evaluating the vibrotactile aids were the subjective tests, the individual questionnaire and the comparative questionnaire. The data for each of these were ranked and are shown in Table 11.12.

What can be said in terms of the initial objectives of this study?

Editor's note: the TAM was not designed as an aid to lipreading, and the signal processing which it incorporates would not seem to make it particularly suitable for this application. It is perhaps disappointing to find that the Minivib and Minifonator, designed with lipreader benefit in mind, do not out-perform the TAM.

Table 11.12 Overall summary of all results

	TAM	Tactaid	Minivib	Minifonator
Test data	2	1	4	3
Individual questionnaire	1	3	2	4
Comparative questionnaire	1	2	3	4
Average rank	1	2	3	4

Vibrotactile aids certainly do give benefit to patients. This is shown by the patient responses, the test data and the fact that seven patients found vibrotactile aids so helpful that they took one home for everyday use. The test procedures that best reflected this benefit were those that gave a statistically significant difference between the aided and unaided conditions. These were the twelve-intervocalic-consonant test, the BKB sentence lists, the connected-discourse tracking and the environmental sounds test.

In comparing the two types of vibrotactile aid (those with single-channel, single-frequency stimulation ('simple') and those with more complex outputs ('complex')), the results become more complicated. The individual questionnaire data came down strongly in favour of the simple aids, which were ranked first and second. Combining the two questionnaires still ranked the TAM device first with the Minivib and Tactaid in equal second place and the Minifonator last. The complex devices do not score at all well until the test data are considered, which rank them first (Tactaid) and third (Minifonator). From experience with hearing aids it is known that the choice made by the patient need not reflect the performance of the aid as measured by speech intelligibility. In this study there are indications that the weight, appearance and ease of use are important factors in the patient's choice and are reflected in the questionnaire answers.

The questionnaire data that most closely reflect the test data results come from two questions: first, asking about people in the home trying to attract the attention of the patient (such as visitors at the door); secondly the one in which the third-party adjudged the patient's ability to control his or her voice and keep it at the appropriate level of loudness.

In the comparison with hearing aids, the simple/complex distinction was also observed. For those patients whose hearing loss is such that they can benefit from hearing aids, their hearing aid gives more benefit than a vibrotactile aid. (It should be noted that most patients who would conventionally be considered for a vibrotactile aid are those who cannot benefit from hearing aids.) When the vibrotactile aid and the hearing aid are used together the more complex aids, Tactaid and Minifonator, give a better result than that from hearing aid alone. The two more simple aids give a result equal to or worse than that from hearing aid alone.

Although not a factor in this study, the relative cost of the devices may be relevant to the comparison. Approximate prices (1990/1991) are: TAM £125 (US$200), Tactaid £595 (US$955), Minivib £285 (US$455), Minifonator £620 (US$995).

There are many factors that patients use in selecting a vibrotactile aid. It is perhaps best to let a patient have the closing word: one commented that the ideal aid would look like the TAM and behave like the Tactaid.

Acknowledgements

The authors gratefully acknowledge the dedicated work and collaboration of their colleagues Jane Day and Sarah Worsfold, of their former colleagues Ian Bell and Stanley Goodsall and thank those who provided test materials.

References

DAY, J., WORSFOLD, S. and THORNTON, A.R.D. (1990). A training programme for vibrotactile aids. *IHR Internal Report Series A, No. 8*.

FAULKNER, A., POTTER, C., BALL, G. and ROSEN, S.M. (1989). Audiovisual speech perception of intervocalic consonants with auditory voicing and voiced/voiceless speech pattern presentation. *Speech Hearing and Language: Work in progress*. 3, 85–106. London: University College, Department of Phonetics and Linguistics.

ROSEN, S.M. and CORCORAN, T. (1982). A video-recorded test of lipreading for British English. *Br. J. Audiol.* 16, 245–254.

ROSEN, S.M., MOORE, B.C.J. and FOURCIN, A.J. (1979). Lipreading with fundamental frequency information. In: *Proceedings of the Institute of Acoustics Autumn Conference* 1979. Edinburgh: Institute of Acoustics, pp. 5–8.

Index